Techniques in
Immunocytochemistry

Techniques in Immunocytochemistry

Volume 2

Edited by

GILLIAN R. BULLOCK

*Research Centre, Ciba-Geigy
Pharmaceutical Division,
Horsham, Sussex, England*

and

PETER PETRUSZ

*Department of Anatomy,
University of North Carolina,
Chapel Hill, USA*

ACADEMIC PRESS

Harcourt Brace Jovanovich Publishers

London   San Diego   New York

Berkeley   Boston   Sydney   Tokyo   Toronto

ACADEMIC PRESS LIMITED
24/28 Oval Road, London NW1 7DX

United States Edition published by
ACADEMIC PRESS, INC.
Orlando, Florida 32887

Third printing 1986
Fourth printing 1989

British Library Cataloguing in Publication Data

Techniques in immunocytochemistry—Vol. 2
   1. Immunochemistry   2. Cytochemistry
   574.2'9   QR183.6

   ISBN 0–12–140402–1
   ISBN 0–12–140405–6 (pbk.)

Printed in Great Britain by Galliard (Printers) Ltd, Great Yarmouth

Contributors

N. J. Atkins *Bland Sutton Institute, Middlesex Hospital Medical School, London W1P 7PN, England*

W. G. Beckman *Departments of Anatomy and Urology, University of North Carolina, Chapel Hill, NC 27514, USA*

D. M. Boorsma *Department of Dermatology, Academic Hospital Free University, de Boelelaan 1117, Amsterdam, The Netherlands*

G. V. Childs *Department of Anatomy, University of Texas Medical Branch, Galveston, Texas 77550, USA*

J. L. Cordell *Haematology Department, John Radcliffe Hospital, Oxford OX3 9DU, England*

R. Cumming *Department of Neurology and the Neurobiology Program, 751 Burnett-Womack Building, University of North Carolina, Chapel Hill, NC 27514, USA*

M. De Brabander *Department of Oncology, Janssen Pharmaceutica Research Laboratories, B-2340 Beerse, Belgium*

J. De Mey *Department of Oncology, Janssen Pharmaceutica Research Laboratories, B-2340 Beerse, Belgium.*

M. De Waele *Department of Haematology, University Hospital of the Free University Brussels (A.Z.-V.U.B.), B-1090 Brussels, Belgium*

A. L. Hartman *Department of Pathology, University of Colorado Health Science Center, 4200 East Ninth Avenue, Denver, Colorado 80262, USA*

J. N. Hayward *Department of Neurology and the Neurobiology Program, 751 Burnett-Womack Building, University of North Carolina, Chapel Hill, NC 27514, USA*

A. J. C. Leathem *Bland Sutton Institute of Pathology, Middlesex Hospital Medical School, London W1 7PN, England*

M. T. Libber *Department of Neurology and the Neurobiology Program, 751 Burnett-Womack Building, University of North Carolina, Chapel Hill, NC 27514, USA*

D. Y. Mason *Haematology Department, John Radcliffe Hospital, Oxford OX3 9DU, England*

M. Moeremans *Department of Oncology, Janssen Pharmaceutica Research Laboratories, B-2340 Beerse, Belgium*

R. S. Molday *Department of Biochemistry, Faculty of Medicine, University of British Columbia, Vancouver, BC V6T 1W5, Canada*

P. K. Nakane *Department of Pathology, University of Colorado Health Science Center, 4200 East Ninth Avenue, Denver, Colorado 80262, USA*

K. A. F. Pulford *Haematology Department, John Radcliffe Hospital, Oxford OX3 9DU, England*

T. A. Reaves, Jr *Department of Neurology and the Neurobiology Program, 751 Burnett-Womack Building, University of North Carolina, Chapel Hill, NC 27514, USA*

J. Roth *Department of Structural Biology, Biocenter, University of Basel, CH-4056 Basel, Switzerland*

M. Sar *Department of Anatomy, Laboratories for Reproductive Biology, University of North Carolina, Chapel Hill, NC 27514, USA*

W. E. Stumpf *Departments of Anatomy and Pharmacology, Laboratories for Reproductive Biology, University of North Carolina, Chapel Hill, NC 27514, USA*

B. Van Camp *Department of Haematology, University Hospital of the Free University Brussels (A.Z.-V.U.B.), B-1090 Brussels, Belgium*

Preface

Although, at the time of writing, only a few months have passed since Volume 1 appeared in print we have been very encouraged by the interest that has been shown in it. The most encouraging comment has been that time has been saved by those using the book as the methods are described in sufficient detail. Therefore, one of our main objectives has been achieved.

This volume is in the same style and has several contributions dealing with cell surface labelling using a wide range of techniques and different instrumentation. Chapters on lectins and the avidin-biotin systems are both felt essential to such a series and, for the same reason, monoclonal antibody preparation has been included. It is also apparent that the use of colloidal gold markers needs proper documentation.

Again, any helpful suggestions would be welcomed by the editors, to add to those already received which will help formulate the contents of Volume 3. We would like to thank all our contributors for the work they have already put in and are delighted that some have felt it possible to write further chapters in this exciting, fast moving field.

February 1983   *Gillian R. Bullock*
Peter Petrusz

Contents of Volume 2

Immunogold Staining Method for the Detection of Cell Surface Antigens with Monoclonal Antibodies

M. DE WAELE, J. DE MEY, M. MOEREMANS,
M. DE BRABANDER and B. VAN CAMP

IMMUNOCYTOCHEMISTRY 2
ISBN 0 12 140402 1

I. INTRODUCTION

In 1971, Faulk and Taylor (1971) introduced their "immunocolloid" method for the study of cell surface antigens. Specific antibodies adsorbed to colloidal gold particles were used to visualize *Salmonella* antigens in transmission electron microscopy (TEM). Since then a large number of studies have documented the potential of colloidal gold as a marker for immunocytochemistry (reviewed in Horisberger, 1979 and 1981; Goodman *et al.*, 1980; De Mey, 1983). Much of the basic methodology for preparing standardized gold sols and stable gold probes has been well established. Colloidal gold particles have been labelled with a variety of macromolecules such as antibodies, enzymes, lectins and polysaccharides (Romano *et al.*, 1974; Geoghegan and Ackerman, 1977; Horisberger and Rosset, 1977; see also Roth this Volume). The smaller sized particles are able to penetrate into whole cultured cells and can be used for pre-embedding labelling of intracellular antigens (De Mey *et al.*, 1981).

Colloidal gold particles are particularly interesting as markers for immunocytochemistry because they can be used both at high and low resolution levels (Horisberger, 1979; 1981; Goodman *et al.*, 1980; De Mey, 1983). Due to their electron dense properties, they are easily detected by TEM. As they are capable of strong emission of secondary electrons, they can be visualized by scanning electron microscopy (Horisberger *et al.*, 1975). In addition, colloidal gold particles strongly absorb visible light (λ max 525–550 nm) and if the density of the gold marker is sufficiently high, the cell labelling can be seen in brightfield microscopy. This approach has been introduced by Geoghegan *et al.* (1978) in a method for the detection of surface immunoglobulin on human B lymphocytes. Brightfield microscopy was also used by Gu *et al.* (1981) for the study of intracellular peptides in gut cells. In their work, the gold labelling was carried out in three ways: an indirect labelling; a bridge procedure, and a combined indirect bridge technique which gave significant amplification of the staining intensity. In addition, they combined this immunogold staining (IGS) procedure with a peroxidase anti-peroxidase (PAP) method for the double immunostaining of gastrin-containing and serotonin-containing cells. Immunogold staining has also been used for the light microscopic localization of tubulin in whole cultured cells (De Mey *et al.*, 1981).

The specificity and sensitivity of an immunocytochemical technique is limited by the specific activity of the antibodies used in the different steps of the procedure. New perspectives in this field have recently been opened by the development of the hybridoma technology, which permits one to raise highly specific monoclonal antibodies against all kinds of antigens. These monoclonal antibodies have so far mainly been applied in immunofluorescence and immunoenzyme techniques, but they also form ideal reagents for colloidal gold labelling procedures (see also Mason *et al.*, this Volume). We have recently described the use of monoclonal antibodies recognizing lymphocyte cell surface antigens, in an immunogold staining procedure for the light microscopical characterization of leukocytes (De Mey *et al.*, 1982; De Waele *et al.*, 1981; 1982a,b). This technique was used to enumerate lymphocyte subpopulations in cell suspensions. The aim of this chapter is to give a detailed description of the technique and to comment extensively on every step of the procedure. Afterwards we will discuss the advantages and possibilities of this method.

II. DESCRIPTION OF THE PROCEDURE

In this procedure, leukocyte cell suspensions are first incubated with monoclonal mouse antibodies directed against lymphocyte cell surface antigens, and then with colloidal gold particles coated with goat antimouse antibodies. The cells are fixed in suspension and cytocentrifuge preparations are made. Monocytes and granulocytes in the preparations are detected by cytochemical staining of their endogenous peroxidase activity. The preparations are examined in brightfield light microscopy.

A. Preparation of the Cell Suspensions

Venous blood is collected in 5% EDTA in phosphate buffered saline (PBS) at pH 7·4. Mononuclear cell suspensions are prepared by Ficoll-Hypaque density gradient centrifugation. The cells are washed three times, for 5 min each in PBS at pH 7·4, containing 1% bovine serum albumin (BSA), 1% heat inactivated normal human AB serum, and 0·02 M sodium azide (PBS-BSA 1%-AB 1%-az: wash buffer). Suspensions of 3×10^{10} cells/l are made in PBS-BSA 5% at pH 7·4, containing 4% AB serum and 0·02 M sodium azide (PBS-BSA 5%-AB 4%-az: incubation buffer).

B. Monoclonal Mouse Antibodies

Monoclonal mouse antibodies raised against lymphocyte cell surface antigens are used (OKT series: Ortho Pharmaceutical Corp. and Ortho Diagnostic Inc., Raritan, N.J.). More information about the specificity of these antibodies can be found in the literature (Reinherz *et al.*, 1979; 1980a,b; Breard *et al.*, 1980; Kung and Goldstein, 1980; Reinherz and

Schlossman, 1981). OKT3, OKT4 and OKT8 respectively identify the mature T-lymphocytes, T-inducer/helper cells and T-cytotoxic/suppressor cells. OKT6 reacts with the majority of thymocytes but not with peripheral blood lymphocytes. OKM1 recognizes an antigen present on monocytes, granulocytes and some null cells. OKIa 1 reacts with a HLA-Dr antigen present on B-lymphocytes, activated T-lymphocytes and some monocytes. The antigen recognized by the OKT10 antibody is present on hemopoietic precursor cells, thymocytes, plasma cells, activated T and B lymphocytes and some null cells. OKT11 reacts with the E-rosette receptor and is used to identify the peripheral T-cells. Also a monoclonal anti-IgM antibody is used (Ortho Diagnostic Inc., Canada). The specificity of this antibody has been demonstrated by immunodiffusion techniques and by indirect immuno-fluorescence on (1) fixed polyclonal and monoclonal bone marrow plasma cells, and (2) normal and leukemic peripheral B-lymphocytes.

These monoclonal antibodies are applied as dilutions of ascitic fluid or of the commercially available reagents. These lyophilized reagents are recon-structed with PBS-BSA 5%. They contain small amounts of sodium azide as preservative. The working dilution of these antibodies, as determined by titration on a leukocyte cell suspension, varies between 1 and 5 μg/ml.

C. Colloidal Gold-labelled Secondary Antibodies

The preparation of the colloidal gold-labelled goat antimouse IgG anti-bodies (GAMG30 reagent) is described in detail elsewhere (De Mey, 1983). Colloidal gold particles with a mean diameter of about 30 nm are obtained by the method of Frens (1973). Just before coupling, the gold sol is brought to pH 9·0 with potassium carbonate. Goat antibodies to mouse immunoglobu-lin G are isolated from goat antimouse IgG serum by affinity chromatogra-phy on mouse IgG-Sepharose-4B. The purified antibodies are dialyzed against 2 mM borax HCl buffer at pH 9·0. Immediately before use, micro-aggregates are removed by centrifugation at 100 000 × g for 1 h at 0 °C.

The amount of antibody necessary for optimal protection of the gold sol against flocculation in salt solutions is determined according to Geoghegan and Ackerman (1977). This antibody is mixed with the gold sol by stirring gently. After 2 min, BSA (BSA-Sigma) fraction V, 10% in borax buffer pH 9·0, is added to achieve a final concentration of 10 mg/ml. Unstabilized marker and free or loosely bound proteins are removed by three cycles of centifugation (14 000 × g, 1 h, 0 °C) and resuspension in 0·02 M Tris-buffered saline at pH 8·2, containing 10 mg/ml BSA and 0·02 M sodium azide (TBS-BSA-az). The GAMG30 preparation used in our work is obtained by resuspending the last pellet (mobile red pool) in the appropriate volume of

TBS–BSA–az to assure that the extinction at 520 nm of a 1/20 reagent dilution is 0·350. When stored at 4 °C this reagent is stable for months. It is centrifuged at low speed before use in order to remove microaggregates.

D. Cell Labelling

Twenty-five microliter (μl) of the cell suspension (approximately 10^6 cells) are incubated for 30 min at room temperature with 25 μl of the monoclonal antibody dilution. The cells are subjected to three 5-min washings with PBS-BSA 1%-AB 1%-az. Thereafter the cells are resuspended in 25 μl of PBS-BSA 5%-AB 4%-az and incubated with 25 μl of the GAMG30 reagent for 1 h at room temperature. During the incubations, the cells are agitated every 10 min. The cells are washed again and are fixed with 0·01% glutaraldehyde in PBS at pH 7·4 for 10 min at room temperature. After subsequent washing, cytocentrifuge preparations are made. These preparations can be stained immediately or may be stored at −20 °C. This does not change the immunogold positivity.

E. Peroxidase Cytochemistry and Counterstain

The cytocentrifuge preparations of immunogold labelled cells are fixed in 4% formaldehyde in absolute ethanol for 2 min at room temperature. Monocytes and granulocytes in the preparations are labelled by cytochemical staining of their endogenous peroxidase activity following the method of Graham and Karnovsky (1966). Therefore the preparations are incubated for 20 min at room temperature in a freshly prepared staining solution containing 0·5 mg/ml 3-3' diaminobenzidine (DAB-HCl) and 0·0006% H_2O_2 in 0·1 M Tris-HCl buffer pH 7·6. Instead of DAB, the Hanker-Yates reagent (Polysciences Inc.) may be used. Good staining results from incubation for 10 min at room temperature in a solution of 1 mg/ml of this reagent and 0·0006% H_2O_2 in 0·1 M Tris-HCl buffer at pH 7·6. The preparations are counterstained with 1% chloroform-extracted aqueous methyl green. After dehydration through ethanol and xylol, they are mounted wth DPX (DPX mountant, Chemical Ltd, England).

F. Examination of the Preparations

We have examined the preparations with a Leitz Dialux 20 EB microscope (objective 100x/1·32 oil, ocular 10x). To enumerate the subsets, 200 lymphocytes are assessed for each specimen and the percentage of labelled cells is determined.

III. RESULTS

A. Appearance of the Preparations

In the immunogold preparations, the leukocytes can be identified by their morphological and cytochemical characteristics. The nuclei of the cells are stained by methyl green. Monocytes and granulocytes have endogenous peroxidase activity in the cytoplasm. In general, this activity is more intensely stained in these preparations than in peripheral blood smears. Lymphocytes are identified as peroxidase negative mononuclear cells. Their cytoplasm is unstained.

Lymphocytes reacting with the monoclonal antibodies have numerous dark granules around the surface membrane. (Plate 1; for the Plate Section see pages between 148–149). A capping phenomenon is not prominent. Most of the negative cells have no granules. A few cells with fewer than three granules are also considered to be negative.

Monocytes are identified by their greater cell size, irregular borders, indented nucleus and endogenous peroxidase activity. Very few of them show fixation of the gold marker on their surface membrane. This is also observed in control preparations where the monoclonal antibody is omitted. Occasionally the monocytes show endocytosis of the gold marker. These cells have an accumulation of dark material in the cytoplasm. This phenomenon is never seen in the lymphocytic cells.

B. Lymphocyte Subsets in Normal Peripheral Blood

The lymphocyte subsets enumerated with immunogold staining in normal peripheral blood are given in Table I (De Waele et al., 1982b). T-cells (OKT3-positive) form 81% of the lymphoid population. T-helper cells (OKT4-positive) and T-cytotoxic/suppressor cells (OKT8-positive) are present at a ratio of 1.75 ± 0.6 (mean value $\pm$ 1 s.d.). The sum of both populations equals the number of OKT 3-positive cells. Thirteen per cent of the lymphocytes display Ia antigens on their surface membrane, while 8% have surface IgM. The Ia antigens are probably not only present on mature B-cells, but also on 20–30% of the null cells (Reinherz et al., 1979). A small number of cells (5%) reacts with the OKM1 antibody but does not show the morphological and cytochemical characteristics of mature monocytes.

TABLE I

Lymphocyte subpopulations in normal peripheral blood.

Reactivity with	% of positive lymphocytes ± 1 s.d.
OKT3	81 ± 6
OKT4	52 ± 6
OKT8	28 ± 5
OKIa1	13 ± 2
anti-IgM	8 ± 1
OKM1	5 ± 2
OKT6	1 ± 0·5
GAMG30[a]	0·5 ± 0·5

Results expressed as the mean percentage for five healthy young adults.
[a] The monoclonal antibody was omitted.

These cells probably correspond to the small nonadherent OKM1 positive cells found by immunofluorescence (Breard *et al.*, 1980). These cells appear to form the majority of the null cell population. They can be promonocytes, precursor cells for other lineages and the major effector cells for antibody-dependent cellular cytotoxicity or natural killing (Breard *et al.*, 1980).

The lymphocyte subsets enumerated by immunogold staining are almost identical to those obtained by immunofluorescence microscopy in the same mononuclear cell suspensions (De Waele *et al.*, 1983a). They are also comparable to those found by others with fluorescence methods (Hoffman *et al.*, 1980; Kung and Goldstein, 1980; Reinherz and Schlossman, 1981). Although the antigen recognized by OKT6 is not present on normal peripheral blood lymphocytes, 1% of the lymphocytes is positive in this negative control experiment. Identical numbers of positive cells are found when the monoclonal antibody is omitted. Therefore, this phenomenon is probably due to non-specific fixation of the colloidal gold-labelled goat antimouse antibodies. It can be found to a similar extent in immunofluorescence microscopy (De Waele *et al.*, 1983a). This small non-specific positivity cannot influence the lymphocyte subsets to a clinically important degree.

IV. COMMENTS

A. Cell Suspensions

1. The Whole Blood-lysis Technique

The immunogold staining procedure can also be performed on the leukocyte suspension obtained by lysis of the red blood cells in whole blood (De Waele

et al., 1983a). For each determination, 25 to 100 μl of whole blood is treated
with 2·5 ml of lysis buffer (8·29 g of NH_4Cl, 37 mg of disodium EDTA and
1 g of $KHCO_3$ per l, pH 7·3 (Hoffman *et al.*, 1980) for 3 min at room
temperature. After centrifugation for 5 min at 200 xg, the supernatant is
decanted. The pellet containing leukocytes, platelets and some erythrocyte
ghosts is washed with PBS-BSA 1%-AB 1%-az. The cells are resuspended in
25 μl of PBS-BSA 5%-AB 4%-az. The immunogold staining procedure is
performed as already described.

The cell density on the cytocentrifuge preparations can be modified by
changing the volume of whole blood used for one determination or by
concentrating or diluting the labelled cell suspension just before making the
cytocentrifuge preparations. On these preparations granulocytes, monocytes, lymphocytes, platelets and some erythrocyte ghosts are found.
Leukocyte morphology is well preserved. The lysis procedure does not
affect the density of the gold marker on the surface membrane of the positive
cells or the endogenous peroxidase activity in granulocytes and monocytes.
The number of OKT3, OKT4, OKT6 or OKT8 positive cells found in these
preparations are nearly identical to those obtained in mononuclear cell
suspensions of the same individuals (De Waele *et al.*, 1983a). Also with cord
blood lymphocytes, where surface antigens may be weakly expressed, no
significant difference is found between the results obtained in the two types
of cell suspensions. The lysis procedure does not change the non-specific
fixation of the GAMG30 reagent on the lymphocytes. The lysis of the red
blood cells may be performed before, in between or after the incubations
with the monoclonal antibody and the colloidal gold reagent.

2. Buffy Coat Cells and Whole Blood

Buffy coat cells and even whole blood (without lysis of red blood cells) may
be used in the immunogold staining procedure (De Waele *et al.*, 1982a). This
simplifies the procedure and reduces the time required for the preparation of
the specimens. However, scanning of the whole blood preparations for
lymphocytes is time consuming due to the high number of red blood cells.

3. Leukocyte Suspensions from Other Sources

Using cell suspensions from other sources than peripheral blood such as
bone marrow, lymphoid organs, pleural effusions and cerebrospinal fluid,
the leukocytes can also be characterized with this method. For complex cell
suspensions such as bone marrow, the peroxidase cytochemistry is of major
importance. With this reaction the granulocytes, monocytes and also the

normoblasts (pseudoperoxidase activity) can be distinguished from the lymphoid cells.

B. Incubation with the Monoclonal Antibody

1. Antibody Dilution Curve

The optimal concentration of the monoclonal antibody in the immunogold staining procedure can be determined by establishing an antibody dilution curve. Therefore, the same amount of mononuclear cells is incubated with graduated concentrations of the monoclonal antibody and the number of positive cells is determined. In Fig. 1, an OKT3 dilution curve is shown. The number of OKT3-positive cells does not vary significantly with OKT3 concentrations varying from 5 μg/ml to 0·625 μg/ml, although the density of the surface labelling on the positive lymphocytes decreases. With further dilutions of the monoclonal antibody the number of OKT3-positive cells rapidly falls. The highest dilution of the antibody with a number of positive cells in the horizontal part of the curve, is used as the working dilution in experiments (e.g. for OKT3: 0·625 μg/ml for 10^6 cells). This antibody dilution curve is nearly identical to that found with immunofluorescence microscopy in the same cell suspensions (see Fig. 1; IF). Therefore, in these experimental conditions, the sensitivity of the colloidal gold detection seems

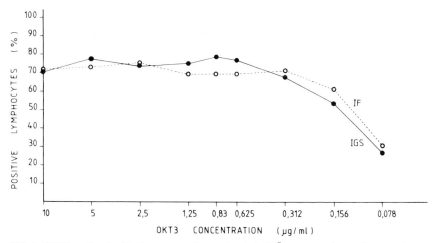

FIG. 1. OKT3 antibody dilution curve. Approximately 10^6 mononuclear cells were incubated with graduated concentrations of the monoclonal antibody (horizontal axis). The percentage of OKT3-positive lymphocytes was determined (vertical axis) by immunogold staining (IGS) and immunofluorescence microscopy (IF).

comparable to that of the immunofluorescence technique (De Waele *et al.*, 1982b). In both procedures, cells with less than three granules on the surface membrane were considered to be negative.

Similar dilution curves have been found for the other monoclonal antibodies. In general, the working concentrations vary between 1 and 5 μg/ml for 10^6 cells. The same concentrations are used for immunofluorescence microscopy.

2. Incubation Time

Variation of the incubation time with the OKT3, OKT4, or OKT8 monoclonal antibodies from 15 min to 1 h does not change significantly the number of positive cells in this immunogold staining procedure. Only a slight increase of the density of the gold marker on the surface membrane of the positive cells is observed. An incubation time of 30 min is used for routine determinations.

3. Monoclonal Mouse IgM Antibodies

As most of the monoclonal mouse antibodies are of the IgG class, an affinity-purified goat antimouse IgG was used for the preparation of the GAMG30 reagent. However, this reagent also shows a strong reaction with monoclonal mouse antibodies of IgM class, e.g. anti-Leu-7 (HNK-1 Becton Dickinson, Sunnyvale, CA 94086), probably through the recognition of the light chains of the immunoglobulin molecules.

C. Incubation with Colloidal Gold-labelled Secondary Antibodies

1. Use of Gamma Fraction of Goat Antimouse Serum

An affinity-purified goat antimouse IgG is used for the preparation of the GAMG30 reagent. When an IgG fraction (gamma fraction) of the goat antimouse serum is coupled to gold, the reaction is weak and consistent results can not be obtained. This is in contrast with the findings of Geoghegan *et al.* (1978). It is possible however that an IgG fraction of a goat serum with a very-high titer of antimouse antibodies would give better results.

2. Diameter of the Gold Particles

In accordance with the findings of Horisberger (1981), we have observed that only gold probes with a particle diameter of 20 nm or more can be used in the light microscopic procedure. With 5 nm probes, no granules are seen on the surface membrane of the positive cells when the preparations are examined with brightfield light microscopy or with darkfield microscopy (see V.C). With increasing diameter of the colloidal gold particles in the probe, the dark granules on the positive cells increase in size but decrease in number. With 20 nm probes a rim of fine red-brown granules is found around the surface membrane. Larger particles give clearly distinguishable dark granules. When the density of the antigen recognized by the mono-clonal antibody on the surface membrane is low, 20 nm probes may give a positive result which is too weak to permit a rapid and accurate enumeration of the positive cells. With 30 and 40 nm probes, no such problems are encountered.

3. Stabilizing Agent

Colloidal gold probes stabilized with BSA give a higher gold density on the surface membrane of the positive cells, than probes with an identical particle diameter, but stabilized with 0·1% polyethylene glycol (Carbowax 20 м). However, with the BSA preparations the background staining is also slightly increased. This latter phenomenon can be reduced by adding heat inacti-vated human AB serum to the incubation and washing buffers.

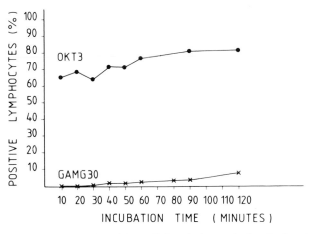

FIG. 2. Number of immunogold-positive cells in relation to the incubation time with the colloidal gold-labelled secondary antibodies. Mononuclear cells were incubated with the OKT3 monoclonal antibody for 30 min and then with the GAMG30 reagent for times ranging from 10 to 120 min at room temperature. The number of OKT3-positive cells was enumerated in the different preparations (OKT3 curve). The influence of the incubation time on the background staining was examined by performing similar experiments in which the monoclonal antibody was omitted (GAMG30 curve).

4. Incubation Time

Prolongation of the incubation time of the cells with the gold probe increases the gold density on the surface membrane of the positive cells, especially during the first 30 min. This is accompanied by an increase in the number of positive cells (Fig. 2; OKT3 curve). With incubations longer than 1 h the background staining becomes more important (Fig. 2; GAMG30 curve) and may contribute significantly to the data obtained. For routine determinations an incubation time of 60 min at room temperature is used. In these conditions a good positivity is obtained while the non-specific staining is still low. The incubation time can be reduced to 30 min for antibodies detecting antigens with a sufficiently high density on the cell surface membrane, such as OKT3.

D. Use of Sodium Azide in the Procedure

Sodium azide is present as a preservative in the monoclonal antibody preparations and in the colloidal gold reagent. It is added to the incubation and washing buffers to prevent capping and internalization of the antigen-antibody-gold probe complexes by blocking the oxidative phosphorylation of the cells. For a complete inhibition of these phenomena, the cells have to be preincubated for 15 min at 37 °C with a 0·01 M concentration of sodium azide and this concentration has to be present during the rest of the experiment (Loor, 1977). In our method the labelling is performed at room temperature in the presence of 0·02 M sodium azide and without pre-incubation of the cells with this reagent. In the OKT preparations, capping is not prominent. It is more obvious when surface IgM is detected with the anti-IgM monoclonal antibody. Endocytosis of the colloidal gold is observed in part of the monocytes, but not in the lymphocytes. The patching of the antigen-antibody-gold probe complexes is not affected by the 0·02 M sodium azide concentration, because it is a passive redistribution process which does not require an active cell metabolism (Loor, 1977).

Capping of the gold marker is slightly enhanced when the concentration of sodium azide in the procedure is reduced by omitting this reagent from the incubation and washing buffers (De Waele *et al.*, 1983b). This reduced azide concentration may also favour internalization or shedding of the antigen-antibody complexes by the unfixed cells. Although the lymphocyte subsets enumerated in these conditions are not significantly different from those found in the presence of 0·2 M sodium azide, it may be advisable to perform the labelling at low temperature (0 °C) to limit all these phenomena.

E. Background Staining

Background staining can be examined by substituting the monoclonal antibody in the procedure by an ascites dilution from a Balb/e mouse injected intraperitoneally with a non-producing hybridoma clone (Kung and Goldstein, 1980). When normal peripheral blood is examined, the OKT6 monoclonal antibody can also be used as negative control (Reinherz *et al.*, 1980b). The determinant defined by OKT6 may, however, be present on circulating abnormal cells, e.g. blasts of T-acute lymphoblastic leukemia (Reinherz *et al.*, 1980a). The non-specific binding of the colloidal gold to the cells can be examined by omitting the monoclonal antibody in the procedure (see Table I; reactivity with GAMG30). In addition, any cross-reactivity of the goat antimouse antibodies of the gold probe with human immunoglobulin molecules has to be excluded, e.g. by immunodiffusion techniques and cytoplasmic immunofluorescence on fixed polyclonal and monoclonal bone marrow plasma cells.

When no human AB serum is added to the incubation and washing buffers, 5% of normal peripheral blood lymphocytes are positive in both negative control experiments (reactivity with OKT6 and with GAMG30 alone; see De Waele *et al.*, 1983a). Therefore the background staining is probably more due to fixation of the colloidal gold probe on to the cells (e.g. on F_c receptors) than of the monoclonal mouse immunoglobulins. It may be influenced by the length of the incubation of the cells with the GAMG30 reagent, by the particle size and by the nature of the stabilizing reagent (BSA or PEG) of the probe.

The background staining can be reduced to 1% of normal peripheral blood lymphocytes by adding heat-inactivated human AB serum to the incubation (2%) and washing (1%) buffers (results in Table I). Fetal calf serum does not produce the same effect as human AB serum in this procedure. Pre-incubation of the cells at 37 °C or fixing the cells with low concentrations of formaldehyde (Schuit and Hymans, 1980) has little effect on the non-specific positivity.

When cells of B-lymphoproliferative disorders in particular are examined, background staining can be important. This non-specific positivity may be diluted out by reducing the concentration of the colloidal gold reagent in the procedures. The use of Fab$_2$ fractions of the goat antimouse serum for the preparation of the gold probe could be advantageous here.

F. Fixation of the Cells in Suspension

In this immunogold staining procedure, the labelled cells are fixed in suspension with glutaraldehyde. This fixation influences the appearance of the labelled cells and their affinity for cytochemical dyes.

On cytocentrifuge preparations, fixed cells appear smaller than unfixed cells. Fixed cells probably retain a more globular shape and are less flattened on the preparations. The intensity of this effect depends on the concentration of the fixative. Fixation with 0·01% glutaraldehyde induces less "cell shrinkage" than a 1% glutaraldehyde concentration. If cellular morphology or cytochemical staining patterns are to be appreciated, the lower concentration should therefore be preferred.

The "cell shrinkage" increases the density of the gold marker on the surface membrane of the positive cells. In unfixed cells, the positivity is seen as a diffuse rim of very fine gold granules. This makes the enumeration of the positive cells difficult and laborious. After fixation with 0·01% glutaraldehyde, distinct dark granules are found around the surface membrane.

Glutaraldehyde fixation enhances the permeability of the cell surface membrane for cytochemical substrates and dyes. To prevent overstaining, the staining times for the cytochemical reaction have to be shorter for fixed cells than for unfixed cells. As an example, the nuclei of unfixed cells are only weakly stained by 1% methyl green and fixed cells are stained very deeply by Giemsa or hematoxylin.

Fixation of the cells with glutaraldehyde before the incubation with the monoclonal antibody induces the same changes in cell shape, labelling density and membrane permeability as described above. However the gold granules on the positive cells are always very fine and have an aspect comparable to that seen on unfixed cells. With electron microscopy (see V. B) colloidal gold particles appear to be dispersed around the surface membrane of the positive cells and almost no patching is observed. When the cells are prefixed with glutaraldehyde concentrations higher than 0·01% the number of OKT-positive cells is lower than normal. These conditions seem to destroy the determinants recognized by the monoclonal antibodies.

G. Enzyme Cytochemistry on Immunogold-labelled Cells

For the routine enumeration of lymphocyte subpopulations, the cytocentrifuge preparations are stained for endogenous peroxidase (Perox) and counterstained with methyl green. Monocytes and granulocytes in the preparations are peroxidase positive and are easily differentiated from lymphocytes which are peroxidase negative.

Other intracellular enzymes can also be detected in the immunogold-labelled cells (De Waele et al., 1982b, 1983a,b). Acid alpha naphthyl acetate esterase (ANAE), acid phosphatase (AP) and beta glucuronidase (BG) have been stained with the classical cytochemical reactions (Goldberg and Barka, 1962; Lorbacher *et al.*, 1967; Mueller *et al.*, 1975). To prevent overstaining the staining times have to be shorter than those for preparations of unlabelled cells. The following times were used: 20 min at room temperature for peroxidase; 35 min at 37 °C, for ANAE (peripheral blood smears 90 min at 37 °C); 45 min at 37 °C for AP and BG (peripheral blood smears: 105 and 150 min at 37 °C respectively). The preparations are rinsed in distilled water and counterstained with methyl green. They are dehydrated and mounted in DPX.

The ANAE, AP and BG activity is present in lymphocytes and monocytes (Plates 2, 3, 4; see between pp. 148–149). The monocytic cells can be recognized by their morphological characteristics. They show an intense diffuse staining pattern for ANAE and AP and a weaker BG activity. The gold labelling on the OKT positive cells is not affected by the cytochemical reactions. The numbers of OKT3, OKT4 or OKT8 positive lymphocytes enumerated in the ANAE, AP and BG preparations are in the same range as those found in preparations of the same cell suspension stained for peroxidase (De Waele *et al.*, 1982a, 1983b). These data prove that the cell identification based on morphological and cytochemical characteristics is accurate in these preparations.

In the lymphoid cells three staining patterns can be distinguished for each enzyme: a localized activity in the form of one or two coarse granules (dot-like activity); an accumulation of smaller granules in the cytoplasm (diffuse granular pattern), or no reactivity at all (negative cells). In the immunogold preparations the staining intensity of the enzymatic activities is higher than in peripheral blood smears of the same individuals, but the staining patterns for the different enzymes and the number of cells showing each pattern in two types of preparations are comparable (De Waele *et al.*, 1982b, 1983b). All these data prove the reliability of this approach.

Combining immunogold staining with enzyme cytochemistry is an ideal method to determine the intracellular enzymatic activities of the lymphocyte subpopulations identified by the different monoclonal antibodies. With this technique, the cytochemical characteristics of the T-lymphocytes (OKT3-positive cells), the T-helper cells (OKT4-positive) and the T-cytotoxic/suppressor cells (OKT8-positive) have been examined (De Waele *et al.*, 1982b, 1983b). T-cells appeared to be characterized by a dot-like activity for the three enzymes. No significant difference was found between the cytochemical staining patterns of T-helper and T-cytotoxic/suppressor cells. They were identical to those of the whole T-cell population. These data are in accordance with the findings of Armitage *et al.* (1982), obtained by performing cytochemistry on T-helper and T-cytotoxic/suppressor cells, identified

by the Leu 3a and the Leu 2a monoclonal antibodies, and purified by cell
sorting.

H. Counterstain

After enzyme cytochemistry, the cells are counterstained with 1% methyl
green in aqua destillata (pH 7·4) for 3 min at room temperature. The methyl
green solution is purified before use by extraction with chloroform. Equal
volumes of 1% methyl green and chloroform are brought in a separation
funnel. After vigorous shaking the two phases are separated. The chloroform containing the impurities is discarded. A new volume of chloroform is
added and the procedure is repeated twice.

With this methyl green counterstain the nuclei of the cells have a green-
blue aspect and the cytoplasm is unstained. The staining is weak in cells not
fixed with glutaraldehyde. There is a good contrast between the green
nuclei, the dark granules on the surface membrane of the OKT-positive cells
and the red or brown colour of the enzyme cytochemistry in the cytoplasm.
Giemsa and hematoxylin solutions stain the glutaraldehyde-fixed cells very
intensely so that all contrast is lost. Therefore, these dyes are not used to
counterstain the immunogold preparations.

When no enzyme cytochemistry is performed, the cells can be stained with
the methyl green-pyronin technique. Methyl green-pyronin stains cellular
DNA green and the RNA red and permits a better appreciation of
cellular morphology than methyl green alone. It can be used in the characterization of leukemias, for example, as the blast cells are easily identified in
these preparations by their intensively red stained nucleoli and cytoplasm
(Plate 5; see between pp. 148–149). There is also good contrast between the
red colour of the cytoplasm and the dark granules on the surface membrane.

I. Examination of the Preparations with Darkfield Microscopy and Polarized Light Epi-illumination Microscopy

The cytocentrifuge preparations of immunogold-labelled cells can also be
examined with darkfield microscopy (De Waele et al., 1982b). The patches
of gold particles on the surface membrane of the positive cells strongly
reflect incident light and appear as bright yellow spots (Plate 6; see between
pp. 148–149). Also for this technique, gold probes with a particle diameter
of 20 nm or more are required. Peroxidase positive cells and erythrocytes
can also be identified.

Immunogold-labelled cells can also be visualized by polarized light epi-illumination microscopy. The equipment used for this purpose is described elsewhere (De Mey, 1983). The patches of gold particles show a strong backscatter of incident polarized light. The polarization of the backscattered light is lost and it will pass the analyzer while other excitation light will be extinguished. This signal is so strong that it is visible against a low background of transmitted non-polarized light which allows identification of the OKT-negative lymphocytes and the peroxidase-positive cells.

V. ELECTRON MICROSCOPY

The immunogold staining method described in this chapter can also be used for electron microscopy (De Waele *et al.*, 1983a,b). In this case, the cell suspension is incubated with the monoclonal antibodies and the colloidal gold reagent as described above. The cells are fixed with 1% glutaraldehyde in 0·1 M cacodylate buffer, pH 7·2, for 30 min at 4 °C. They are treated with osmium tetroxide and stained with uranyl acetate. They are dehydrated and embedded in epon. Thin sections are stained with lead citrate.

With this procedure the cellular ultrastructure is well preserved, but the mitochondria may be affected by the sodium azide (Fig. 3). The gold particles appear as patches on the surface membrane of the OKT-positive cells. One such patch is probably seen as a dark granule in light microscopy. When the azide concentration in the procedure is reduced (De Waele *et al.*, 1983b), rare pinocytotic vesicles containing a few gold particles may be found in some of the lymphocytes. Larger accumulations of gold in phagosome-like organelles are only seen in monocytic cells.

This approach has been used by Matutes and Catovsky (1982) to determine the ultrastructural characteristics of the normal lymphocyte subpopulations defined by the OKT monoclonal antibodies. In this study the cells were fixed, before labelling, for 5 min in 1% glutaraldehyde in 0·1 M cacodylate buffer (pH 7·4). The labelling was performed as described by De Mey *et al.* (1983). Due to the short prefixation, the disposition of the gold was more uniform over the whole surface of the positive cells. A cell was said to be labelled (positive) if it had several gold particles (at least three) attached to the surface membrane. Distinct morphological characteristics were found for the T and B cells and the OKT4-positive and OKT8-positive subpopulations. However, different results were obtained with other methods. Using electron microscopical examination of purified T-helper and T-suppressor cells (respectively Leu 3a and Leu 2a positive cells), Armitage *et al.* (1982) could not find any significant morphological difference between these functional T-cell subpopulations. Additional information seems to be needed in this field.

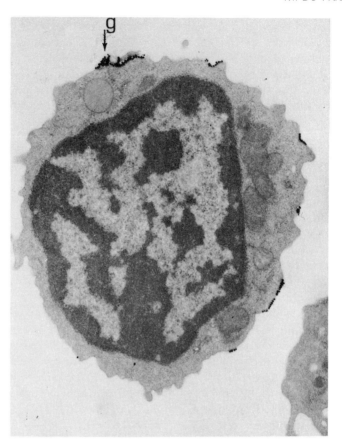

FIG. 3. Thin section of a lymphocyte, labeled with OKT3 and GAMG30. The gold particles (g) are found in patches at the surface membrane of the cell (magnification 18 000×).

Also at the electron microscopical level, the immunogold staining can be combined with enzyme cytochemistry. The lead-containing reaction product of the cytochemical reaction in the cytoplasm of the cells can easily be distinguished from the gold particles on the cell surface. This approach was used by Bain *et al.* (1981) to characterize the abnormal circulating cells in some cases of acute myelofibrosis. These cells were identified as megakaryoblasts by the presence on their surface membrane of a platelet antigen, recognized by the AN51 monoclonal antibody, and by a positive platelet peroxidase reaction in the nuclear envelope and endoplasmic reticulum.

Acid phosphatase can also be demonstrated in immunogold-labelled cells at the ultrastructural level (De Waele *et al.*, 1983b). In normal lymphocytes,

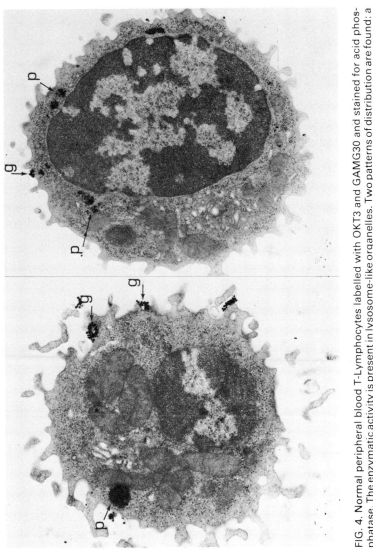

FIG. 4. Normal peripheral blood T-Lymphocytes labelled with OKT3 and GAMG30 and stained for acid phosphatase. The enzymatic activity is present in lysosome-like organelles. Two patterns of distribution are found: a dot-like (left) or a scattered acid phosphatase activity (right), g: colloidal gold; p: acid phosphatase activity; (magnification 24 000×).

this enzymatic activity is present in lysosome-like organelles. They are localized in one or two groups (Fig. 4; left) or are more numerous and dispersed in the cytoplasm of the cells (Fig. 4; right). These distribution patterns could explain the dot-like and diffuse granular acid phophatase activity seen in lymphocytes in light microscopy.

VI. CONCLUSIONS

In the past ten years, colloidal gold has been used as a marker for the immunocytochemical detection of a large variety of cell surface and intracellular antigens and receptors, both at low (photonic microscopy) and high resolution levels (TEM and SEM) (reviewed by Horisberger, 1979; 1981; Goodman et al., 1980; De Mey, 1983). During this period, the methodology for preparing standardized gold sols and stable colloidal gold reagents has been well established. Colloidal gold has several advantages when compared to other cytochemical markers such as ferritin or enzymes (Horisberger, 1979; 1981; Goodman et al., 1980; De Mey, 1983). In addition colloidal gold probes are cheap and are rapidly prepared with only small amounts of specific macromolecules, which show little change in their bioactivity.

In the antibody-gold techniques, mainly antisera or relatively pure antibodies have so far been used, with the concomitant problems of staining specificity. New perspectives in this field have been opened by the development of the hybridoma technology, which allows one to raise highly specific monoclonal antibodies to all kinds of antigens.

In this chapter, an immunogold staining method is described for the characterization of leukocytes with monoclonal antibodies raised against cell surface antigens. In this method cells reacting with the monoclonal mouse antibodies (OKT series) are detected in light microscopy after incubation with colloidal gold-labelled goat antimouse antibodies. Patches of antigen-antibody gold complexes on the surface membrane of the positive cells are seen as red-blue granules, without any additional cytochemical reaction. This immunogold staining procedure is a reliable tool for the enumeration of T-lymphocytes and their subclasses (De Waele et al., 1982a, 1983a). The preparations are stable and the immunogold-labelled lymphocytes can be identified by their morphological and cytochemical characteristics in light microscopy. This permits a rapid and accurate cell counting without special equipment. The method can also be applied on small volumes of whole blood, providing a microtechnique for the enumeration of lymphocyte subsets, e.g. in pediatric patients.

This immunogold staining procedure forms a general method for the study of lymphocyte subpopulations in all kinds of cell suspensions. It has been used to enumerate the lymphocyte subsets in bone marrow, lymph node and tonsil. It was also applied in the detection of malignant lymphoid cells in cerebrospinal fluid and pleural effusions from patients with leukemia and lymphoma.

With this method, the immunological detection of cell surface antigens can be combined with the cytochemical staining of intracellular enzymatic activities (De Waele *et al.*, 1983b). In the immunogold-labelled lymphocytes acid alpha-naphthyl acetate esterase, acid phosphatase and beta-glucuronidase can be detected by the classical cytochemical reactions. This seems to be an ideal approach to establish a correlation between the stage of differentiation, the state of activation or the functional characteristics of the cells and their enzymatic content.

Cells labelled with this procedure can also be examined with electron microscopy. The morphology is well preserved and ultrastructural cytochemistry can be performed. Parallel use of different monoclonal antibodies, directly coupled to colloidal gold particles of different sizes would permit the detection of multiple antigens on the same cell at the ultrastructural level.

The patches of gold particles on the immunogold-labelled cells can be visualized with darkfield and polarized light epi-illumination microscopy. This approach could offer the potential of quantitation of labelled cells by automated equipment.

Monoclonal antibodies will probably soon be used instead of antisera or purified antibodies in the different antibody-gold procedures for the detection of intracellular antigens in tissue sections and cultured cells. Whether the gold marker can also be applied to detect cell surface antigens in tissue sections remains under investigation. A variety of monoclonal antibodies against all kinds of cell surface antigens, e.g. HLA-related antigens, tumor markers etc will become available shortly. Immunogold staining provides a general procedure for their use in light and electron microscopy.

VII. ACKNOWLEDGEMENTS

We are indebted to G. Goldstein (Ortho Pharmaceutical Corp., Raritan, N.J. 08869) and J. Rogers (Ortho Diagnostic Systems, Inc., Raritan, N.J. 08869) for providing the monoclonal antibodies. We are also grateful to L. Broodtaerts and L. Smet (Department of Hematology, AZ-VUB, Brussels) for excellent technical assistance, to M. Borgers and F. Thone (Janssen Pharmaceutica Research Laboratories, Beerse, Belgium) for performing the ultrastructural cytochemistry and to C. Verellen for typing the manuscript. This work was partly supported by a grant (to J.D.M. and M.D.B.)

from the Instituut ter Bevordering van het Wetenschappelijk Onderzoek in Landbouw en Nijverheid (IWONL), Brussels, Belgium, and by grants No 3.0041.81 (to B.V.C.) and No 3.0076.83 (to M.D.W.) from the "Fonds voor Geneeskundig Wetenschappelijk Onderzoek", Brussels, Belgium.

VIII. REFERENCES

Armitage, R. J., Linch, D. C., Worman, C. P. and Cawley, J. C. (1982). *Br. J. Haemat.* **51**, 605–613.

Bain, B. J., Catovsky, D., O'Brien, M., Prentice, H. G., Lawlor, E., Kumaran, T. D., McCann, S. R. Matutes, E. and Galton, D. A. G. (1981). *Blood* **58**, 206–213.

Breard J., Reinherz, E. L., Kung, P. C., Goldstein, G. and Schlossman, S. F. (1980). *J. Immun.* **124**, 1943–1948.

De Mey, J., Moeremans, M., Geuens, G., Nuydens, R. and De Brabander M. (1981). *Cell Biol. Int. Rep.* **5**, 889–899.

De Mey, J. (1983). *In* "Immunocytochemistry: Practical Applications in Pathology and Biology" (J. Polak and S. Van Noorden, eds), pp. 82–113. J. Wright and Sons Ltd, London.

De Mey, J., Moeremans, M., De Waele, M., Geuens, G. and De Brabander, M. (1982). *In* "Protides of the Biological Fluids" (H. Peeters, ed.), Vol. 29, pp. 943–947, Pergamon Press, Oxford.

De Waele, M., De Mey, J., Moeremans, M. and Van Camp, B. (1981). *In* "Leukemia Markers" (W. Knapp, ed.), pp. 173–176. Academic Press, London.

De Waele, M., De Mey, J., Moeremans, M. and Van Camp, B. (1982a). *In* "Protides of the Biological Fluids" (H. Peeters, ed.), Vol. 29. pp. 949–953. Pergamon Press, Oxford.

De Waele, M., De Mey, J., Moeremans, M., Broodtaerts, L., Smet, L. and Van Camp, B. (1982b). *J. Clin. Immun.* **2** (Suppl.), 24S–31S.

De Waele, M., De Mey, J., Moeremans, M., De Brabander, M. and Van Camp, B. (1983a). *J. Histochem. Cytochem.* **31**, 376–381.

De Waele, M., De Mey, J., Moeremans, M., Smet, L., Broodtaerts, L. and Van Camp, B. (1983b). *J. Histochem. Cytochem.* **31**, 471–478.

Elias, J. M. (1969). *Stain Techn.* **44**, 201.

Faulk, W. P. and Taylor, G. M. (1971). *Immunochemistry* **8**, 1081–1083.

Frens, G. (1973). *Nature Phys. Sci.* **241**, 20–22.

Geoghegan, W. D. and Ackerman, G. A. (1977). *J. Histochem. Cytochem.* **25**, 1187—1200.

Geoghegan, W. D., Scillian, J. J. and Ackerman, G. A. (1978). *Immunol. Commun.* **7**, 1–12.

Geuze, H., Slot, J., Van der Ley, P., Schuffer, R. and Griffith, J. (1981). *J. Cell Biol.* **89**, 653–665.

Goldberg, A. F. and Barka, T. (1962). *Nature* **195**, 297.

Goodman, S. L., Hodges, G. M. and Livingston, D. C. (1980). *In* "Scanning Electron Microscopy" (O. Johari, ed.), Vol. II. pp. 133–145. IITRI, Chicago.

Graham, R. C. Jr. and Karnovsky, M. J. (1966). *J. Histochem. Cytochem.* **14**, 291–302.

Gu, J., De Mey, J., Moeremans, M. and Polak, J. M. (1981). *Regulatory Peptides* **1**, 365–374.
Hoffman, R. A., Kung, P. C., Hansen, W. P. and Goldstein G. (1980). *Proc. Natn. Acad. Sci. USA.* **77**, 4914–4917.
Horisberger, M., Rosset, J. and Bauer, H. (1975). *Experientia* **31**, 1147–1149.
Horisberger, M. and Rosset, J. (1977). *J. Histochem. Cytochem.* **25**, 295–305.
Horisberger, M. (1979). *Biologie Cell.* **36**, 253–258.
Horisberger, M. (1981). *In* "Scanning Electron Microscopy" (O. Johari, ed.) Vol. II. pp. 9–31. IITRI, Chicago.
Kung, P. C. and Goldstein, G. (1980). *Vox Sang.* **39**, 121–127.
Larsson, L. I. (1979). *Nature* **282**, 743–746.
Loor, F. (1977). "Progress in Allergy", Vol. 23. pp. 1–153. Karger, Basel.
Lorbacher, P., Yam, L. T. and Mitus, W. J. (1967). *J. Histochem. Cytochem.* **15**, 680–687.
Matutes, E. and Catovsky, D. (1982). *Clin. Exp. Immunol.* **50**, 416–425.
Mueller, J., Brun del Re, G., Buerki, H., Keller, H. U., Hess, M. W. and Cottier, H. (1975). *Eur. J. Immunol.* **5**, 270–274.
Reinherz, E. L., Kung, P. C., Pesando, J. M., Ritz, J., Goldstein, G. and Schlossman, S. F. (1979). *J. Exp. Med.* **150**, 1472–1482.
Reinherz, E. L., Kung, P. C., Goldstein, G., Levey, R. H. and Schlossman, S. F. (1980a). *Proc. Natn. Acad. Sci. USA* **77**, 1588–1592.
Reinherz, E. L., Moretta, L., Roper, M., Breard, J. M., Mingari, M. C. Cooper, M. D. and Schlossman, S. F. (1980b). *J. Exp. Med.* **151**, 969–974.
Reinherz, E. L. and Schlossman, S. F. (1981). *Immunology Today* (April), 69–75.
Romano, E. L., Stolinski, C. and Hughes-Jones, N. C. (1974). *Immunochemistry* **11**, 521–522.
Romano, E. L. and Romano, M. (1977). *Immunochemistry* **14**, 711–715.
Roth, J., Bendayan, M. and Orci, L. (1978). *J. Histochem. Cytochem.* **26**, 1074–1081.
Schuit, H. R. E. and Hymans, W. (1980). *Clin. Exp. Immunol.* **41**, 567–574.
Van Camp, B., Thielemans, C., Dehou, M. F., De Mey, J. and De Waele, M. (1982). *J. Clin. Immunol.* **2**, (Suppl.), 67S–74S.

Localization of Steroid Hormones and their Receptors. A Comparison of Autoradiographic and Immunocytochemical Techniques

W. C. BECKMAN, Jr, W. E. STUMPF and M. SAR

I. INTRODUCTION

Steroid receptor assays have been used for determination of the receptor content of various tissues (Godefroi and Brooks, 1973; Jensen and De Sombre, 1973; Lippman and Huff, 1976, McGuire, 1973; Thompson et al., 1980.) Since tissues must be homogenized in preparation for the assay, the inaccuracy of these biochemical approaches increases with the heterogeneity of the tissue upon which they are performed. Hence, a high receptor content within individual cells and tissues which comprise a small proportion of the sample may not be identifiable with an assay which averages all cell types. The problem of tissue heterogeneity is of particular significance to clinicians who are using *in vitro* receptor assays as diagnostic

IMMUNOCYTOCHEMISTRY 2
ISBN 0 12 140402 1

tools for breast cancer. The mechanism of action of steroid hormones within cells containing steroid receptors is understood to involve binding to the cytosolic receptor followed by translocation to the nucleus where binding to chromatin occurs (Grody *et al.*, 1982). Cytosolic estrogen receptor (ER) concentrations in breast tumors are widely held to be predictive of the eventual course of endocrine thereapy (Osborne *et al.*, 1978). Patients whose tumors contain less than 15 fmol of cytoplasmic ER are not as likely to respond to anti-estrogen therapy as those whose tumors contain greater than 10–15 fmol of ER per mg of tissue. In most cases, patients whose tumors are found to be receptor positive are treated with anti-estrogens such as tamoxifen, yet between 55 and 60% of such tumors do not respond to this treatment.

It has been suggested (Lippman and Allegra, 1978; Pertschuk *et al.*, 1980b) that the ambiguity of biochemical receptor assays as predictors of the outcome of endocrine therapy may be related to heterogeneity of tumor cell types. Since homogenization of the tumor averages all cell types, the problem of heterogeneity must be resolved by another diagnostic approach. A morphological technique which could define the distribution of receptor-containing cells within the tumor mass would provide important information regarding tumor heterogeneity both before and after anti-estrogen therapy.

Histochemical techniques for the localization of steroid hormones or their receptors have several potential advantages over biochemical receptor assays. They are relatively inexpensive, permit evaluation of tissues at the cellular level and this can be performed rapidly after the tissue has been obtained. The histochemical approaches currently in use differ on the basis of their use of:

1. Radioactive or fluorescent labels attached to steroid molecules

2. Antisera directed against steroid receptors

3. Antisera directed against steroid hormones.

II. HISTOCHEMICAL TECHNIQUES UTILIZING STEROIDS LABELED WITH RADIOACTIVE OR FLUORESCENT TRACERS

A. *In Vivo* Uptake of Steroids

1. Radioactive Compounds

Steroid target sites may be identified by autoradiography after *in vivo* injection of ^{3}H or ^{125}I labeled steroid. Dry-mount and thaw-mount autoradiography were developed for the localization of diffusible compounds (Stumpf and Roth, 1966) and have been utilized by numerous investigators for the cellular and subcellular localization of steroid hormones in normal tissues (Stumpf and Sar, 1976a) and mammary tumors (Stumpf, 1969). Results from autoradiographic studies employing these techniques have consistently shown nuclear concentration and retention of the hormone or its metabolites, with lesser and variable amounts in the cytoplasm, depending on the time after the application of the labeled steroid and the amount of endogenous hormone present.

2. Fluorescent Compounds

Uptake of fluoresceinated estradiol 17 β in vivo has been reported by Barrows et al., (1980). These investigators injected fluoresceinyl-estrone into intact 16 week old female rats. Frozen sections of uterus were thawed onto slides, dried, dipped for 5 sec in 100% ethanol and then mounted in xylene. This procedure revealed nuclear fluorescence of uterine stromal and epithelial cells, a pattern similar to that observed by autoradiography. Nuclear uptake was observed by these authors in cells of uterus, pituitary, testis and prostate after in vitro incubations, but was absent in other known estradiol target tissues (Stumpf and Sar, 1976a,b) such as brain, kidney, and skin. Since μM quantities of unlabeled estradiol were unable to completely inhibit the observed nuclear labeling in vitro, and since tissues were dehydrated in ethanol, it is unlikely that the observed fluorescence in the studies of Barrows et al. was directly related to binding to the estrogen receptor.

In vivo approaches with radioactive and perhaps with fluorescent compounds as well, have the advantage of more nearly approximating physiological conditions than studies performed in vitro, since the circulatory system of the animal is an important factor in the transport of steroids and their penetration into and removal from tissues in a living animal. This factor is difficult to reproduce in vitro. Certain experimental procedures, however, cannot be carried out in vivo. In such cases, the use of labeled steroids under appropriate in vitro conditions utilizing cell cultures or tissue explants may be considered.

B. *In Vitro* Uptake of Steroids

1. Radioactive Compounds

The smear-mount autoradiographic technique was developed for the study of cell suspensions or cultured cells (Stumpf and Sar, 1975; 1982.) In addition to this approach, cell suspensions can be pelleted and cut on a cryostat for autoradiographic analysis (Sheridan et al., 1979). In vitro incubation of living tissue slices with radioactive steroids was introduced by Stumpf (1968) and has subsequently been modified and used to determine the presence of estrogen or androgen receptors in dog prostrate (Leav *et al.*, 1978; Ofner *et al.*, unpublished) and estradiol receptors in breast tumors (Buell and Tremblay, 1981; Beck *et al.*, 1982). When thin tissue slices are used, penetration problems are minimized and localization of steroid hormones in target cells approaches that obtained in tissues following *in vivo* application. When steroid concentrations are kept in a physiological range (10^{-11} to 10^{-9} M), a distinct nuclear uptake of steroids can be recognized and the general tissue radioactivity is relatively low.

2. *Fluorescent Compounds*

In vitro incubation of living cells or tissues with fluorescein-conjugated estrogens has been reported by several groups (Barrows *et al.*, 1980; Rao *et al.*, 1980a; Nenci *et al.*, 1980a; 1981; Fisher *et al.*, 1982) Neither Rao *et al.* nor Fisher *et al.* were able to correlate their findings with biochemical assays of receptor content. Nenci *et al.* (1980c; 1981), utilizing a preparation in which estradiol and fluorescein were conjugated to bovine serum albumen (fluorescein-BSA-estradiol), reported cell surface membrane binding, capping and internalization following *in vitro* incubation with isolated cell suspensions from human breast cancers. This compound, previously applied topically to frozen sections by Pertschuk *et al.*, (1976), did not appear to penetrate the intact cell surface membrane to bind to steroid receptors in the cytosol.

Nenci *et al.*, following the technique of Dandliker *et al.*, (1978), synthesized 17-fluoresceinyl estrone and studied its binding to dispersed breast tumor cells and cell lines at 4 and 37 °C. These investigators reported temperature dependent translocation of the estrone-fluorescein compound, although nuclear uptake was mainly restricted to the nucleolus, a pattern not observed with autoradiographic studies. Nucleoli of normal target cells do not retain ^{3}H estradiol after either *in vivo* or *in vitro* incubation. After long autoradiographic exposure times, the nuclear region of receptor containing cells becomes heavily labeled, with the exception of the nucleolar region which is conspicuously devoid of silver grains (Stumpf *et al.*, 1969; 1976a).

Barrows *et al.* (1980) reported temperature-dependent nuclear translocation of cytosol-bound estradiol-fluorescein conjugates following incubation of tissue slices from endometrium and mammary tissues. When frozen sections from tissues which had been incubated at 4 °C were permitted to warm for 60 sec, translocation to the nucleus occurred. Translocation of fluorescein-estradiol did not result in permanent binding of labeled estrogen in nuclei, since cell specific fluorescence could not be demonstrated after 2 min of thawing on the slide. The observation of temperature dependent translocation of the fluorescein-estrogen compound to the nucleus without pronounced nucleolar binding is similar to the pattern observed with auto-radiography and in contrast to the observation of predominately nucleolar binding reported by Nenci *et al.* (1980a). Considerable question remains regarding the significance of the observations, by Barrows *et al.* (1980), who were not able to obtain optimal competition with a saturated solution of estradiol alone. A mixture of equinolone, estrone, estradiol and diethylstil-bestrol (concentrations not specified) was required in order to displace binding of the fluorescinyl-estrone compound in competition studies. In their studies, in order to obtain optimal demonstration of fluorescence, dried sections mounted on slides were dipped for 5 sec in 100% EtOH before mounting in xylene. In this context, it is important to note that similar section incubation with ^{3}H estradiol, followed by dipping in liquid photo-graphic emulsion, does not show nuclear concentrations of radioactivity in uterine target cells (Tchernitchin, 1967), in contrast to results obtained with the dry-mount and thaw-mount autoradiographic techniques.

To date, results with fluorescein-estrogen compounds have not yielded reproducible results which are consistent with the known mechanism of action of steroid hormones. The ability to demonstrate translocation of steroids to the nucleus remains the final criterion for histochemical detection of steroid sensitive tissues.

C. Topical Application of Labeled Steroids to Frozen Sections

1. Radioactive Steroids

In vitro incubation of frozen sections mounted on slides with ^{3}H-estradiol was applied by Tchernitchin. The results from these studies did not show nuclear uptake in uterine cells, but yielded only labeling of cytoplasm of eosinophils (Tchernitchin, 1967; Brokelman, 1969). Such cytoplasmic label-ing of eosinophils could not be reproduced *in vivo* (Stumpf *et al.*, 1976b).

2. Fluorescent Steroids

Topical application of fluorescein-conjugated estradiol to histological sec-tions was utilized by Lee (1978) and Pertschuk *et al.* (1978). Pertschuk *et al.* (1978a) employed a fluorescein-BSA-estradiol compound conjugated at position 17. These investigators applied 50 pmol of this compound to each section. Lee (1978) and other groups using his preparations incubated sections in a solution of 2 μM estradiol-BSA-fluorescein conjugated at position 6 (Lee, 1978; 1980; 1981; Kalland and Forsberg, 1980; Hanna *et al.*, 1982). These investigators reported primarily cytoplasmic labeling of breast tumors (Lee, 1978; 1980), myometrium (Hanna *et al.*, 1982) and thymus (Kalland and Forsberg, 1980). All investigators using Lee's preparation reported that non-target tissues such as skeletal muscle did not show similar cytoplasmic retention of the estradiol-fluorescein compound. Competition with estradiol conjugated to BSA did not prevent cytoplasmic fluorescence, and BSA-flourescein conjugates alone did not bind to the cytoplasm. Only Hanna *et al.* (1982) reported successful competition with diethylstilbestrol (1×10^{-4} M). Investigators using fluorescein-conjugated estrogen concluded that the observed binding was specific for the cytosolic estrogen receptor. Only Pertschuk *et al.* (1980b) and Hanna *et al.* (1982) reported correlation of results from histochemical and biochemical studies.

The concentrations of steroid hormones used in these histochemical studies are likely to saturate non-specific (Type II and III) binding sites (Clark *et al.*, 1978; Chamness *et al.*, 1980; Mercer *et al.*, 1981), and therefore, further correlation between the cytosolic receptor identified biochemically and the observed cytoplasmic fluorescence will be necessary before the validity of these techniques can be assessed.

Steroids conjugated to fluorescein, if proved to be reliable and reproducible indicators of the presence of steroid receptors, would have the advantage of providing a more rapid diagnosis of the presence or absence of receptors than radioactive steroids. However, due to extinction of fluorescence and the difficulty of recognizing cellular characteristics under fluorescent light, photographs of the tissue would often have to be taken under both fluorescent and bright field illumination for purposes of comparison. On the other hand, autoradiographic preparations permit the sections to be viewed repeatedly under bright field illumination with a variety of histological stains for differentiation of the morphology and histochemical characteristics of the tissues and lend themselves more readily to quantitative analysis. For clinical and research applications in which time is not as important a factor as the need for optimal assessment of histological characteristics and repeated viewing of the material with bright field microscopy, autoradiography will remain the technique of choice. If techniques for *in vitro* and *in vivo* application of fluoresceinated compounds can be demonstrated to be reproducible and reliable, there may be clinical or laboratory situations in which the rapidity and safety of these techniques would be preferred. However, the specificity, reliability and reproducibility of results obtained *in vivo* and *in vitro* with conjugated hormones does not warrant their use for clinical or routine laboratory investigations of steroid-sensitive tissues at the present time.

III. HISTOCHEMICAL TECHNIQUES UTILIZING ANTISERA TO STEROID HORMONE RECEPTOR MOLECULES

Several recent reports of antisera to proteins which can be demonstrated to bind steroid hormones have appeared in the literature (Greene *et al.*, 1977; Wrange *et al.*, 1979; Radanyi *et al.*, 1979). Preliminary reports of the use of these antisera for immunohistochemistry are appearing at meetings and in conference proceedings (Gustafsson *et al.*, 1981). Morel *et al.*, (1981) used antibodies to uterine cytosolic estradiol receptors to demonstrate receptor localization by means of electron microscopic immunohistochemistry. These authors reported the presence of immunostaining in the cytoplasm and nucleus of all anterior pituitary cell types except corticotropes. Because of problems related to specificity, several laboratories have produced monoclonal antisera to steroid receptor proteins (Green *et al.*, 1980. It is too early to determine whether these antisera will be of value for the histochemical detection of steroid sensitive tissues.

IV. HISTOCHEMICAL TECHNIQUES UTILIZING ANTISERA TO STEROIDS

Immunohistochemical detection of steroids in endocrine tissues has been attempted by several investigators. Immunohistochemical localization of testosterone (Bubenik *et al.*, 1975) was reported in frozen sections of rat and monkey testis. Kawaoi *et al.* (1978) showed both immunofluorescent and immunoperoxidase localization of progesterone in a progesterone-secreting mouse adrenocortical adenoma cell line. Dornhorst and Gann (1978) reported the immunolocalization of cortisol in cat adrenal and pituitary glands which were fixed in Bouin's fluid and embedded in paraffin. These studies have not been reproduced by other investigators. This technique may be useful in demonstrating steroid secreting cells. However, immunostaining of steroids in source tissues is hampered by diffusion of unbound steroid molecules.

Nenci (1976) and Pertschuk (1976) reported that antibodies to estradiol, in conjunction with the immunoperoxidase method, could be used to demonstrate the presence of estradiol on frozen and paraffin sections of estrogen target tissues. Numerous articles on the subject of immunohistochemical localization of estradiol have followed these initial reports (Ghosh *et al.*, 1978; Kurzon and Sternberger, 1978; Pertschuk *et al.*, 1978b; Nenci, 1978; Nenci and Marchetti, 1978; Nenci *et al.*, 1980b; 1980d; Walker *et al.*, 1980; Taylor *et al.*, 1981; Farley *et al.*, 1982).

In response to these reports, claiming the validity of immunohistochemical procedures for localization of estradiol in tissue sections, a number of authors have questioned the validity of the immunohistochemical approach (Mercer *et al.*, 1980; Morrow *et al.*, 1980; Chamness *et al.*., 1980; Penney and Hawkins, 1980; Zehr *et al.*, 1981; McCarty *et al.*, 1982; Underwood *et al.*, 1982). Two primary criticisms have been advanced. Firstly, it has been known for nearly a decade that steroid antibodies are not able to bind to steroid molecules which are already bound to a high-affinity receptor site (Fishman and Fishman, 1974; Castaneda and Liao, 1975; Morrow *et al.*, 1980). Thus, antibodies to steroids are not likely to be able to visualize the antigen in sections of frozen or paraffin embedded tissues. Nenci (1976b,c) has argued that his technique of immunolocalization of estradiol works because of conformational changes in the receptor which occur during drying in the cold, permitting estrogen molecules to become accessible to antibodies. Although considerable question exists concerning the significance of immunohistochemical localization of steroids which are already bound to a high-affinity binding site, Nenci did perform the required steroid competition and immunochemical controls. Thus some degree of specificity is claimed for this approach.

Pertschuk has attempted to circumvent the problem of localizing receptor-bound steroids by utilizing polyestradiol phosphate (PEP), which was initially considered to be capable of binding to the receptor while leaving an immunologically identifiable estradiol molecule available for binding by the antiserum (Pertschuk, 1976; 1978b). Morrow *et al.* (1980) and Zehr *et al.*, (1981) were unable to reproduce the binding of anti-estradiol antiserum to polyestradiol phosphate after *in vivo* injection or in a competitive binding assay. Further, Morrow *et al.* have shown that 200-fold excess polyestradiol phosphate was unable to compete with ^{3}H-estradiol for binding sites in the calf uterus. This suggests that the compound does not have as high an affinity for the receptor as does monomeric estradiol and may be binding non-specifically to other proteins. A second concern is the presence in estrogen-sensitive cells of several types of binding sites for estradiol. Clark *et al.* (1978) provided evidence for the existence of an additional non-translocatable low affinity, high capacity type of binding site which was termed "Type II". These sites are not detected when the concentration of estradiol is below 10 nM, but if the concentration of estradiol is increased, as is necessary for immunofluorescent demonstration of binding, the Type II sites become a factor to be considered (Mercer *et al.*, 1981). Pertschuk has noted that in some cases it is possible to demonstrate translocation to the nucleus, which would not be the case if Type II receptors are being observed (Pertschuk *et al.*, 1982). The translocation of receptors has also been demonstrated to be a temperature associated factor involved in the handling of frozen tissue after cutting (Barrows *et al.*, 1980). Barrows observation that estradiol fluorescence was translocated to, but not retained by, the nucleus for longer than two minutes raises considerable doubt that Pertschuk *et al.*, (1976; 1978) could be visualizing the active estradiol receptor after thawing, air drying and exposing the section to acetone fixation. Underwood *et al.* (1982) and Penney and Hawkins (1980) reported that acetone fixation virtually eliminated specific estradiol binding to estrogen receptors from MCF-7 cells and rat uterus. Some of the unanswered questions regarding the utility of these techniques will await standardization of the conditions under which tissues are processed for immunohistochemistry.

V. CONCLUSION

Comparison of studies utilizing dry- and thaw-mount autoradiography with ^{3}H-estradiol and immunohistochemistry with antibodies to estradiol show that there remain significant differences in the results obtained with these methods. While in the autoradiographic studies after *in vivo* and *in vitro* administration of ^{3}H-estradiol concentration of radioactivity is consistently observed in nuclei of target tissues, in immunohistochemical studies with antibodies to estradiol, cytoplasmic staining prevails and only occasional nuclear staining is reported. In our autoradiograms, there is no labeling of nucleoli and of cytoplasm of eosinophils which, however, are strongly stained with antibodies to estradiol and with estradiol conjugates. Further, centrioles of target and non-target cells are strongly stained with antibodies to estradiol, an observation which is difficult to explain in light of the deviations mentioned above. There is good agreement between the results obtained with biochemical techniques and those obtained with dry- and thaw-mount autoradiography (Stumpf, 1968; Stumpf *et al.*, 1981) in respect to the nuclear concentration. There is accumulating evidence that the histochemical section incubation techniques with radiolabeled estradiol, estradiol antibodies, or conjugated to estradiol do not show true receptor sites.

Since estradiol is noncovalently bound to its receptors and easily translocatable, any step in the histochemical preparation must be carefully controlled in order to prevent redistribution and loss (Stumpf and Roth, 1966). The importance of technique in the localization of estradiol has been clearly demonstrated in earlier reviews of the autoradiographic literature and must not be ignored. According to these reviews, preparations of autoradiograms by different investigators with five different techniques yielded results which differed from each other, but were characteristic of and reproducible within each technique. In studies designed to assess the effects of solvents or embedding media as applied in the above autoradiographic techniques, results obtained with six different techniques similarly deviated from each other, but were reproducible within each technique (Stumpf and Roth, 1966; Stumpf, 1968).

In most of the current histochemical studies with steroid antibodies and conjugates, redistribution and loss of the ligand or the "receptor" have not been controlled. The validity of histochemical techniques is now being challenged by numerous groups (Mercer *et al.*, 1980; Morrow *et al.*, 1980; Chamness *et al.*, 1980; Penney and Hawkins, 1980; Zehr *et al.*, 1981; McCarty *et al.*, 1982; Underwood *et al.*, 1982; Stumpf and Sar, 1982). Results obtained with these techniques must be interpreted with caution. The term receptor must not be applied, unless there is evidence that the localization represents the site of action. Even though the results derived from immunohistochemical approaches with estradiol antibodies probably do not show receptor sites, some utility for clinical diagnosis of hormone responsive tumors cannot be excluded and may be tested further. Cytoplasmic binding proteins other than receptors may be present in target cells and their localization may prove to be sufficiently specific.

A careful extrapolation suggests that a higher utility and reliability can be expected in the future use of antibodies to nuclear receptors, which may supercede the less reliable use of antibodies to steroid hormones or of conjugated steroids. Steroid autoradiography with radioactively labeled hormones probably will retain its informative value and continue to be used in identifying steroid hormone target sites both *in vivo* and *in vitro*.

VI. ACKNOWLEDGEMENTS

Supported by USPHS grants NS09914 and NS05911.

VII. REFERENCES

Barrows, G. H., Stroupe, S. B. and Riehm, J. D. (1980). *Am. J. Clin. Path.* **73**, 330–339.
Beckman, Jr, W. C. , Newsome, J. F. and Stumpf, W. E. (1982). Abstract, Symposium on Breast Cancer, San Antonio, TX, November, 1982.
Brokelman, J. (1969). *J. Histochem. Cytochem.* **17**, 394–407.
Bubenik, G. A., Brown, G. M. and Grota, L. J. (1975). *Endocrinology* **96**, 63–69.
Buell, R. H. and Tremblay, G. (1981). *J. Histochem. Cytochem.* **29**, 1316–1321.
Castaneda, E. and Liao, S. (1975). *J. Biol. Chem.* **250**, 883–888.
Chamness, G. C., Mercer, W. D., and McGuire, W. L. (1980). *J. Histochem. Cytochem.* **28**, 792–798.
Clark, J. H., Hardin, J. W. and Upchurch, S. (1978). *J. Biol. Chem.* **253**, 7630–7634.
Dandliker, W. B., Brawn, R. J., Hsu, M.-L., Brawn, P. N., Levin, J., Meyers, C. Y. and Kolb, V. M. (1978). *Cancer Res.* **38**, 4212–4224.

Dornhorst, A. and Gann, D. S. (1978). *J. Histochem. Cytochem.* **26**, 909–913.
Farley, A. L., O'Brien, T., Moyer, D. and Taylor, C. R. (1982). *Cancer* **49**, 2153–2160.
Fisher, B., Gunduz, N., Zheng, S. and Saffer, E. A. (1982). *Cancer Res.* **42**, 540–549.
Fishman, J. and Fishman, J. H. (1974). *J. Clin. Endocr. Metab.* **39**, 603–606.
Ghosh, L., Ghosh, B. C. and Das Gupta, T. K. (1978). *J. Surg. Oncol.* **10**, 221–224.
Godefroi, V. C. and Brooks, S. C. (1973). *Anal. Biochem.* **51**, 335–344.
Greene, G. L., Closs, L. E., Fleming, H., De Sombre, E. R. and Jensen, E. V. (1977). *Proc. Natn. Acad. Sci. USA* **74**, 3681–3685.
Greene, G. L., Nolan, C., Engler, J. P. and Jensen, E. V. (1980). *Proc. Natn. Acad. Sci. USA* **77**, 5115–5119.
Grody, W. W., Schrader, W. T. and O'Malley, B. W. (1982). *Endocr. Rev.* **3**, 141–163.
Gustafsson, J.-A., Carlstedt-Duke, J., Fuxe, K., Carlstrom, K., Okret, S. and Wrange, O. (1981). *In* "Steroid Hormone Regulation of the Brain" (K. Fuxe, J.-A. Gustafsson and L. Wetter berg, eds, Vol. 34. pp. 31–40.) Wenner-Gren Symposium Series.
Hanna, W., Ryder, D. E. and Mobbs, B. G. (1982). *Am. J. Clin. Path.* **77**, 391–95.
Jensen, E. V. and De Sombre, E. R. (1973). *Science* **182**, 126–134.
Kalland, T. and Forsberg, J. G. (1980). *Immunol. Lett.* **1**, 293–297.
Kawaoi, A., Uchida, T., Okano, T., Matsumoto, K. and Shikata, T. (1978) *Acta Histochem. Cytochem.* **11**, 1–12.
Kurzon, R. M. and Sternberger, L. A. (1978). *J. Histochem. Cytochem.* **26**, 803–808.
Leav, I., Merk, F. B., Ofner, P., Goodrich, G., Kwan, P. W. L., Stein, B. M., Sar, M. and Stumpf, W. E. (1976). *Am. J. Path.* **93**, 69–85.
Lee, S. H. (1978). *Am. J. Clin. Path.* **70**, 197–203.
Lee, S. H. (1979). *Cancer* **44**, 1–12.
Lee, S. H. (1980). *Am. J. Clin. Path.* **73**, 323–329.
Lee, S. H. (1981). *Histochemistry* **71**, 491–500.
Lippman, M. E. and Allegra, J. C. (1978). *New Engl. J. Med.* **299**, 930–933.
Lippman, M. E. and Huff, K. (1976). *Cancer* **38**, 868–74.
McCarty, K. S. Jr, Reintgen, D. S., Seigler, H. F. and McCarty, K. S. Sr, (1982). *Horm. Breast Cancer* (in press).
McGuire, W. L. (1973). *J. Clin. Invest.* **52**, 73–77.
Mercer, W. D., Wahl, T. M., Carlson, C. A., Wahl, D. A., Lippman, M. E., Lezotte, D. and Teague, P. O. (1980). *Cancer* **46**, 2859–2868.
Mercer, W. D., Edwards, D. P., Chamness, G. C. and McGuire, W. L. (1981). *Cancer Res.* **41**, 4644–4652.
Morel, G., DuBois, P., Benassayag, C., Nunez, E., Radanyi, C., Redeuilh, G., Richard-Foy, H. and Baulieu, E. (1981). *Exp. Cell Res.* **132**, 249–257.
Morrow, B., Leav, I., DeLellis, R. A. and Raam, S. (1980). *Cancer* **46**, 2872–2879.
Nenci, I., Beccati, M. D., Piffanelli, A. and Lanza, G. (1976a). *J. Steroid Biochem.* **7**, 505–510.
Nenci, I., Beccati, M. D., Piffanelli, A. and Lanza, G. (1976b). *In* "Research on Steroids" (A. Vermeulen *et al.*, eds), Vol. VII. pp. 137–147. Elsevier, Amsterdam.
Nenci, I., Piffanelli, A. Beccati, M. D. and Lanza, G. (1976c). *J. Steroid Biochem.* **7**, 883–890.
Nenci, I. (1978). *Cancer Res.* **38**, 4204–4211.

Nenci, I., and Marchetti, E. (1978). *Cell Biol.* **76**, 255–260.

Nenci, I., Dandliker, W. B., Meyers, C. Y., Marchetti, E., Marzola, A. and Fabris, G. (1980a). *J. Histochem. Cytochem.* **28**, 1081–1088.

Nenci, I., Fabris, F., Marchetti, E. and Marzola, A. (1980b). *Virchows Arch. B. Cell Path.* **32**, 139–145.

Nenci, I., Fabris, G., Marchetti, E. and Marzola, A. (1980c). *In* "Perspectives in Steroid Receptor Research" (F. Bresciani, ed.), pp. 61–72. Raven Press, New York.

Nenci, I., Fabris, G., Marzola, A. and Marchetti, E. (1980d). *In* "Pharmacological Modulation of Steroid Action" (E. Genazzini *et al.*, eds), pp. 99–110.

Nenci, I., Marchetti, E., Marzola, A. and Farris, G. (1981). *J. Steroid Biochem.* **14**, 1139–1146.

Osborne, C. K. and Lippman, M. E. (1978). *In* "Breast Cancer: Advances in Research and Treatment" (W. L. McGuire, ed.), Vol. 2, pp. 103–154.

Panko, W. B., Mattioli, C. and Wheeler, T. (1980). Worcester Foundation Symposium on Cancer and Hormones, March, 1980.

Penney, G. C. and Hawkins, R. A. (1980). *Lancet* **1**, 930.

Pertschuk, L. P. (1976). *Res. Commun. Chem. Path. Pharmacol.* **14**, 771–774.

Pertschuk, L. P., Zava, D. T., Gaetjens, E., Macchia, R. J., Brigati, D. J. and Kim D. S. (1978a). *Res. Commun. Chem. Path. Pharmacol.* **22**, 427–430.

Pertschuk, L. P., Tobin, E. H., Brigati, D. J., Kim, D. S., Bloom, N. D., Gaetjens, E., Berman, P. J., Carter, A. C. and Degenshein, G. A. (1978b). *Cancer* **41**, 907–911.

Pertschuk, L. P., Gaetjens, E., Carter, A. C., Brigati, D. J., Kim, D. S. and Fealey, T. E. (1979). *Am. J. Clin. Path.* **71**, 504–508.

Pertschuk, L. P., Di Maio, M. F. and Gaetjens, E. (1980a). *J. Steroid Biochem.* **13**, 1121–1124.

Pertschuk, L. P., Tobin, E. H., Tanapat, P., Gaetjens, E., Carter, A. C., Bloom, N. D., Macchia, R. J. and Eisenberg, K. B. (1980b). *J. Histochem. Cytochem.* **28**, 799–810.

Pertschuk, L. P., Rosenthal, H. E., Macchia, R. J., Eisenberg, K. B., Feldman, J. G., Wax, S. H., Kim, D. S., Whitmore, W. F., Abrahams, J. I., Gaetjens, E., Wise, G. J., Herr, H. W., Karr, J. P., Murphy, G. P. and Sandberg, A. A. (1982). *Cancer* **49**, 984–993.

Poulsen, H. S. (1981). *Eur. J. Cancer* **17**, 495–501.

Radanyi, C., Redeuilh, G., Eigenmann, E., Lebeau, M. C., Massol, N., Secco, C., Baulieu, E. E. and Richard-Foy, H. (1979). *Compt. Rend. Acad. Sci. Paris* **288**, 255–263.

Rao, B. R., Fry, C. G., Hunt, S. Kuhnel, R. and Dandliker, W. B. (1980a). *Cancer* **46**, 2902–2906.

Rao, B. R., Patrick, T. B. and Sweet, F. (1980b). *Endocrinology* **106**, 336–362.

Sheridan, P. J., Buchanan, J. M., Anselmo, V. C. and Martin, P. (1979). *Nature* **282**, 579–582.

Stumpf, W. E. and Roth, L. J. (1966). *J. Histochem. Cytochem.* **14**, 274–287.

Stumpf, W. E. (1968). *In:* "Radioisotopes in Medicine: *In Vitro* Studies" (R. L. Hayes *et al.*, eds), AEC Symposium Series No. 13 (CONF-671111), pp. 633–660. AEC, Oak Ridge, Tennessee.

Stumpf, W. E. (1969). *Endocrinology* **85**, 31–37.

Stumpf, W. E. and Sar, M. (1975). *In* "Hormone Action, Part A. Steroid Hormones" (B. W. O'Malley and J. G. Hardman, eds), Methods in Enzymology, Vol. XXXVI. pp. 135–156. Academic Press, New York.

Stumpf, W. E. and Sar, M. (1976). *J. Steroid Biochem.* **7**, 1163–1170.

Stumpf, W. E. and Sar, M. (1976). *In* "Receptors and Mechanism of Action of Steroid Hormones" (J. Pasqualini, ed.), Modern Pharmacology-Toxicology, Vol. 8. pp. 41–84. Marcel Dekker, New York.

Stumpf, W. E. and Sar, M. (1982). *Acta Histochem. Jap.* (in press).

Taylor, C. R., Cooper, C. L., Kurman, R. J., Goebelsmann, U. and Markland, F. S. (1981). *Cancer* **47**, 2634–2640.

Tchernitchin, A., (1967). *Steroids* **10**, 661–668.

Thompson, J. A., Haven, M. C., Langdon, S. M. and Haven G. T. (1980). *Am. J. Clin. Path.* **73**, 340–344.

Underwood, J. C. E., Sher, E., Reed, M., Eisman, J. A. and Martin, T. J. (1982). *J. Clin. Path.* **35**, 401–406.

Walker, R. A., Cove, D. H. and Howell, A. (1980). *Lancet* **1**, 171–173.

Wrange, O., Carlstedt-Duke, J. and Gustafsson, J.-A. (1979). *J. Biol. Chem.* **254**, 9284–9290.

Zehr, D. R., Satyaswaroop, P. G. and Sheehan, D. M. (1981). *J. Steroid Biochem.* **14**, 613–617.

Lectin Binding to Paraffin Sections

A. J. C. LEATHEM and N. J. ATKINS

I. INTRODUCTION

Lectins are proteins or glycoproteins of non-immune origin derived mostly from plants but also from some animals, which bind specifically to carbohydrate groups. Their value in histochemistry lies in their ability to localise, identify and distinguish tissue carbohydrates with great sensitivity and specificity.

Stillmark is credited with being the father of lectins with his publication of a plant extract (termed Ricin from *Ricinus communis*) reacting with sub-

IMMUNOCYTOCHEMISTRY 2
ISBN 0 12 140402 1

stances in serum, in his thesis of 1888. There has been a revival of interest in the last 20 years, especially by biologists and immunologists for fractionation of cell subpopulations in suspension (Edelman, 1971; Reisner and Sharon, 1980), and more recently selection of populations by their resistance to lectin toxicity (Briles, 1982), by biochemists for fractionation of the cell components by affinity chromatography (Ogata *et al.*, 1975; Lotan *et al.*, 1977) and electrophoresis (Bjerrum and Bog-Hansen, 1976; Bog-Hansen *et al.*, 1978; Horejsi *et al.*, 1979).

The great variety of lectin applications is best appreciated by perusing some of the review articles on lectins (Lis and Sharon, 1973; Nicolson, 1974; Sharon, 1977; Brown and Hunt, 1978; Lotan, 1979).

The term "lectin" was proposed by Boyd and Shapleigh, in 1954, from the Latin Lego/lectum meaning I choose or pick out, as being more appropriate than such previous terms as phytotoxins and phytohaemagglutinins, since similar carbohydrate-binding substances can be isolated from animal as well as plant sources. The term "lectin" is now generally accepted to mean a "sugar binding protein of non-immune origin which agglutinates cells and/or precipitates glycoconjugates" (Goldstein *et al.*, 1980), but because this does not distinguish them from enzymes with sugar-specific binding sites, the term "affinitins" has been proposed as a collective term for lectins, enzymes and antibodies with a high affinity for specific chemical structures (Franz and Ziska, 1981). The term "receptor-specific protein" has also been introduced by Gold and Balding (1975). However, the term "lectin" is currently the best known to cover these non-immune entities.

Lectins have been detected in a vast range of organisms, especially plants, and a comprehensive source list has been published by Gold and Balding (1975). As all lectins possess at least two carbohydrate binding sites they can agglutinate cells bearing surface glycoconjugates. Most work on lectins has been directed towards finding blood-group-specific reagents; thus most lectins have been identified by their ability to agglutinate red blood cells, either untreated or enzymatically modified (e.g. by neuraminidase).

Lectins are generally followed during their purification by their haemagglutinating property but they can agglutinate other cells in suspension depending on the expression of oligosaccharides at the cell surface. The removal of terminal groups such as sialic acids by enzymes (e.g. trypsin and neuraminidase) frequently reveals carbohydrates not normally exposed. Although such carbohydrates may normally be sequestered by terminal groups, changes in cell behaviour and function may be reflected by a failure to form the typical terminal sugar groups. During changes in the cell cycle (Shoham and Sachs, 1974), transformation (Talmadge *et al.*, 1974; Lis and Sharon, 1973), tumour development (Nicolson, 1980), metastatic potential (Pearlstein *et al.*, 1980) and in normal cell differentiation (Newman *et al.*,

1979; Galili *et al.*, 1981) there are surface changes in the sugars detectable by lectins. Although at present there are no lectins which are cell specific or tumour specific, there is great interest in using lectins as a tool to aid in the determination of differentiation, metastatic potential and functional as opposed to simple morphological transformation.

More recently cytoplasmic oligosaccharides have been identified by lectins in tissue sections and this provides a new and potentially enormously useful tool for assessing cell differentiation and function in normal and histopathological formalin fixed paraffin sections.

We wish to provide details here of several different approaches to showing lectin binding to paraffin sections.

A. Abbreviations

Fuc, fucose; Gal, galactose; GalNAc, N-acetyl galactosamine; Glc, glucose; GlcNAc, N-acetyl glucosamine; Man, mannose; NANA, N-acetyl neuraminic acid; CEA, carcino-embryonic antigen.

II. LECTINS TO IDENTIFY TISSUE CARBOHYDRATES

Markers of tissue function generally fall into 3 main groups:

1. Antigens (mainly proteins)—recognised by antibodies, detectable in frozen and in paraffin sections.
2. Enzymes—recognised by their function on substrate, usually require unfixed, frozen sections.
3. Receptors—recognised by their function of binding to their ligand, require unfixed, frozen sections.

We describe here a fourth major group, the carbohydrates:

4. Carbohydrates—recognised by lectins, detectable in frozen and in paraffin sections.

Carbohydrates occur conjugated to lipids (as glycolipids) and to proteins (as glycoproteins) in all animal cells. As they confer stability and recognition groups they are found predominantly at the surface of normal cells, particularly on the luminal surface of epithelial cells and in their secretions. However, in cells involved in active secretion, in undifferentiated cells and in cells undergoing dysplastic and neoplastic change, there is an accumulation of glycoconjugates in the cytoplasm. It is for these changes that lectins have a particular value to the histologist and histopathologist.

By applying lectins as stains to frozen and paraffin sections of tissues, we can identify many cells and their alterations in function and behaviour by changes in glycosylation. Using a panel of several lectins, such functional changes can be detected before any morphological change.

Lectins have two major advantages over any other histochemical method for demonstrating carbohydrates; they can be extremely sensitive and specific. Because of this specificity, only a small proportion of the carbohydrates present may be identified unless "cocktails" of lectins are used.

III. SUGAR SPECIFICITIES OF LECTINS

It is important to realise that the soluble simple sugar which inhibits lectin binding and haemagglutination may not be the same as the sugar group to which the lectin *preferentially* binds in the tissue. This is largely because each binding site may lock into a combination of sugars more tightly than into a single sugar. Further, although the polysaccharide preferred may be of identical units (e.g. of GlcNAc polymers see Table I, as preferred by wheatgerm) the units may be different (heteroglycans, such as α-L-fucose (1–2) α-D-galactose (1–4) GalNAc which is preferred to α-L-fucose by Lotus, see Table I).

Therefore, two lectins with apparently similar simple sugar specificities, e.g. concanavalin A and lentil lectin, each with binding sites for α-D-mannose > glucose > GlcNAc (see Table I) do not bind to identical tissue components; although each may bind to terminal mannose groups, lentil lectin binds to α-mannose-fucosyl groups at dilutions (or in the presence of weak mannose, glucose or GalNAc) where concanavalin A shows no binding.

Table I shows a selection of lectins which are either fairly readily available or which give interesting tissue binding specificities. We have attempted to distinguish those simple sugars (*simple sugar specificity*), which at 0·1 M concentration should inhibit specific lectin binding (but not of non-specific hydrophobic binding), from those complex polysaccharides which are present in animal tissues and may represent the actual binding complex for the lectin (*preferred sugar binding group*). By the use of several lectins exhibiting similar simple sugar binding properties it will be possible to identify precisely complex carbohydrates and distinguish cell populations. At present the polysaccharide specificities for most lectins are not known.

IV. SOURCES OF LECTINS

There are many commercial sources of lectins, those we have used are listed in the Appendix, and some, e.g. concanavalin A are so cheap and reliable

TABLE I
Lectins which are readily available or have interesting binding specificities.

Lectin	Source	Simple sugar specificity	Preferential tissue binding group
Abrin	*Abrus precatorius* (Jequirty bean)	Gal $\beta > \alpha$	Gal-GalNac . . . (terminal)
Bandeiraea	*Bandeiraea* or *Griffonia simplicifolia* (5 isolectins)	α-D-Gal $\beta > \alpha$ GlcNAc	α-D-Gal . . . (terminal) β-GlcNAc . . . (terminal only; not internal)
Bauhinia	*Bauhinia purpurea* (2 isolectins)	GalNAc > Gal	β-galactopyranosyl (1 → 3) 2 acetamindo-2 deoxy-D-galactosyl-
Broad bean	*Vicia fava*	α-D-Man > α-D-Glc	c.f. lentil
Concanavalin A	*Canavalia ensiformis* (Jack bean)	α-Man > α-Glc > α-GlcNAc > α-methyl mannoside	
Crotolaria	*Crotolaria juncea* (Sunn hemp)	Gal	
Cystisus	*Cystisus sessilifolius*	β-GlcNAc	β-GlcNAc (1 → 4)β-GlcNAc
Eel	*Anguilla rostrata*	L-Fuc	L-fucosyl . . .
Erythrina	*Erythrina cristagalli*	Gal	β-D-galactose (1 → 3) N-acetyl-D-galactosaminyl-c.f. peanut
Gorse	*Ulex europeus* isolectin 1 isolectin 2	L-Fuc GlcNAc	fucose (1 → 2) D-Gal (1 → 4)- GlcNAc (1 → 6)-
Helix aspersa	*Helix aspera* (Garden snail)	GalNAc	?
Helix pomatia	*Helix pomatia* (Roman snail)	α-GalNAc	?
Horse gram	*Dolichos biflorus*	α-GalNAc	α-D-GalNAc . . . (terminal)
Horseshoe crab	*Limulus polyphemus*	Sialic acid	N-acetyl neuraminic acids also phosphoryl choline
Kidney bean	*Phaseolus vulgaris* (5 isolectins)	GalNAc	NANA-β-D-Gal (1 → 3, 4) β-D-Gal (1 → 2) D-Man-
Laburnum	*Laburnum alpinum*	GlcNAc	GlcNAc-GlcNAc
Lentil	*Lens culinaris* (2 isolectins A and B)	α-methyl Man > Glc > GlcNAc	. . . β-GlcNAc-α-mannosyl and α-Man-fucosyl . . . (c.f. pea, con A)
Lima bean	*Phaseolus limensis* or *lunatus* (2 isolectins)	GalNAc	?

TABLE I—continued

Lectin	Source	Simple sugar specificity	Preferential tissue binding group
Locust bean	*Robinia pseudoaccacia*	?GlcNAc	?
Lotus	*Lotus tetragonolobus* (3 isolectins A, B and C)	α-L-Fuc	α-L-fuc(1 $\rightarrow$ 2)α-D-Gal (1 $\rightarrow$ 4)GalNAc c.f. Gorse/Ulex 1
Mistletoe	*Viscum album*	Gal	?
Modeccin	*Adenia digitata*	Gal	?
Osage orange	*Maclura pomifera*	α-D-Gal	? (terminal) c.f. Bandeiraea 1
Pea	*Pisum sativum* (2 isolectins)	α-methyl Man > Glc > GlcNAc	α-fucosyl-Asn-linked oligosaccharides c.f. con A, pea, lentil.
Peanut	*Arachis hypogaea*	Gal	β-D-Gal(1 $\rightarrow$ 3)N acetyl-D-galactosaminyl- c.f. Erythrina
Pokeweed	*Phytolacca americana* (5 isolectins)	?	(1 $\rightarrow$ 4)N acetyl-D-glucosaminyl-
Potato	*Solanum tuberosum*	GlcNAc	(1 $\rightarrow$ 4)N acetyl-D-glucosaminyl-
Ricin	*Ricinus communis* RCA 1	Gal	Gal-GlcNAc-Gal . . .
Ricinin	(castor oil bean) RCA 2 (2 isolectins)	Gal	(terminal) ?
Slug	*Limax flavus*	Sialic acid	Sialic acid
Sophora	*Sophora japonica*	GalNAc	?
Soya bean	*Glycine soya* or *max*	GalNAc Gal	?
Wheatgerm	*Triticum vulgaris* or *aestivum* (isolectins)	GlcNAc	GlcNAc-GlcNAc-GlcNAc . . .
Wistaria	*Wistaria floribunda* 1 (2 isolectins) 2	GalNAc GlcNAc	? ?

that it is hardly worth isolating one's own. However, if large amounts of any lectin are to be used, if the lectin of interest is not readily available or if it is prohibitively expensive, then it is necessary to isolate and purify them. In addition, a great attraction of lectins is their binding sugar may be known and the site can be specifically blocked as a control; to do this, it is helpful to understand the principles of lectin affinity purification.

The simplest method for isolating lectins is by affinity chromatography, using a suitable sugar immobilised on an insoluble support, e.g. beads. A lectin source, e.g. a bean, is homogenised in saline, applied to a column of appropriate immobilised sugar and, after washing the column, the lectin is eluted off the column by the soluble appropriate sugar, which is dialysed out to leave "pure" lectin. The binding of lectin to sugars is reversible and soluble sugars compete with the immobilised sugar for the binding sites.

Some of the solid supports used in gel chromatography are themselves sugar polymers, such as Sephadex (a dextran polymer of glucose) and Agarose, Bio-Gel A or Sepharose (galactose polymers) and thus can be used for the purification of glucose binding lectins (such as concanavalin A, lentil, *Pisum sativum*) or galactose binding lectins without further modification of the support. Most naturally ocurring polysaccharides are found as sugar mixtures and may not be suitable for isolating lectins with a single sugar specificity from crude plant extracts unless isolectins are sought. Some natural insoluble polysaccharides can be used without modification. Chitin, for example, the polysaccharide exoskeleton of insects, crabs etc., is readily available commercially and provides a solid matrix for the isolation of N-acetylglucosamine binding lectins.

The most convenient source of immobilised sugars for affinity chromatography is to buy them (see Appendix for suppliers). As simple carbohydrates are very small molecules, they are much more effective if bound to an insoluble matrix via a spacer (which physically places the sugar away from the matrix and thus allows the lectin to bind more easily, giving higher yields). An alternative to using the specific sugar is to use an immobilised glycoprotein. This is particularly useful for lectins which bind to heteropolysaccharides (heteroglycans) or polysaccharides containing two or more different monosaccharide units (such as connective tissue mucins, e.g. hyaluronic acid = D-glucuronic acid and N-acetyl-D-glucosamine).

Blood group substance has been used by several workers after coupling to some support but for most people the isolation of blood group substance would be too arduous. However, many lectins bind to erythrocytes, frequently without species specificity, and whole, washed blood cells can be used, either fresh or formalinised and stored, as a solid phase, and the lectins eluted with specific soluble sugars.

The external carbohydrate of the major blood groups is N-acetyl-D-galactosamine for group A, D-galactose for group B and L-fucose for group O. Therefore, cells from these major groups can be used to isolate lectins binding to the exposed carbohydrate simply by mixing cells with crude lectin extract, washing and eluting off lectin with 0·2 M soluble sugar. After dialysing out the sugar, the presence of the lectin can be confirmed by haemagglutination.

Some major points to consider in purification of lectins are:

1. Many lectins require the presence of heavy metals, in particular calcium, manganese and magnesium, to maintain an active binding site. If washing and eluting buffers are devoid of such trace components the lectin may lose activity and become denatured. The problem is exacerbated if some sequestering salts are present, in particular phosphates (which are insoluble with these heavy metals) and therefore phosphate-buffered-saline (PBS) should be avoided for lectins. We prefer to use plain saline or Tris-buffered-saline (TBS, see Appendix).

2. Most lectins have preferential binding sites for complex carbohydrates, thus peanut lectin will preferentially bind to b-D-gal (1–3) GalNAc rather than to galactose and wheatgerm lectin will preferentially bind to polymers of GlcNAc-GlcNAc-GlcNAc rather than to simple N-acetyl-D-glucosamine (GlcNAc). Thus lectin bound to an affinity column of immobilised complex carbohydrate may not easily elute using the simple soluble sugar. This equally applies to tissue sections and is considered further under Section VIII.

3. The binding of lectins is not purely by interaction with carbohydrates but may be through hydrophobic bonds (Ochoa *et al.*, 1981). This varies with different lectins from insignificant to marked (in the red bean, *Phaseolus vulgaris*) and may require incorporation of a detergent, such as Tween 20, into the elution buffer.

For some staining procedures described here (antibody method and sugar-lectin-sugar sandwich) pure lectin is not needed, and either the inexpensive blood-grouping reagents or even crude saline extracts of plant material may be used effectively.

V. STAINING METHODS

In tissue sections we are seeking binding of lectin and not the effects of cross-linking such as agglutination, thus lectins which fail to haemagglutinate can still bind to and stain tissues.

In a similar way to immunofluorescence and immunoperoxidase, fluorescein (FITC) and such enzymes as peroxidase and alkaline phosphatase are used as labels to localise lectin binding sites.

The binding of lectin to tissue sections can be demonstrated in two main ways:

1. Direct staining; with conjugation of a label such as fluorescein or an enzyme to the lectin.

2. Indirect; localising bound lectin either with an antibody directed against the lectin, by an avidin-biotin reaction or by applying labelled sugar to unoccupied binding sites on the lectin.

Direct staining is the most convenient but lacks sensitivity particularly for paraffin sections, unless high concentrations are used.

To increase sensitivity in an indirect system, antibodies to the lectin can be used or lectin biotinated and then an avidin label used to localise it.

But perhaps the most elegant indirect system involves a sugar-lectin-sugar sandwich: most lectins have at least two binding sites and up to 8 or 10 on each molecule (unless an artificial monomer is used such as a succinylated lectin). The agglutinating property of lectins is proportional to these cross-linking or binding sites. However, when lectins bind to carbohydrates in

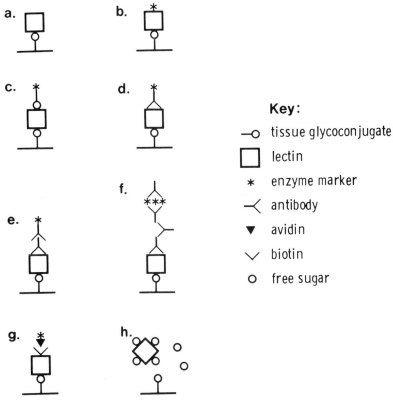

Key:

—o tissue glycoconjugate

☐ lectin

∗ enzyme marker

⤙ antibody

▼ avidin

∨ biotin

○ free sugar

FIG. 1. (a) Lectin binding to tissue glycoconjugate; (b) Lectin labelled with a fluorescent or enzyme marker; (c) sandwich technique using a labelled glycoconjugate; (d) direct immunoenzyme technique; (e) indirect immunoenzyme technique; (f) peroxidase anti-peroxidase immunoenzyme technique; (g) biotin-avidin method; (h) competitive inhibition by free sugar.

tissue sections, several binding sites on the lectin remain unoccupied. These spare binding sites can be used to bind free sugars conjugated to a label, e.g. peroxidase.

Each of these approaches is described in detail below and see Fig. 1.

A. Direct Lectin Staining

Lectin conjugated to fluorescein or an enzyme is incubated on the section and the label visualised under a fluorescence microscope or after incubating in enzyme substrate.

A large variety of lectins conjugated to fluorescein, rhodamine (for double staining) and horseradish peroxidase are commercially available (see Appendix) and although expensive, kits with small amounts of conjugate are very convenient to assess any particular system or tissue.

Direct staining procedure (see Fig. 2):

1. Dewax section.
2. Incubate in appropriate dilution of lectin-conjugate (e.g. 100 μg/ml) for 30 min at room temperature.
3. Wash in 3 changes of buffer, 2 min each.
4. Examine under fluorescence microscope or incubate in substrate, counterstain, mount.

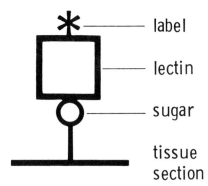

FIG. 2. Direct staining.

Notes: The optimum dilution of each new batch of lectin-conjugate is determined by incubation on sections for a fixed time. A range of doubling dilutions, e.g. 1000, 500, 250, 125, 62, 31, 16, 8 μg/ml should be tried, diluting them in a buffer containing trace metals (see Appendix).

Frozen sections of unfixed material are ideal to start the investigation of any tissue for lectin binding, as carbohydrates have not been masked by fixation and glycolipids not dissolved out by processing. Initially, plain air dried, frozen sections (30 min at room temperature with a hair-drier) are used as any attempts to promote adhesion of sections to the slide (heat, albumenising the slides, dipping in alcohol or acetone) may introduce arti-facts into lectin staining. Sections of compound blocks containing an assort-ment of organs are used. A mixture of kidney, stomach, lung, mammary gland, bladder, fallopian tube, salivary gland and pancreas has shown stain-ing of some of the cells with every lectin we have so far used (see Figs. 3–12 for examples of staining). Tissues from a wide variety of animals give similar (though not always identical) distribution of lectin binding and rat or mouse tissues provide good positive control tissues.

Fluorescein conjugated lectins are excellent for direct staining of cryostat sections, they often work at high dilution, e.g. 10 μg/ml and the method is simple and reliable. If enzyme-lectin conjugates must be used then blocking of endogenous tissue enzymes may be required; this should be considered with caution as the action of blocking agents (e.g. hydrogen peroxide in dilute HCl or methanol) on carbohydrates may alter the lectin binding pattern. Tissues low in endogenous enzymes may not need blocking.

Paraffin sections are not as satisfactory as cryostat sections for direct lectin

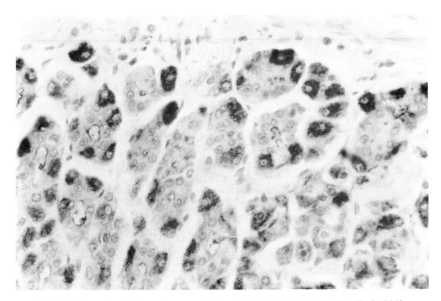

FIG. 3. Normal rat stomach; soya bean lectin staining parietal cells (×320).

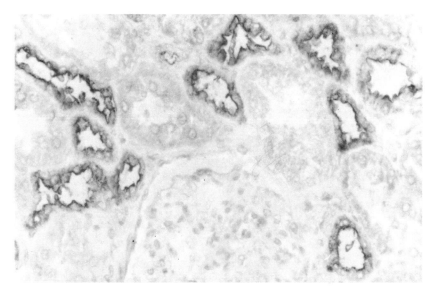

FIG. 4. Normal human kidney; helix pomatia lectin staining luminal surface and cytoplasm more weakly of distal tubule cells (×250).

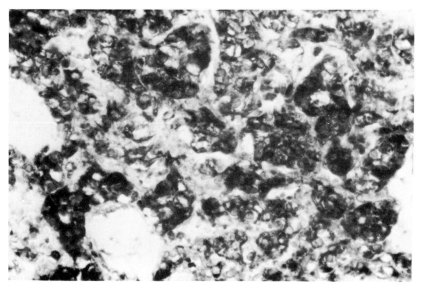

FIG. 5. Carcinoma of human kidney; helix pomatia staining cytoplasm of cancer cells
(×250).

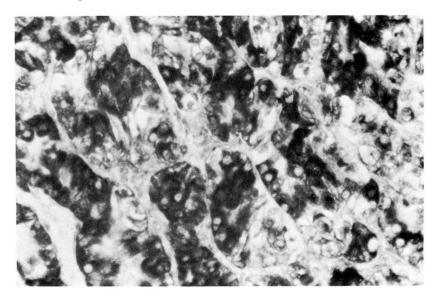

FIG. 6. Carcinoma of human kidney; peanut lectin staining cytoplasm of cancer cells (×250).

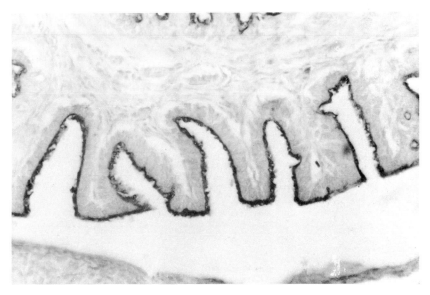

FIG. 7. Rat fallopian tube; Bauhinia lectin staining cilia (×200).

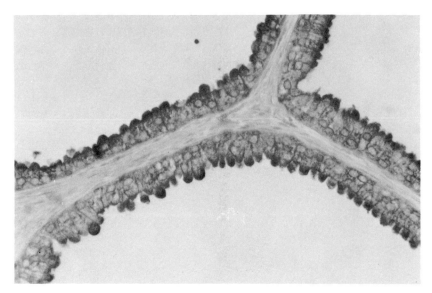

FIG. 8. Normal human prostate; pokeweed lectin staining epithelium (×250).

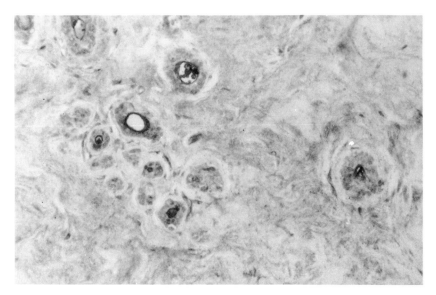

FIG. 9. Normal human breast; helix pomatia lectin staining luminal surface and secretion of normal acini (×200).

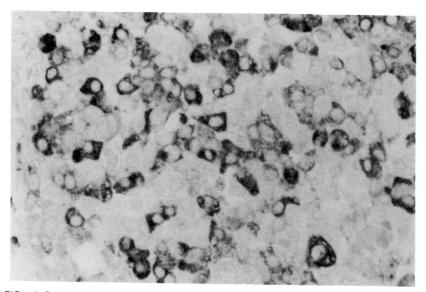

FIG. 10. Carcinoma of human breast; helix pomatia lectin staining a sub-population of cancer cells (×250).

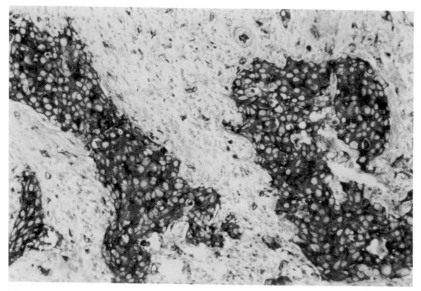

FIG. 11. Carcinoma of human breast; Bandeiraea 1 lectin staining cytoplasm of cancer cells (×200).

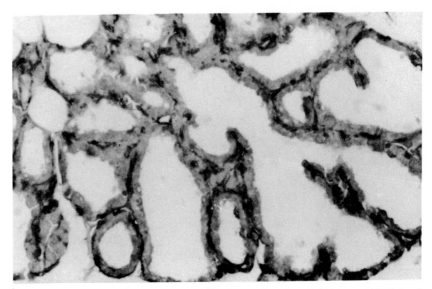

FIG. 12. Lactating mouse mammary gland; pokeweed lectin staining myoepithelial cells (×200).

staining since the denaturing action of fixatives may mask carbohydrates and processing fluids leach out glycolipids. Thus detection of binding sites for lectins may require very high concentrations of lectin (e.g 100–1000 µg/ml) or prolonged staining and although direct staining is excellent for frozen sections, paraffin sections require some amplification as described in the following sections.

B. Indirect Staining

There are currently 4 main approaches to this:

1. An antibody directed against the lectin, in an indirect antibody type stain. This can either be by using an anti-lectin antibody conjugated to a label.

2. A slightly more prolonged but more convenient (as each anti-lectin can be used unconjugated) method is to incubate with anti-lectin antibody after incubating with lectin and finally to incubate with a second antibody conjugated to a label.

3. An avidin-biotin system, which requires biotinated lectin and then avidin conjugated to a marker.

4. A glycosylated marker added to the section, after incubation with lectin, to attach to unoccupied binding sites.

1. One Step Antibody

For this, an antibody is raised to a lectin and conjugated with a label. It has a particular advantage that expensive lectin can be used in very low concentration and the native, unconjugated lectin can be used. Further, it is much more sensitive than direct lectin-conjugates. Double staining can be achieved by using two monospecific antilectins. Although this method generally requires conjugating our own antiserum (Hudson and Hay, 1980), there are some commercial sources of conjugated anti-lectin antisera (see Appendix).

1. Dewax.
2. Block endogenous peroxidases by 3% hydrogen peroxide in methanol, 10 min.
3. Incubate with lectin, e.g. 10 μg/ml for 30 min.
4. Wash 3 times in buffer, 2 min each.
5. Incubate with conjugated antibody to lectin e.g. 1/100 or 10 μg/ml for 30 min.
6. Wash 3 times in buffer.
7. Examine under fluorescence microscope or incubate in substrate, counterstain and mount.

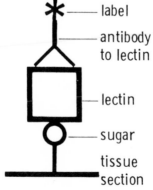

FIG. 13. One step antibody method (direct immunoenzyme).

Notes: Antibody to lectin can be raised by the method below or purchased. The neat antiserum or its IgG fraction can be tested against lectin by an Ouchterlony gel diffusion. If whole serum is used, it may be necessary to incorporate soluble sugar into the gel to prevent lectin precipitating serum glycoproteins. The IgG fraction is obtained from most mammalian serum using protein A bound to Sepharose beads (Pharmacia Ltd, who supply the reagent and working instructions). This is a very rapid and convenient procedure.

Antibodies conjugated to FITC or to enzymes work equally well. The optimum dilution is determined by draught-board dilutions of both lectin and conjugate, e.g. using lectin at 10, 20 and 40 μg/ml for 30 min against antibody diluted 1/50, 1/100, 1/200 etc. for 30 min (or 20 μg antibody/ml, 10, 5 etc.). As a rough indication we find 10 μg lectin/ml and conjugated antibody diluted 1/100 a frequently effective combination.

If direct staining with lectin has been attempted unsuccessfully, we have found it possible to perform a one step antibody stain subsequently on the same section and reveal the bound lectin.

This method appears 5–10 times more sensitive than direct staining.

2. Two Step Antibody

This is a slightly more prolonged staining technique but it has the advantage of increasing sensitivity and, as only one conjugate is required, it is much more convenient and versatile. We find this a very useful method as the lectin and primary antibody may be used unconjugated.

1. Dewax.
2. Block endogenous peroxidases as appropriate with 3% hydrogen peroxide in methanol for 10 min.
3. Incubate in lectin, e.g. 10 μg/ml for 30 min.
4. Wash 3 times in buffer, 2 min each.

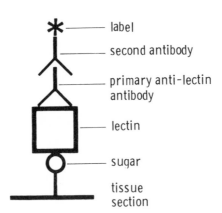

FIG. 14. Two step antibody method (indirect immunoenzyme).

5. Incubate in primary anti-lectin antibody 10 μg/ml or in anti-lectin serum 1/100 for 30 min.
6. Wash 3 times in buffer, 2 min each.
7. Incubate in conjugated second antibody 1/50–1/100 for 30 min.
8. Examine under fluorescence microscope or incubate in substrate, counterstain, mount.

Notes: We have used rabbit antisera to a variety of lectins and although they often stain to very high dilutions, we find a dilution of 1/100 or an IgG fraction (prepared by immobilised protein A) at about 10 μg/ml produces strong staining.

The conjugated anti-rabbit IgG we use comes from a variety of sources and we have found FITC and peroxidase conjugated anti-rabbit IgG from Dakopatts to be very reliable (diluted 1/50) and alkaline phosphatase conjugated anti-rabbit IgG from Sigma equally good (diluted 1/50).

The peroxidase-anti-peroxidase (PAP) method may be used in this system. Because of the extra step involved we have used most often the indirect antibody method but the increased sensitivity achieved with PAP may be required for some lectins.

Varying with the lectin used, we have found an increase in sensitivity of 10–50 fold by this indirect antibody system over the direct lectin-conjugate (Atkins and Leathem, 1982). This is more than we expected and might result from binding forces such as hydrophobic lectin-antibody interaction in addition to antibody-antigen.

Although serum glycoconjugates present in whole antiserum to lectins might be expected to compete for and displace lectins bound to tissue section this effect is insignificant using serum diluted to 1/100 or more for 30 min. The use of IgG fraction produces cleaner staining but is not essential.

3. Avidin-biotin Lectin Method

The lectin is biotinated and after incubating on the section, avidin conjugated to an enzyme or fluorescein is added. The avidin binds tightly and specifically to the biotin.

1. Dewax section.
2. Block endogenous peroxidases with 3% hydrogen peroxide in methanol for 10 min.
3. Incubate section with biotinated lectin 10 μg/ml for 30 min.
4. Wash 3 times in buffer, 2 min each.
5. Incubate with avidin-enzyme or -fluorescein conjugate, 10 μg/ml for 30 min.

6. Wash 3 times in buffer, 2 min each.
7. Examine under fluorescence microscope or incubate in substrate, counterstain and mount.

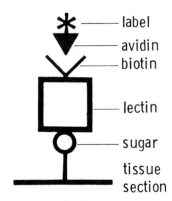

FIG. 15. Avidin-biotin lectin method.

Notes: This is theoretically both very sensitive (comparable to PAP) and specific but suffers from several teething problems and we cannot claim much success with it yet. The two major problems appear to be background staining with avidin-conjugates and difficulty in obtaining biotinyl-lectin which binds effectively. We include it here for completeness in the hope that others might have more success with what seems to be a potentially good approach.

4. Sugar-lectin-sugar Sandwich Method

This is potentially the most elegant, specific and sensitive method available for localising lectin binding sites on tissues, but is still at an adolescent stage, for the reagents are not yet readily available.

In principle, after incubating excess lectin on the section and washing, unoccupied binding sites on the lectin are used to link a glycosylated enzyme label. Lectins have at least 2 binding sites and some 10 or more, i.e. plenty of unoccupied binding sites should be available.

1. Dewax section.
2. Block endogenous peroxidases in 3% hydrogen peroxide in methanol for 10 min.
3. Incubate with lectin, 10 μg/ml for 30 min.
4. Wash 3 times in buffer, 2 min each.

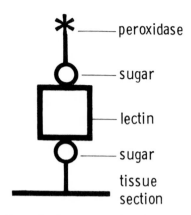

FIG. 16. Sugar-lectin-sugar method (lectin sandwich).

5. Incubate with glycosylated peroxidase 10μg/ml or simple peroxidase 50 μg/ml for 30 min.
6. Wash 3 times in buffer, 2 min each.
7. Incubate in substrate, counterstain and mount.

For controls, use lectin diluted in 0·1 M solution of appropriate and of inappropriate sugar for step 3. This should almost completely block specific staining sites. For total removal of lectin related staining, it may be necessary to omit the lectin step (3) altogether, since lectins preferentially bind to immobilised sugars and more particularly to carbohydrate chains (e.g. to Gal-b-1-3-GalNAc in preference to galactose by peanut lectin). Because of this and the hydrophobicity of many lectins, total inhibition by soluble simple sugars may be difficult to achieve.

Horseradish peroxidase contains mannose and thus will bind to concanavalin A, lentil and pea lectins without any alteration. To enable peroxidase to bind to other lectins, a suitable carbohydrate group has to be inserted onto the peroxidase (glycosylation). The method published by Lee *et al.* (1976) is comprehensive but complicated and there is a much more convenient method described by Keida *et al.* (1977) which we have modified. Alternatively a small number of new glycosylated peroxidase products are becoming commercially available.

The glycosylation of proteins is relatively straightforward using the method of Keida *et al.* (1977) since nitrophenyl-carbohydrate derivatives are readily and cheaply obtainable (Serva, Koch-Light). The procedure for glycosylation of peroxidase as published by Keida *et al.* is equally applicable to other proteins including enzymes and electron microscopy labels.

Briefly, the method is in two steps: p-nitrophenyl-sugar is reduced to p-aminophenyl-sugar; this is converted to a diazo derivative which is stable and reacts with tyrosyl, histidyl, lysyl, tryptophanyl and arginyl residues in proteins (McBroom et al., 1972).

The following is a method modified after Keida et al. (1977).

Step one. 30 mg p-nitrophenyl-sugar (Serva, Koch-Light) is reduced by dissolving it in 10 ml methanol with 20 mg of 5% palladium on charcoal. It is then mixed for 30 min at room temperature, filtered and freeze dried. This produces the p-aminophenyl-sugar derivative. Some stable p-aminophenyl-sugars are commercially available.

Step two. p-aminophenyl-sugar is dissolved in 3 ml of 0·1 M HCl with 3 mg KBr in ice bath, 10 mg of sodium nitrite in 1 ml distilled water is added very slowly, a drop at a time, and then left mixing for 1 h at 0 °C. This produces the diazophenyl-sugar derivative. For glycosylation of horseradish peroxidase, 10 mg of peroxidase RZ 3·3, dissolved in 7·5 ml of 0·2 M NaHCO$_3$ pH 10, is slowly added at 0 °C. The reaction is stopped after 30 min mixing by slowly adding 0·5 M HCl to produce a slightly acid pH (6·0).

The glycosylated-peroxidase is passed through a well washed Sephadex G-25 column equilibrated with Tris buffered saline pH 7·4 and the conjugate stored in the dark at 4 °C. It is diluted for use in Tris-buffered saline and should give good results at 10–100 μg/ml for 30 min at room temperature.

A monosaccharide coupling reagent, cyanomethyl-1-thioglycoside, based upon the method of Lee et al. (1976) is available from E-Y Laboratories.

As a rough guide, peroxidase (not treated in any way) will link to mannose-binding lectins, such as concanavalin A, lentil and pea. Lactose-peroxidase will link to galactose-binding lectins, such as peanut, soya bean and ricin. Fucosyl-peroxidase will link to fucose-binding lectins, such as Ulex 1 and lotus. Chitobiose-peroxidase will link to gulcosamine-binding lectins such as wheatgerm and Ulex 2.

A very simple test to find which lectins will bind to a particular enzyme or glycosylated enzyme is to perform an Ouchterlony-type gel diffusion and seek either a precipitate in the gel (using serial dilutions of both lectin and glycosylated-enzyme) or, as a more sensitive method, after pressing the gel and washing, incubating in enzyme substrate.

A great attraction of this method is that, unlike the avidin-biotin method, the lectin does not need to be altered in any way, with consequent denaturing, and, unlike the antibody method, there are only carbohydrate binding ligands involved. For fixed, processed material the technique above presents few problems, but if unfixed or frozen section material is used, some caution is required for the glycosylated-enzyme may bind to tissue lectin-like substances (Gros et al., 1982).

VI. EXPOSURE OF LECTIN BINDING SITES BY PROTEOLYTIC AND OTHER ENZYMES

Although many carbohydrate groups remain exposed and detectable in paraffin sections after the distortion imposed by fixation and processing, a sensitive method for their demonstration is needed and simple direct lectin staining may not be sufficient, necessitating an indirect or antibody sandwich method. Tissue antigens, carbohydrates and other markers which have been sequestrated during fixation and processing can often be revealed by treating tissue sections with proteolytic enzymes, e.g. trypsin and pronase (Curran and Gregory, 1977; Mepham *et al.*, 1979; Hautzer *et al.*, 1980). These act by breaking up the protein matrix and rendering the tissue antigens and markers more accessible to ligands.

The effect of proteolytic enzymes on revealing otherwise undetectable sequestered tissue markers can be dramatic and this applies equally to carbohydrates. Many proteolytic enzymes are available and are worth trying but trypsin and pronase are most likely to work when starting a new system. Most of our experience has been with trypsin. This enzyme works fastest at pH 8–9 but, in alkaline pH, undergoes considerable autodigestion and thus may be more efficient overall if used at a neutral or slightly acid pH. Trypsin hydrolyses the carboxyl groups of lysine and arginine in particular and most preparations of trypsin are contaminated with chymotrypsin and their precursors, but chymotrypsin hydrolyses the carboxyl groups of tyrosine and phenylalanine and therefore different sources of trypsin may give different results.

The methods described by Mepham *et al.* (1979) can establish the role of chymotrypsin in revealing such binding sites. We use a practical grade of trypsin (Sigma 11, not too pure, on grounds of cost and also effectiveness), try to keep to the same source and test each new batch on control sections using a constant concentration (0·1%) but varying the incubation time.

It is likely that part of the reduction in lectin binding to paraffin sections is due to extraction of glycolipids by the solvents used in processing (chloroform, toluene) and if it is practical, it is worth keeping exposure times to such solvents as brief as possible. However, carbohydrates incorporated into glycoproteins should remain in processed tissues.

The amount of proteolysis required will depend upon the type, strength and duration of fixation; the longer the fixation the longer the incubation required in trypsin. Trypsin may also be used at a higher concentration. Therefore each laboratory needs to work out its own optimal trypsinisation. But as a rough guide, assuming 24–48 h of fixation in 10% formal-saline, the trypsin incubation might be as follows.

Trypsin solution. 1. Pre-warm 100 ml of distilled water to 37 °C.

2. Dissolve 200 mg of $CaCl_2$ and 200 mg of trypsin, and correct to pH 7·0 with 0·1 M NaOH. Filter, since some of the trypsin may not dissolve. Use at once.

Calcium appears to aid in dissolving trypsin and act as an activator by inhibiting autodigestion of trypsin.

The linkage of glycoconjugates to cell structures may be through those amino groups which are digested by trypsin or other enzymes. An advantage of using trypsin is the digestible sites are limited, although other enzymes may work well. Until we know more about the complex carbohydrates and their peptide linkages in different cells it is worth taking a pragmatic approach to the choice of proteolytic enzyme.

Other enzymes may produce different and more specific results. Glycosydic enzymes are available as a wide variety of exoglycosidases (for revealing the sequence and α or β configuration of the oligosaccharide chains) and endoglycosidases (for cleaving off complex carbohydrates):

Man
Man --- Man b(1–4) GlcNAc b(1–4) GlcNAc --- Asparagine-Protein
                                    ↑
          site of action of endoglycosidase D

Glycosydic enzymes can be used to cleave off sugars sequentially and either stop specific lectin binding or, by revealing adjacent carbohydrate, show a different staining pattern.

Sialic or neuraminic acids are commonly found as terminal groups on cell surface glycoconjugates and their removal by sialidase or neuraminidase may reveal sub-terminal lectin binding carbohydrates. The differences between malignant and non-malignant or between well and poorly differentiated cancer cells as revealed by lectin binding may be due partly to changes in sialation. Digestion of sialic acid can nullify such differences, thus neuraminidase may be of limited value. However, staining of some normal cells cannot be achieved without neuraminidase treatment and its use should be considered. Similarly, hyaluronidase reveals staining patterns not otherwise obtained.

Neuraminidase. This enzyme is available derived from different organisms, in particular *Vibrio cholerae,* influenza virus and several *Clostridia,* their main differences lie in variations of activity. A wide range of drastic and expensive treatments with neuraminidase have been reported for analysis of glycoconjugates (e.g. 100 units/ml for 48 h at 37 °C), but such enthusiasm is rarely needed on tissue sections and while the conditions required will vary with processing and tissue, the method below works on our paraffin sections. The effects are enhanced if the section is briefly pre-treated in trypsin.

Neuraminidase treatment.

1. Dewax sections to warm water.
2. Incubate in neuraminidase solution for 30 min at 37 °C.
3. Wash in running tapwater 5 min.
4. Incubate with lectin and proceed as above for localisation of lectin.

Neuraminidase solution. Pre-warm 10 ml of sodium acetate buffer 0·05 M pH 5·5 to 37 °C, dissolve 1 unit of neuraminidase (Hoechst, Sigma, BDH, Calbiochem, Worthington) and 100 μl of 1% $CaCl_2$. Use at once.

Where small volumes of precious reagents are to be used, the slide may be inverted (resting on matches) over a drop of solution in a petri dish, or a drop of solution simply overlaid with a cover slip in a humid petri dish.

VII. PRODUCTION OF ANTISERA TO LECTINS

Methods for raising antibodies to lectins are similar to producing antisera to any other proteins but with two main differences:

1. Lectins are often very toxic and their toxicity may need to be attenuated.
2. One needs to block the lectin binding sites to reduce antibody production to them, i.e. prevent competitive inhibition.

As a general principle of antibody production, the less soluble or more particulate a protein, the more likely it is to induce a good antibody response. We have achieved good antibody titres in rabbits immunising with lectins immobilised on Sepharose beads, and recommend this as being most convenient.

A good range of sugars covalently attached to beads are commercially available and are ideal for preparing lectins in a highly immunogenic form. We have developed the following method for producing rabbit antisera to lectins (Atkins and Leathem 1982).

The principle is as follows: After a lectin is added to beads bearing the appropriate sugar the lectin is fixed to the sugar irreversibly through its sugar receptor by a mixture of formalin and heat. Unoccupied binding sites are saturated with soluble sugar. After washing the beads they are injected into multiple subcutaneous sites using 2 rabbits for each lectin. For example

1. 1 ml of agarose-lactose beads (Sigma Ltd., binding capacity 12 mg lectin/ml) mixed with 1 mg of peanut lectin, mixed for 1 h at room temperature.

2. 10 ml of 10% formalin added, heated to 60 °C in waterbath for 10 min.

3. Beads washed by centrifuging in saline, divided into aliquots of 100 μl of beads stored at −20 °C.

4. Subcutaneous injections into multiple sites over the back of 2 rabbits using 100 μl of beads on each occasion. Injections are repeated at 3 weekly intervals. 40–50 ml of blood are taken from the marginal ear vein prior to each immunisation. The serum is pooled and stored at −20 °C.

We evolved this method following several rabbit fatalities and it offers several advantages over using lectin alone or just with adjuvant.

Many lectins are highly toxic in very small doses, in particular abrin, ricin and mistletoe lectin and others, while not being so toxic, can induce sickness in rabbits. All lectins should therefore be treated with respect as their toxic effects may be delayed. Storage in solution is less hazardous than storing powder. Immunisation of an animal with native lectin may produce a high mortality or morbidity unless the lectin is denatured before injection.

Any denaturing may well destroy antigenic sites important in recognition of the native lectin or induce formation of new antigenic sites. We have found that a mixture of formalin fixation together with heat reduces the toxic effects of all lectins so far investigated by ourselves, including abrin and ricin, and that the antibodies induced continue to react very satisfactorily with the native lectins as tested by Ouchterlony gel-diffusion.

In addition to reducing the toxicity of the lectins, formalin and heat denature lectins sufficiently to prevent their dissociation by soluble sugars; therefore the lectins remain particulate after immunisation.

Finally, as the lectin is immobilised through the binding site, the site is sequestered from the rabbit immune recognition system. Therefore antibodies are not produced to the lectin-carbohydrate binding site. This is important since such antibodies might compete with carbohydrate for the sites.

VIII. CONTROLS

Simple blocking sugars for the majority of lectins are already known and the precise binding specificities are becoming understood, therefore it is increasingly feasible to specifically inhibit the binding of lectins and demonstrate their specificity. To do this we can incorporate both positive and negative controls in each staining run.

A. Positive

A positive control is required to show that the stain should work under these conditions.

The majority of lectins bind to erythrocytes, sometimes with considerable blood group specificity but more often with no group or even species specificity. This feature is of value for monitoring the steps in isolating pure lectins. Thus erythrocytes in tissues will commonly stain positively as will the endothelium of blood vessels. Kidney provides a source of epithelium which commonly stains with lectins (mostly luminal surface of distal tubule epithelium) and if blood-group substance/erythrocytes fail to stain, kidney (of many species) provides a useful positive control tissue.

Specific carbohydrates immobilised onto the surface of beads (e.g. Sepharose) are commercially available from several sources (E-Y Labs, Sigma Ltd) and these as well as being invaluable for the isolation of lectins, can be suspended or embedded in albumen (as this has no glycoconjugates) and either smears made on slides or blocks processed in parallel with tissues into paraffin section as positive controls for staining.

B. Negative

A particular attraction of lectins as probes is that, with few exceptions, the simple sugar specificity of each is known and these can be used to specifically inhibit or compete with lectin binding to tissues. Such competition is used in the elution of lectins from affinity chromatography columns of immobilised sugars.

If pairs of tissue sections are incubated with lectin solution and then one of each pair is washed in the appropriate specific sugar solution, the lectin should elute off the section into the sugar solution. However, the more complex the binding carbohydrate and the longer a lectin is incubated, the tighter the binding appears to become (perhaps depending on the exposure of the tissue sugar) and the bound lectin is subsequently eluted with a variable degree of ease. Stepwise elution, with progressively stronger sugar solutions, appears to elute lectins from different cell components at different rates, and this can produce differential staining. This may also occur if elution is performed with soluble complex carbohydrates.

However, this also means that complete elution of lectin, and thus demonstration of specificity of binding can be difficult. To overcome this, we attempt to prevent lectin binding to tissues in the first place. This is done by diluting the lectin in appropriate (and, to show the sugar specificity, also with inappropriate) sugar solution at 100 mM for 60 min prior to using the solution to "stain" a section. If the lectin binding is specific, it should be completely inhibited in the presence of the appropriate sugar solution but not by the inappropriate sugar. Ideally every section stained should have its adjacent, serial section "stained" with the lectin dissolved in the appropriate sugar as a negative control for specificity.

Even these controls may not totally abolish lectin binding owing to non-specific binding such as hydrophobic interactions between lectins and tissues. However, it will show whether the staining is specific or not.

IX. ACKNOWLEDGEMENTS

We would like to thank Jenny Gardner and Gail Watts for their technical assistance and Professor Neville Woolf for his support.

X. REFERENCES

Atkins, N. J. and Leathem, A. J. (1982). *J. Clin. Path.* (in press).
Bernhard, W. and Avrameas, S. (1971). *Exp. Cell Res.* **64**, 232–236.
Bjerrum, O. J. and Bog-Hansen, T. C. (1976). *Biochem. Biophys. Acta* **455**, 66–89.
Bog-Hansen, T. C., Prahl, P. and Lowenstein, H. (1978). *J. Immunol. Methods* **22**, 293–307.
Boyd, W. C. and Shapleigh, E. (1954). *Science* **119**, 419.
Briles, E. B. (1982). *Int. Rev. Cytol.* **75**, 101–165.
Brown, J. C. and Hunt, R. C. (1978). *Int. Rev. Cytol.* **52**, 277–349.
Curran, R. C. and Gregory, J. (1977). *Experientia* **33**, 1400.
David, G. and Reisfeld, R. (1974). *J. Natn. Cancer Inst.* **53**, 1005–1010.
Edelman, G. M., Rutishauser, U. and Millette, C. F. (1971). *Proc. Natn. Acad. Sci. USA* **68**, 2153–2157.
Franz, H. and Ziska, P, (1981). "Lectins—Biology, Biochemistry, Clinical Biochemistry" (T. C. Bog-Hansen, ed.,), Vol. I. pp. 17–21. Walter de Gruyter and Co., Berlin.
Franz, H., Mohr, J. and Ziska, P. (1982). "Lectins — Biology, Biochemistry, Clinical Biochemistry" (T. C. Bog-Hansen, ed.,), Vol.II pp.553–562 Walter de Gruyter and Co., Berlin.
Galili, U., Galili, N., Or, R. and Polliak, A. (1981). *Clin. Exp. Immunol.* **43**, 311–318.
Gold, E. R. and Balding, P. (1975). "Receptor Specific Proteins — Plant and Animal Lectins". Excerpta Medica, Amsterdam.
Goldstein, T. J., Hughes, R. C., Monsigny, M., Osawa, T. and Sharon, N. (1980). *Nature* **285**, 66.
Gros, D., Bruce, B., Challice, C. E. and Schrevel, J. (1982). *J. Histochem. Cytochem.* **30**, 193–200.

Hautzer, N. W., Wittkuhn, J. F. and Elliott McCaughey, W. T. (1980). *J. Histochem. Cytochem.* **28**, 52–53.

Holthofer, H., Virtanen, I., Pettersson, E., Tornroth, T., Alfthan, O., Linder, E. and Miettinen, A. (1981). *Lab. Invest.* **45**, 391–399.

Horejsi, V., Ticha, M. and Kocourek, J. (1979). *Trends in Biochemical Science* **1**, n6–n7.

Hudson, L. and Hay, F. C. (1980). "Practical Immunology". 2nd edn., p.237. Blackwell Scientific Publishing Company, Oxford.

Keida, C., Delmotte, F. and Monsigny, M. (1977). *Febs Letters* **76**, 257–261.

Kinzel, V., Richards, J. and Kubler, D. (1977). *Exp. Cell Res.* **105**, 389–400.

Klein, P. J., Vierbuchen, M., Wurz, H., Schulz, K. D. and Newman, R. A. (1981). *Br. J. Cancer* **44**, 746–748.

Lee, Y. C., Stowell, C. and Krantz, M. J. (1976). *Biochemistry* **15**, 3956–3963.

Lis, H. and Sharon, N. (1973). *Ann. Rev. Biochem.* **42**, 541–574.

Lotan, R., Beattie, G., Hubbell, W. and Nicolson, G. L. (1977). *Biochemistry* **16**, 1787–1794.

Lotan, R. (1979). *Scanning Electron Microscopy* **3**, 549–564.

Marshall, R. D. (1972). *Ann. Rev. Biochem.* **41**, 673–702.

McBroom, C. R., Samanen, C. H. and Goldstein, I. J. (1972). *Methods Enzymol.* **28**, 212.

Mepham, B. L., Frater, W. and Mitchell, B. S. (1979). *Histochem. J.* **11**, 345–357.

Newman, R. A., Klein, P. J. and Rudland, P. S. (1979). *J. Natn. Cancer Inst.* **63**, 1339–1346.

Nicolson, G. L. (1974). *Int. Rev. Cytol.* **39**, 89–190.

Nicolson, G. L. (1980). "Cancer Markers" (S. Sell, ed.), pp. 403–443 Humana Press, New Jersey.

Ochoa, J-L., Sierra, A. and Cordoba, F. (1981). "Lectins — Biology, Biochemistry, Clinical Biochemistry" (T. C. Bog-Hansen, ed.), Vol. I. pp. 73–80. Walter de Gruyter and Co., Berlin.

Ogata, S., Muramatsu, T. and Kobata, A. (1975). *J. Biochem.* **78**, 687–696.

Pearlstein, E., Salk, P. L., Yogeeswaran, G. and Karpatkin, S. (1980). *Proc. Natn. Acad. Sci. USA* **77**, 4336–4339.

Reisner, Y. and Sharon, N. (1980). *Trends in Biochemical Science* **5**, 29–31.

Sharon, N. (1977). *Scient. Am.* **236**, 108–119.

Shoham, J. and Sachs, L. (1974). *Cold Spring Harbor Symposium.* **1**, 297–304.

Spengler, G. A. and Weber, R. M. (1981) "Lectins — Biology, Biochemistry, Clinical Biochemistry" (T. C. Bog-Hansen, ed.), Vol.I. pp.231–240. Walter de Gruyter, Berlin.

Stillmark, H. (1888). Uber Ricin, ein giftiges Ferment aus den Samen von Ricinus communis L. und einigen anderen Euphorbiaceen. Inaug. Diss., Dorpat.

Stoddart, R. W., Collins, R. D. and Jacobson, W. (1980). *J. Path.* **131**, 321–332.

Stoward, P. J., Spicer, S. S. and Miller, R. L. (1980). *J. Histochem, Cytochem.* **28**, 979–990.

Talmadge, K. W., Noonan, K. D. and Burger, M. M. (1974). *Cold Spring Harbor Symposium* **1**, 313–325.

Yogeeswaran, G. (1980). "Cancer Markers" (S. Sell, ed.), pp.371–401. Humana Press, New Jersey.

XI. APPENDIX

Buffer Solutions

Tris buffered saline (TBS) is generally very useful, easy to make up and store. The main precaution with this buffer is that it should be avoided in any procedures involving conjugations of amino groups, since Tris has free amino groups itself.

TBS Formula

0·15 M NaCl 0·05 M Tris, corrected to neutral pH (we use 7·4) with 0·1 M HCl.

e.g.: Tris 60·57 g, NaCl 87 g, $H_2O \rightarrow 10$ l.

Phosphate Buffered Saline

PBS is often used in histochemistry but has distinct problems in lectin histochemistry since the phosphate groups can complex with and sequester heavy metals such as calcium and manganese, and therefore inhibit the binding of those lectins requiring metal ions (e.g.) concanavalin A, lima bean, horseshoe crab, pea, erythrina, etc.). We aim at tight binding of lectin to tissue. Phosphate buffered saline has been used with metal-dependent lectins in affinity chromatography (David et al., 1974; Kinzel et al., 1977), e.g. for concanavalin A purification of CEA from metastases, and perhaps here it has some value in decreasing the tightness of binding and allowing more easy elution.

Unbuffered saline can be used as a diluent or for washing, but the pH varies considerably with the source of distilled water and acid pH tends to break lectins into their subunits.

The addition of a non-glycosylated protein (e.g. albumen) to the dilute lectin may stabilise it. We do not use albumen routinely but reports exist on its use (normally BSA) at concentrations varying from 0·1% BSA to 10% BSA. The purity of the albumen is important as although albumen has no carbohydrate, traces of glycoprotein contaminant might compete for the binding sites on the lectin.

The pH of the lectin solution does not appear critical as long as it is near neutral and anything between 6·8–7·8 is acceptable. We find pH 7·4 works well. Acid pH should be avoided as lectins may dissociate into subunits or monomers.

The addition of detergent to the lectin solution may decrease non-specific binding (such as through hydrophobic bonds) and a variety of detergents can be used for this, such as 0·1% Triton X100, 0·1% Tween 20 and 0·1% Nonidet P40. However, just as with antibody-antigen reactions, detergents may inhibit binding of some lectins and non-ionic detergents are generally preferable to ionic. In addition, detergents may solubilise glycolipids and thus alter the lectin-binding patterns.

Many lectins require heavy metal ions to maintain an active binding site and depletion of essential ions can severely limit the binding capacity of a lectin. To avoid this and in an attempt to optimise the conditions, we add a cocktail of calcium, magnesium and manganese chloride to Tris buffered saline to give 1 mM of each. This "general lectin buffer" is used for diluting lectins and washing sections.

Enzyme Labels

The choice of enzyme label is largely determined by the particular application of our staining. Diaminobenzidine as a substrate for peroxidase gives a product which can be localised in the electron microscope and allows high resolution light microscopy, important for examining single cells as in lymph nodes. An alternative substrate for peroxidase is aminoethyl carbazole, which may be attractive to laboratories not wishing to use benzidine derivatives. Since it produces a red colour, it is easier to photograph in black and white than the brown colour from diaminobenzidine. The red colour produced by alkaline phosphatase on fast red TR is even more photogenic (particularly for colour photography) but as with that from aminoethyl carbazole, is soluble in alcohol/xylol and requires water soluble mountant with a reduction in resolution.

Peroxidase Substrates

Diaminobenzidine: 0·5 mg/ml of Tris buffered saline 0·05 M Tris, 0·15 M sodium chloride, pH 7·6 + 10 μl/ml of 20 volume hydrogen peroxide. Incubate for 10 min at room temperature. If needed for longer periods, make up fresh substrate.

Aminoethylcarbazole: To make a stock solution, dissolve 1 g of 3-amino-9-ethyl carbazole (Sigma no A 5754) in 10 ml of dimethylformamide and make up to 1 l with distilled water. Store on the bench. Add 5 ml of this to 100 ml of acetate buffer pH 5·0, 0·05 M and 100 μl of 20 volume hydrogen peroxide. Incubate for 15–20 min at room temperature. This produces a red colour, soluble in alcohol and xylene, therefore one must use aqueous mountant. The red colour is particularly brilliant if the stock solution is matured on the bench.

Alkaline phosphatase substrate: (Azo method): 20 mg of naphthol AS-TR or AS-MX, phosphoric acid, sodium salt, is dissolved in 100 μl of dimethylformamide together with 40 mg of fast red TR and made up to 100 ml with Gomori Tris buffer pH 9·0, 0·05 M. 100 μl of 1 M magnesium chloride is added as activator and the mixture filtered. Slides are incubated for 10 min at room temperature. More prolonged incubations may be necessary, with renewal of fresh substrate, but these tend to impart a yellow background. Unfixed frozen or Carnoy-fixed paraffin sections of breast tissue or of animal kidney provide good positive controls for the enzyme reaction.

Photography

Colour photography of lectin sections presents no problem and we use high speed Ektachrome daylight film for immunofluorescence rating it 1 stop slower (i.e. 18 Din instead of 21 Din) to account for poor penetration of the emulsion.

Black and white photography is more difficult, particularly if the brown colour from diaminobenzidine is to be recorded as brown imparts no contrast. To enhance the brown colour we use a dense cyan filter (Kodak 44A), rate Pan F film at 15 Din instead of 18 Din and overdevelop the film by 50% (using ID 11). This is necessary because of the effect of filters. For the red colour of aminoethyl carbazole or fast red TR we use a green filter. The illustrations in this chapter were photographed using the above conditions and printed on Multigrade paper with Multigrade filter number 4 and Ilfospeed developer diluted 1 + 5.

List of Suppliers of Lectins and Related Products

Telephone numbers are in parentheses.

BDH Ltd (0202–745520)
Bethesda Research Labs (0223–315504)
Boehringer Ltd (07916–71611)
Calbiochem Ltd (0279–56081)
E-Y Labs (Tissue Culture Services [75–36068])
Fluka Ltd (04574–62518)
LKB Ltd (657–8822)
Medac GmbH (Hamburg) (010–49–40–3590851)
Miles Ltd (369–2151)
Pharmacia Ltd (01–572–7321)
P-L Biochemicals (0604–499325)
Polysciences Ltd (0604–46496)
Serva Ltd (Uniscience [0223–64623])
Sigma Ltd (0202–733210)
Worthington Ltd (Flow Labs [0294–74242])

Immunocytochemical Identification of Intracellularly Dye-marked Neurons: A Double-labelling Technique for Light and Electron Microscopic Analysis

T. A. REAVES, Jr, R. CUMMING, M. T. LIBBER and J. N. HAYWARD

I. INTRODUCTION

Immunocytochemical studies of the nervous system using specific antisera to a host of neuroactive substances reveal that more than one chemical type of neuron usually occurs within each nucleus examined. For example, within the hypothalamic paraventricular nucleus there are several different chemical types of neurons: vasopressin, oxytocin, enkephalin, neurotensin, cholecystokinin, dynorphin and others. This heterogeneity of cell type within a single nucleus necessitates a systematic analysis of individual neurons to relate neurophysiological properties with morphological and immunocytochemical identities (Hayward, 1977).

IMMUNOCYTOCHEMISTRY 2
ISBN 0 12 140402 1

During our electrophysiological studies of the hypothalamic magnocellular neuroendocrine system, we developed a double-labelling technique for the study of single neurons to resolve this problem (Reaves and Hayward, 1979a,b; 1980; Reaves et al., 1982b,c,d). This double-labelling method combines the techniques of intracellular neurophysiology, dye-marking and immunocytochemistry of single neurons. Thus, electrophysiological, light microscopic and ultrastructural properties of a single chemically-identified neuron can be directly correlated.

This double-labelling technique can be applied to the study of a variety of cell types within different systems: nervous (Reaves and Hayward, 1979 a,b; 1980; Reaves et al., 1982b,c,d), endocrine (Michaels and Sheridan, 1981) and others. This chapter should provide readers with a detailed outline of our procedures in order for them to apply this technique to their own studies of chemically identified cells.

II. METHODOLOGY

A. Animal Preparation

Our studies involve the goldfish, in vivo, and an in vitro explant preparation of the rat hypothalamo-neurohypophysial complex (HNC; Sladek and Knigge, 1977). Details of the goldfish preparation have been described previously (Reaves and Hayward, 1980). The rat HNC explant with attached neurohypophysis is excised according to Sladek and Knigge (1977) and then placed on a nylon net in a tissue culture chamber and allowed to equilibrate in oxygenated, perfused (0·38 ml/min) Yamamoto's media (Yamamoto, 1972) at 36 °C for 30–60 min before electrical recordings (Reaves et al., 1982c,d).

B. Electrophysiology and Dye-Injection (Single-label)

For intracellular recordings, neurons of the goldfish preoptic nucleus (NPO) and rat HNC supraoptic nucleus (NSO) are impaled with glass micropipettes filled with a solution of either 2–3% Lucifer Yellow-Ch (LY; Stewart, 1978) in 0·1 M Tris/HCl with 0·15 M lithium chloride or 4% Procion Yellow-M4RS (PY; Hayward, 1974) in 0·1 M Tris/HCl with 0·15 M KCl, both at pH 7·4. Electrodes are bevelled to an impedance of 6–40 megohm (Brown and Flaming, 1975). An AB Transvertex electronically-controlled stepping microdrive is used to guide the microelectrode to its target. The neurosecretory neurons of the NPO or NSO are antidromically activated by electrical stimulation of the pituitary gland with insulated tungsten bipolar stimulating electrodes with exposed sharpened tips of less than 0·5 mm. An isolated constant-current stimulator delivers bipolar pulses of 0·1–5·0 mA and 0·5–1·0 msec duration at 1/sec intervals. The anionic fluorescent dyes (LY or PY) are iontophoretically injected intracellularly by 5–10 nA of hyperpolarizing DC current for 0·3–6·0 min. Only one cell per nucleus is marked for subsequent localization.

C. Tissue Fixation and Microtomy

In the goldfish, the brain is fixed by intracardial perfusion with teleost physiological solution (Young, 1933) containing 0·3% sodium nitrite and 0·1% heparin followed by various aldhyde fixatives. We currently fix with 30–100 ml of 1% paraformaldehyde in 0·075 M phosphate buffer (PB; pH 7·4) followed by 50–100 ml of 4% paraformaldehyde in PB containing 0·25% glutaraldehyde (pH 7·4). In the rat HNC, the explant is fixed by immersion in 4% paraformaldehyde containing 0·1% glutaraldehyde in 0·1 M PB (pH 7·4). The goldfish brain and the HNC explant are both post-fixed overnight at 4 °C in fresh fixative. After post-fixation, some goldfish brains are embedded in paraffin, sectioned serially at 6–10 μm in the frontal plane and the sections mounted on glass slides to dry. The brains of other fish and the rat HNC are embedded in 5·0% agar in saline and sectioned serially (30 μm, vibratome) in the frontal plane. Sections are collected in cold PB saline (PBS), rinsed several times in cold PBS and then scanned under incident UV light (495 nm) to select those sections containing LY- or PY-filled somata.

D. Immunocytochemistry (Double-label)

Using the indirect immunofluorescence technique (Coons, 1958), we apply the second label (tetramethylrhodamine-isothiocyanate; TRITC) to sections containing dye-filled somata. PBS-rinsed sections with dye-filled somata are incubated sequentially in a series of solutions: (1) PBS containing 1% normal sheep serum (NSS, 10 min); (2) rabbit anti-rat neurophysin antiserum (1:100–1:200 in PBS/NSS, room temperature, 2–24 h; Lot RN#4, compliments of Dr. A. G. Robinson, University of Pittsburgh, Pittsburgh, PA) or with one of three rabbit antisera diluted 1:100 against met[5]-enkephalin (anti-met[5]-enkephalin, Lot #22Tu8, ImmunoNuclear Corp., Stillwater, MN) or arginine vasotocin (anti-arginine vasotocin, Lot G2, a gift from Dr John Fernstrom, MIT, Boston, MA) or oxytocin (anti-oxytocin, Lot K22, a gift from Dr R. R. Dries, Ferring Pharmaceuticals,

Kiel, West Germany); (3) PBS/NSS, 10 min, room temperature; (4) TRITC-conjugated goat anti-rabbit IgG antisera (1:50 in PBS/NSS, 1–2 h, room temperature; Cappel Labs); (5) PBS.

To retard evaporation, all antisera incubations were under conditions of high humidity. Specificity of the antisera is determined by conventional methods of substituting normal rabbit serum for the primary antiserum, omitting the primary antiserum step, and by absorbing (liquid or solid phase) the primary antibodies with excessive amounts of their respective antigens (Sternberger, 1979). Sections were scanned for immuno-fluorescence under incident light at 580nm.

E. Identification of Double-labelled Cells

Double-labelled neurons are identified first by observing the section under incident light at 495 nm for dye-marker fluorochrome fluorescence and then at 580 nm for TRITC-fluorochrome fluorescence. Only one cell (double-labelled) in the field will show corresponding fluorescence of unique cell profiles at both wavelengths of light. For verification, double-labelled neurons can then be photographed at 495 and 580 nm using Kodak Tri-X Pan or similar type film. Camera lucida drawings of adjacent sections permit reconstruction of the soma and processes of chemically identified neurons.

In situations where the dye-marked neuron is not chemically identified on the first attempt, the section can be rinsed in PBS/NSS and then restained with one of the other primary antisera following the procedures outlined in the section on immunocytochemistry. This procedure can be repeated until the cell in question is chemically defined.

Another variation of the double-label method is depicted in Fig. 1. When using thin sections (paraffin, cryostat, etc.) the dye-marked neuron will usually appear in more than one consecutive serial section. Here, three serial sections are observed to contain a dye-marked neuron (top row, Fig. 1). Each section is then stained immunocytochemically but each with a different primary antisera (bottom row, Fig. 1), followed by the TRITC-tagged secondary antisera. In this example, corresponding fluorescence of the intracellular dye marker and of TRITC occurs only in section 81, indicating that the dye-injected neuron was enkephalinergic.

F. Preparation for Electron Microscopy

Unmounted sections containing Lucifer Yellow (LY) injected double-labelled neurons are rinsed in Tris buffer (0·1 M, pH 7·6, 10 min), soaked in a

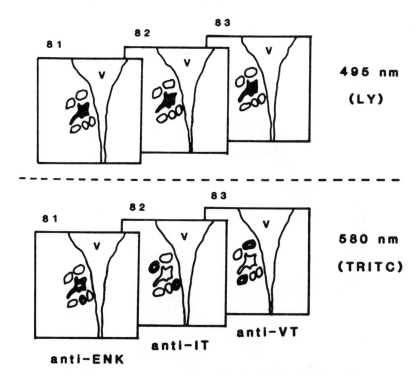

FIG. 1. Identification protocol for double-labelled neurons. Fluorescence microscopy (495 nm; top row) or paraffin sections (10 μm) show the soma of a hypothetical neuron (black) which was injected intracellularly with Lucifer Yellow (LY) and found on sections 81, 82 and 83. Bottom row shows the same sections (81, 82, 83) when viewed at 580 nm after applying a different primary antisera (ENK, enkephalin; IT, oxytocin; VT, vasotocin) to each section with the indirect immunofluorescence technique using a rhodamine-tagged secondary antibody. The LY injected neuron is identified as enkephalinergic since corresponding fluorescence profiles at 495 and 580 nm occur only on section 81. V, ventricle.

solution of diaminobenzidine (DAB; 1·5 mg/ml of Tris buffer; 15 min) and irradiated under light (495 nm, epi-illumination with a 25 × objective) in DAB until the LY-fluorescence fades below visibility (Maranto, 1981; Reaves *et al.*, 1982). Irradiated sections are then rinsed in Tris buffer, osmicated (2% OsO_4 in PB), dehydrated, infiltrated with Epon and sand-wiched between Teflon-coated cover-slips. After photographing stained neurons under the light microscope, we cut ultrathin sections for observation with a Zeiss EM 109 electron microscope. Selected grids can then be contrasted with uranyl acetate and lead citrate.

III. LIGHT MICROSCOPY OF DOUBLE-LABELLED NEURONS

In our experimental system, neurons showing antidromic activation following electrical stimulation of the neurohypophysis are iontophoretically
injected with either LY or PY for subsequent localization with fluorescence

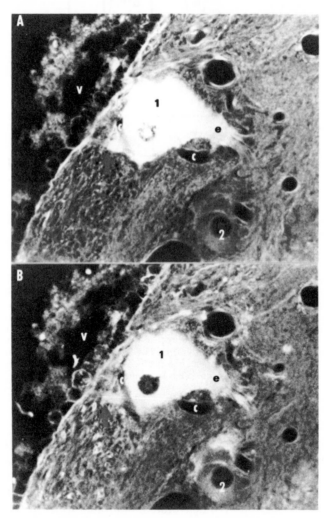

FIG. 2. Double-labelled isotocin neuron in goldfish preoptic nucleus. (A) Lucifer Yellow
(LY) fluorescence (495 nm) in physiologically studied cell 1 (injected with LY). An
adjacent cell is not LY filled (cell 2). V, ventricle; c, capillary. (B) Rhodamine
immunofluorescence (580 nm) after an anti-oxytocin antisera confirms chemical
identity of cell 1 (from Reaves and Hayward, 1979a).

microscopy. To aid in matching the electrophysiological characteristics of an individual neuron with its morphology, only one cell (or one cell/fluorescent dye) is dye-injected per nucleus. The chemical identity of dye-filled, physiologically studied neurons is established immunocytochemically by comparing cell location, size, contour, and processes on the same tissue section first at 495 nm (Fig. 2A) for LY/PY fluorescence and then at 580 nm (Fig. 2B) for fluorescence.

Figures 2–4 illustrate the results of double-labelling from 10 μm thick paraffin-embedded sections of the goldfish preoptic nucleus (NPO). An isotocinergic neuron is shown in Fig. 2A with intense fluorescence of LY within the cytoplasm and the nucleolus while immunoreactivity (Fig. 2B) is limited to the cytoplasm. A double-labelled enkephalinergic neuron is shown in Fig. 3 along with other enkephalin neurons in the NPO near the LY-injected cell (Fig. 3B). By tracing the LY-fluorescent profiles from several adjacent sections, this enkephalinergic neuron was reconstructed and is shown in two-dimensional profile in Fig. 3C. A third type of magnocellular NPO neuron found in goldfish, i.e. vasotocinergic (Fig. 4), can also be double-labelled. This cell is situated abutting another vasotocinergic cell (Fig. 4B, C).

A double-labelled magnocellular supraoptic neuron of the rat HNC is seen in Fig. 5. This bipolar configured neuron lies at the dorsal crest of the supraoptic nucleus (NSO; Fig. 5A). The same section viewed at 580 nm for

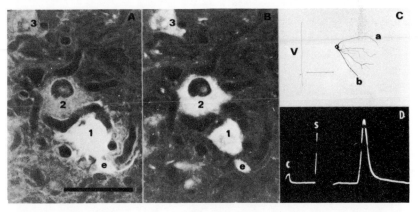

FIG. 3. Electrophysiological, morphological and chemical identity of an enkephalin neuron (cell 1) in the goldfish preoptic nucleus. (A) Lucifer Yellow (LY) fluorescence (495 nm) of cell 1. Cells 2 and 3 do not contain LY. Bar = 50 μm. (B) Rhodamine fluorescence (580 nm) of the LY marked cell 1 after using anti-met[5]-enkephalin antiserum on tissue section in A. Cells 2 and 3 are also enkephalin positive. (C) Reconstruction of dye-filled neuron 1 from A. Bar = 200 μm. (D) Antidromically activated intracellular action potential from cell 1. c, calibration pulse; s, stimulus artifact (from Reaves and Hayward, 1979b).

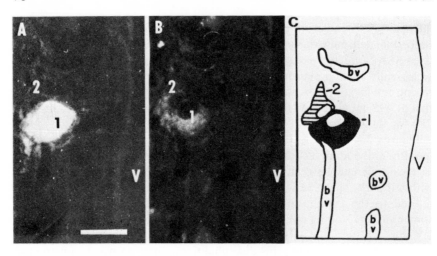

FIG. 4. Vasotocin neuron (cell 1) in goldfish preoptic nucleus. (A) Lucifer Yellow (LY) filled cell 1 (495 nm) near an unmarked cell (2). V, ventricle. Bar = 25 μm. (B) Rhodamine fluorescence (580 nm) provides the double -label for cell 1. Cell 2 also contains vasotocin. (C) Drawing of profiles seen in A and B. bv, blood vessel. Black cell (1) is double-labelled (from Reaves and Hayward, 1980).

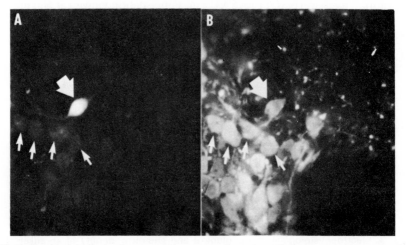

FIG. 5. Double-labelled rat supraoptic neuron from hypothalamo-neurohypophysial complex. (A) Large arrow denotes Lucifer Yellow (LY) filled (495 nm) antidromically-identified neuron. For orientation purposes, the faint rhodamine fluorescence of adjacent non-LY filled cells (small arrows) can be seen at 495 nm. (B) After staining with anti-neurophysin antisera and the rhodamine-tagged second antibody, the LY-marked cell (large arrow) is positive for neurophysin as are several nearby neurons (small arrows; 580 nm).

TRITC fluorescence reveals a positive immunofluorescence for neurophysin (a carrier protein for oxytocin and vasopressin). Many other neurophysinergic neurons are visible in the NSO and show beaded fibres extending within and outside of the NSO (Fig. 5B). It is interesting to note that TRITC

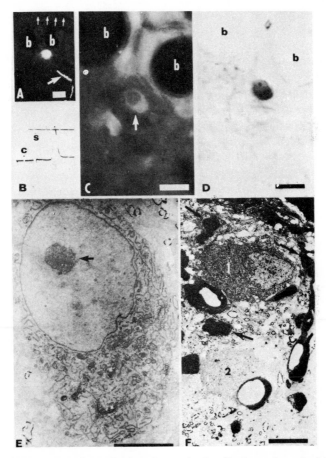

FIG. 6. Light microscopic and ultrastructural visualization of a double-labelled neurophysin neuron from the goldfish preoptic nucleus. (A) Lucifer Yellow (LY) filled (495 nm), physiologically-studied neuron. Large arrow denotes axon. Small arrows outline the ventricular lining. b, blood vessel. Bar = 50 μm. (B) Intracellular antidromically-invaded action potential of cell in A. (C) Arrow denotes rhodamine immunofluorescence of the LY-filled neuron in A. Bar = 25 μm. (D) Same cell as in A and C after irradiation in DAB (see methods). Embedded in Epon, bar = 25 μm. (E) Electron micrograph of ultrathin section cut from cell in D. Not contrasted. Arrow denotes densely stained nucleolus. Bar = 5 μm. (F) Electron micrograph of cell in D after contrasting. Cell 1 is same cell as in (A), (C), (D), (E). Bar = 5 μm (from Reaves et al., 1982b).

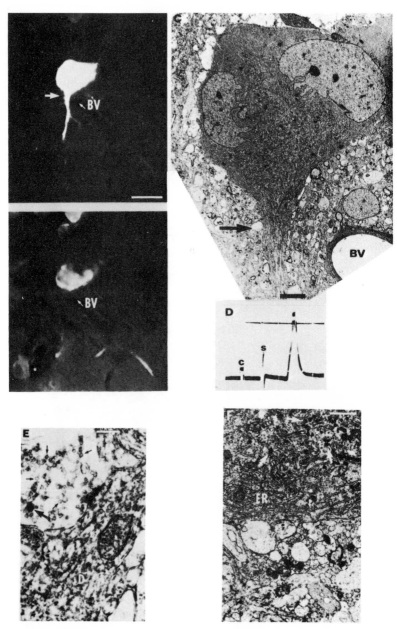

FIG. 7. Light- and electron-microscopy of a double-labelled neuron in goldfish preoptic nucleus. (A) Lucifer Yellow (LY) injected cell (495 nm) with axon (large arrow). Small arrow points to blood vessel (BV). Bar = 25 μm. (B) Neurophysin immunofluorescence (580 nm) of LY-filled neuron of A. (C) Low magnification electron micrograph of cell in A

immunofluorescence is visible not only at 580 nm (Fig. 5B) but also at 495 nm (Fig. 5A, small arrows). At 495 nm, TRITC immunofluorescence is very faint, appearing dull reddish orange in colour which is easily distinguished from the brilliant yellow or orange-yellow fluorescence of LY or PY, respectively. This ability to visualize TRITC fluorescence at 580 nm and at 495 nm is convenient for viewing other immuno-stained cells as landmarks while localizing double-labelled neurons.

IV. ULTRASTRUCTURAL ASPECTS

If ultrastructural analysis of an LY-injected (Fig. 6A, 7A) immuno-cytochemically identified (Fig. 6C, 7b) neuron is desired, a dark in-soluble osmiophilic polymer (diaminobenzidine photo-oxidation product, DAB-POP Fig. 6D) can be produced within that LY-marked cell by irradia-tion (495 mm) in the presence of DAB. Osmication makes the DAB-POP more intense and electron dense (Fig. 6E, 7C), resembling the DAB reac-tion product in the somata of an HRP-filled neuron (Fig. 6D).

At the ultrastructural level, the DAB-POP stained goldfish NPO soma stands out clearly from the surrounding neuropil (Fig. 6E, 7C). The granular DAB-POP is distributed throughout the cytoplasm of LY-double-labelled neurons. Contrasting with uranyl acetate and lead citrate greatly increases the electron density of DAB-POP stained somata (Fig. 6F, 7C). The ultra-structural features of many DAB-POP stained neurons are well preserved (Fig. 6E, 7F). Some DAB-POP stained neurons however, show other features: swollen mitochondria or endoplasmic reticulum having the appearance of vacuoles within the cytoplasm; electron-dense intranuclear spots; and a reactive zone surrounding the injected neuron of numerous polymorphonuclear leukocytes and scattered large empty spaces (Fig. 6F, 7C). Neurosecretory granules, peripheral arrays of endoplasmic reticulum in the somata and the neuropil adjacent to the injected neuron are visible in Fig. 7F. An asymmetric synaptic junction on a dendrite from a DAB-POP stained cell is shown in Fig. 7E.

V. DISCUSSION

Since the fluorescence of the intracellular dye-marker and of the rhodamine-tagged antibody can be visualized on the same tissue section at different

and B. Arrow points to axon (see A). Bar = 5 μm. (D) Action potential for antidromic identification of cell in A. (E) Axon terminal innervating a small dendrite (D) from cell in C. Bar = 250 nm. (F) Neurosecretory granules (arrows) and peripherally situated endo-plasmic reticulum (ER) from double-labelled neuron in C. Bar = 1 μm.

wavelengths of light, the double-labelling technique described here allows for the direct chemical characterization of electrophysiologically studied cells. The morphology of these functionally-studied, chemically-defined cells can be examined both at the light- and at the electron-microscopic levels. The union of this chemical identification procedure to the study of cells with known physiological and anatomical features adds a new dimension to the analysis of single cells, cellular ensembles, tissues and organ systems.

Since our introduction of this technique, in 1979, for studies of the nervous system, others have successfully applied this procedure to their own studies. Michaels and Sheridan (1981) were able to demonstrate heterologous coupling between types A, B and D (glucagon-, insulin- and somatostatin-producing cells, respectively) cells of the rat pancreas islet of Langerhans. They established cell chemical identity using the indirect immunoperoxidase technique on $1 \cdot 0$ μm thick Epon sections. Kayser et al., (1982) used a different double-labelling procedure which utilized the indirect immunoperoxidase PAP (peroxidase-anti-peroxidase complex) technique to chemically identify LY-injected rat supraoptic neurons in vitro on the same tissue section. Their chemical identification step produced a brown peroxidase-DAB (diaminobenzidine) complex which masks the fluorescence of cytoplasmic LY but does not interfere with nuclear bound LY which is used to localize the injected cell. Double-labelled cells were found with LY fluorescence and which reacted with either vasopressin or oxytocin antiserum. Variations of the double-labelling technique have been successfully employed with neuroanatomical pathway studies which incorporate fluorescent dyes (Sawchenko and Swanson, 1981) or horseradish peroxidase (Bowker et al., 1981) markers for the retrograde labelling of neurons.

Ultrastructural studies of double-labelled cells will allow quantitative analysis of the synaptic innervation impinging upon those cells. Although indirect ultrastructural studies of non-chemically defined dye-filled neurons have been reported (Berthold et al., 1979; Purves and McMahan, 1972; Stewart, 1981), direct ultrastructural analysis of dye-marked cells has not been technically feasible since these dyes are not electron dense. However, the new photo-oxidation process developed by Maranto (1981) in which DAB forms an electron-dense reaction product within the confines of an LY-injected structure now allows the direct ultrastructural visualization of LY-marked cells. When combined with our double-labelling technique, the irradiation procedure allows for the light microscopic and ultrastructural examination of physiologically defined, chemically identified cells (Reaves et al., 1982b).

The general ultrastructural features of double-labelled cells appear similar to that of other adjacent cells and the DAB-POP reaction product resembles the DAB reaction product seen in cells marked intracellularly with horseradish peroxidase (Reaves *et al.*, 1982a) or by the immunoperoxidase method of immunocytochemistry (Cumming *et al.*, 1982). We must point out, however, that some double-labelled cells display ultrastructural alterations characteristic of mammalian (Berthold *et al.*, 1979) and invertebrate (Purves and McMahan, 1972) PY-injected neurons. These alterations (see Section IV) presumably result as a consequence of the dye injection.

We feel that combinations of identification techniques such as electrophysiological study, intracellular cell marking with a fluorescent dye (preferably LY), immunocytochemistry and quantitative ultrastructural analysis will result in precise descriptions of specific functional subsets of neurons or cellular groups. An important addition to this double-labelling technique will be the development of post-embedding immunocytochemical staining methods which will allow the chemical nature of the synaptic input onto these cells to be established. Also, the development of new marking dyes, fixatives and fixation procedures, and immunocytochemical methods should allow further use of this double-labelling technique to study a myriad of cellular systems throughout the body.

VI. ACKNOWLEDGEMENTS

We wish to thank Dr W. W. Stewart for supplying Lucifer Yellow, Dr A. G. Robinson for antisera against rat neurophysin (RN#4; Grant AM-16166) and Dr J. D. Fernstrom for antisera against synthetic arginine vasotocin (Lot G2). We also thank Ms D. Cronce for her skilful technical assistance and S. Curtis for editorial comments. Supported, in part, by NIH Grant NS-13411 and Neurobiology Fellowships to R.C. and M.T.L.

VII. REFERENCES

Berthold, C.-H., Kellerth, J.-Q. and Conradi, S. (1979). *J. Comp. Neurol.* **184**, 709–740.
Bowker, R. M., Steinbusch, H. W. M. and Coulter, J. D. (1981). *Brain Res.* **211**, 412–417.
Brown, K. T. and Flaming, D. G. (1975). *Brain Res.* **86**, 172–180.
Coons, A. H. (1958). *In* "General Cytochemical Methods" (J. F. Danielli, ed.), pp. 399–422. Academic Press, New York.
Cumming, R., Reaves, T. A., Jr and Hayward, J. N. (1981). *Neurosci. Letters* **27**, 313–318.
Hayward, J. N. (1974). *J. Physiol. (Lond.)* **239**, 103–124.
Hayward, J. N. (1977). *Physiol. Rev.* **57**, 574–658.

Kayser, B. E. J., Muhlethaler, M. and Dreifuss, J. J. (1982). *Experientia* **38**, 391–393.

Maranto, A. R. (1981). *Soc. Neurosci. Abstr.* **7**, 418.

Michaels, R. L. and Sheridan, J. D. (1981) *Science* **214**, 801–803.

Purves, D. and McMahan, V. J. (1972). *J. Cell Biol.* **55**, 205–220.

Reaves, T. A., Jr, Cumming, R. and Hayward, J. N. (1982a). *Neuroscience* **7**, 1545–1557.

Reaves, T. A., Jr, Cumming, R., Libber, M. T. and Hayward, J. N. (1982b). *Neurosci. Letters* **29**, 195–199.

Reaves, T. A., Jr and Hayward, J. N. (1979a). *Cell Tissue Res.* **202**, 17–35.

Reaves, T. A., Jr and Hayward, J. N. (1979b). *Proc. Natn. Acad. Sci. USA* **76**, 6009–6011.

Reaves, T. A., Jr and Hayward, J. N. (1980). *J. Comp. Neurol.* **193**, 777–788.

Reaves, T. A., Jr, Hou-Yu, A., Zimmerman, E. A. and Hayward, J. N. (1982c). *Physiologist* **25**, 316.

Reaves, T. A., Jr, Libber, M. T. and Hayward, J. N. (1982d). *Soc. Neurosci. Abstr.* **8**, 531.

Sladek, C. D. and Knigge, K. M. (1977). *Endocrinology* **101**, 1834–1838.

Sternberger, L. A. (1979). "Immunocytochemistry". John Wiley and Sons, New York.

Stewart, W. W. (1978). *Cell* **14**, 741–759.

Stewart, W. W. (1981). *Nature* **292**, 17–21.

Sawchenko, P. E. and Swanson, L. W. (1981). *Brain Res.* **210**, 31–51.

Yamamoto, C. (1972). *Exp. Brain Res.* **14**, 423–435.

Young, J. Z. (1935). *Pubbl. Staz. Zool. Napoli* **12**, 425–431.

The Application of the Avidin-biotin Peroxidase Complex Technique to the Localisation of Anterior Pituitary Hormones on Plastic Sections and Cell Monolayers

GWEN V. CHILDS

I. INTRODUCTION

The avidin-biotin peroxidase complex (ABC) technique was developed and introduced first by Hsu *et al.* (1981a) and applied to the localization of antigens in the thyroid. Hsu and his colleagues reported that the technique was more sensitive and rapid than immunoperoxidase techniques that employ peroxidase-antiperoxidase complexes (PAP) (1981a,b) or protein A labeled with peroxidase (1981b). The background was lower and the ABC method could be used with higher dilutions of specific antisera.

IMMUNOCYTOCHEMISTRY 2
ISBN 0 12 140402 1

Figure 1 illustrates the steps of the ABC technique diagrammatically. The primary antibody is applied first to etched sections of chemically fixed or frozen fixed tissues (Step 2). It is then localized with biotinylated goat anti-rabbit immunoglobulin G (Step 3). The avidin DH is then combined with biotinylated horseradish peroxidase and the complex is formed for 30 min prior to its use in the stain (Step 4). The ABC complex is then applied to the section (Step 5). Finally, the peroxidase in the ABC complex is localized with a solution containing its substrate diaminobenzidine (DAB) and hydrogen peroxide. The reaction product (precipitated DAB) may then be stabilized with OsO_4 (Step 6).

In ongoing studies of the localization of pituitary antigens during the past decade, we have utilized the PAP complex techniques and established stains for adrenocorticotropin (ACTH) (Moriarty and Halmi, 1972), luteinizing hormone (LHβ) and follicle stimulating hormone (FSHβ) (Moriarty, 1975). Thyroid stimulating hormone (TSHβ) (Moriarty and Tobin, 1976); and prolactin (PRL) in the rat pituitary. These stains employ working dilutions of primary antisera in the range of 1:5000–1:125 000 depending on the type of fixative and the physiological state of the animal. The incubation times required to produce stain with these high dilutions were usually 48 h.

During the past year, we applied the ABC method to the localization of the pituitary hormones and found that it produced a more rapid, sensitive,

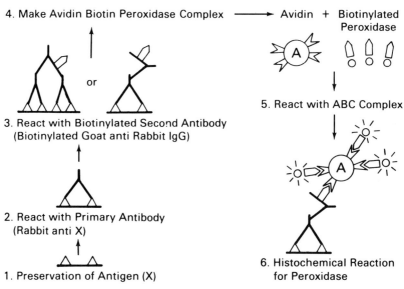

FIG. 1. Diagram of the avidin-biotin complex technique. The Steps are described in the text in more detail.

and reliable stain (Childs and Unabia, 1982a,b). The purpose of this report is to describe and discuss the ABC techniques that we have used both on embedded pituitaries, and on dissociated cells that were fixed and stained immunocytochemically before embedding.

II. PREPARATION OF PITUITARY TISSUES (STEP 1; FIG.1)

A. Removal, Fixation or Freezing, Embedding

Pituitaries removed from anesthetized, decapitated male and female rats were immersed in 1% glutaraldehyde fixative at room temperature. The neurointermediate lobes were gently removed and fixed separately, also in glutaraldehyde only. The anterior lobes were then minced in 1 mm^3 pieces, divided, and placed into various fixatives including 1% glutaraldehyde; 4% p-formaldehyde; or picric acid-formaldehyde for 1 h at room temperature. The fixatives were diluted in 0·1 M phosphate buffer, pH 7·4, and the osmolality was measured with a Wescor microoosmometer. Glutaraldehyde was 318 (1%) or 418 (2·5%) mosmol/l; 4% p-formaldehyde was 1405 mosmol/l and picric acid formaldehyde was 757 mosmol/l. The pituitaries were then washed in 0·1 M Sorensens phosphate buffer containing 4·5% sucrose (pH 7·4, osmolality 327). They were then dehydrated in ethanol, infiltrated with propylene oxide and embedded in Araldite 6005 according to our standard protocol (Moriarty, 1974).

A second group of male rat pituitaries were rapidly frozen and freeze-dried in vacuo according to Dudek *et al.* (1982). They were then embedded in Araldite 6005. Some of these blocks were also exposed to OsO_4 vapor prior to the embedding.

A third group of male or female rat pituitaries were dissociated with 0·5% trypsin according to Denef *et al.* (1968) and grown for 2–4 days in monolayer culture on plastic coverslips. The cells were then fixed in 1% glutaraldehyde for 30 min at room temperature (diluted in 0·1 M phosphate buffer, 370 mosmol/l).

The cells were then washed by several changes of the 0·1 M phosphate buffer containing 5% sucrose (375 mosmol/l). The fixed cells were first treated with 1:100 normal goat serum and then exposed to primary antiserum for 12 h, diluted in 0·1 M phospate buffer + 2·5 mg/ml human serum albumin. The primary antiserum was then removed, and the monolayers were stained with the avidin-biotin complex (ABC) technique. No pretreatment with Saponin, H_2O_2 or Triton X-100 was necessary. The immunoreactants appeared to penetrate the fixed cells without membrane solubilization.

A final group of pituitaries were dissociated, grown for 12 h, fixed in 1% glutaraldehyde as above, and then centrifuged in a pellet containing 4% agar (40 °C). The agar-cell pellet was hardened and then dehydrated and embedded in Araldite 6005 as in the above studies.

Semithin (0·5-1 μm) or ultrathin sections of the embedded blocks were cut and prepared for staining as described in the following sections.

B. Preparation of Semithin Sections for Staining

Semithin (0·5-1 μm) sections were cut, located with a diamond pen, and dried for 1 h on slides on a warming tray. They were then etched with saturated sodium ethoxide for 10–15 min at room temperature. The sodium ethoxide was made 2–3 days prior to its use in the stain by placing a monolayer of sodium hydroxide pellets in absolute ethanol. The solution turns yellow-orange and was used for 1–2 months. The saturated sodium ethoxide removes plastic from the section and will damage fragile tissue. Therefore, precautions must be taken to test its applicability to each tissue system.

The sections were washed by running a stream of absolute ethanol gently over the slide that is held at a 45° angle (jet washing). They were then rehydrated by gentle jet-washing in a sequence of solutions containing 95%, 70%, 50% ethanol, distilled water, and 0·05 M phosphate buffer (pH 7·4).

The excess buffer was blotted around the area containing the sections and 10% H_2O_2 was added for 8–10 min. This solution unmasks antigenic sites and abolishes endogenous peroxidase activity. It may, however, cause damage to the tissue so its use should be tested in the individual tissues to be stained. It may be omitted with no obvious change in the staining pattern.

The sections were then jet-washed with 0·05 M phosphate buffer and the excess buffer was blotted and replaced with 1:100 normal goat serum for 10 min. This solution was blotted around the sections to remove excess, replaced with diluted primary antiserum and the slides incubated for up to 12 h at room temperature in a moisture chamber, which is a polypropylene (refrigerator type) tray lined with moist paper towels and has a tight-fitting lid.

C. Preparation of Ultrathin Plastic-embedded Sections for Staining

Ultrathin light gold sections were cut and mounted on bare nickel grids (200 mesh). They are stored indefinitely in dust proof boxes. They were etched prior to staining by floating the grid (section face down) on a drop of 10%

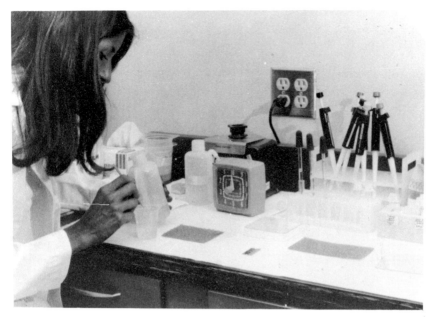

FIG. 2. Jet washing is performed by gently running a stream of millipore filtered buffer or distilled water across the grids held with a forceps at a 45° angle. Also shown are wax sheets on which drops of the staining solution (antibody, etc.) are placed. The grids are floated on these drops while covered by the square plastic petri dish lid.

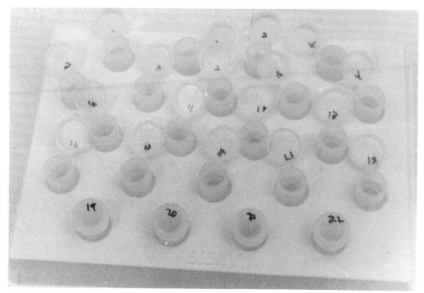

FIG. 3. Grids are incubated in 50 μl of diluted primary antibody in individual BEEM capsules which are number or letter coded. Covers are snapped on tightly during the 2–12 h incubation. BEEM capsules are heat sterilized in an embedding oven (50–60 °C) prior to their use.

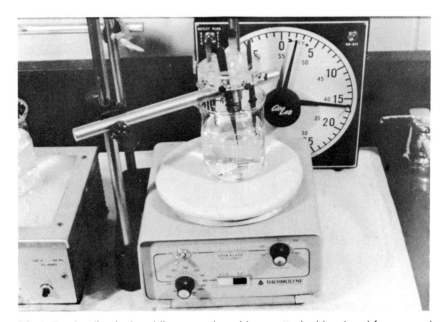

FIG. 4. For the diaminobenzidine step, the grids are attached by closed forceps and inserted in a lucite ring. The entire unit is then lowered into the moving diaminobenzidine H_2O_2 solution on the magnetic stirrer. After 3–4 min, the beaker of DAB is quickly replaced by a beaker of millipore filtered water which is also stirred to wash the grids. The forceps are removed individually, the grid is jet washed (Fig. 2) and allowed to dry on filter paper.

H_2O_2 and then jet washed in 0·05 M phosphate buffer (Fig. 2). The grids were floated on drops of 1:100 normal goat serum for 3 min (Fig. 3) and then gently blotted on torn filter paper to remove excess serum. The grids were placed in microtiter wells or BEEM capsules containing the diluted (>1:5000). primary antiserum (Fig. 4). Incubation continued in these capsules for 2–12 h at room temperature.

III. PREPARATION OF PITUITARY CELL MONOLAYERS FOR STAINING

The glutaraldehyde-fixed pituitary cells were attached to coverslips in multiwell dishes (Falcon Plastics). They were first pre-treated in the dishes with 1:100 normal goat serum for 10 min at room temperature. This was poured off and replaced with diluted primary antiserum (>1:5000). The multiwell dish lid was then replaced and the cells incubated for 12 h at room temperature. Our experiments have demonstrated that there are no endogenous avidin binding sites on the fixed, unembedded pituitary cells. Also, no pre-solubilization or etching steps were needed to promote penetration of immunoreactants. Therefore, we did not apply Saponin or Triton X-100 in our buffer, nor is pre-treatment with 10% H_2O_2 necessary.

A. Application of the Primary Antibody (Step 2, Fig. 1)

Our initial tests of the stain on the semithin sections or cell monolayers showed that the optional incubation time in primary antibody was 12–16 h. Optimal working dilutions for the antisera (applied to normal rat pituitary cells) were as follows:

1. 1:10 000 – 1:60 000 anti-bovine LHβ (J. G. Pierce)
2. 1:5000 – 1:60 000 anti-human FSHβ (NIADDK)*
3. 1:5000 anti-rat prolactin (NIADDK)
4. 1:20 000 – 1:50 000 anti-$^{25-39}$ ACTH (produced in our laboratory)
5. 1:16 000 – 1:24 000 anti-rat TSHβ (NIADDK)

Changes in these dilutions were required when they were applied to rats in different physiological states. For example gonadotropes 12–24 h after castration required a 1:5000 – 1:10 000 dilution of anti-LHβ and a 1:2500 dilution of anti-FSHβ. Often the FSHβ stain was optimal only after a 48-h incubation. Developing thyrotropes from neonatal rats were stained optimally after a 1:8000 dilution of anti-rTSHβ was applied for 12–16 h.

One could decrease the time in the diluted primary antibody to as little as 4 h, however only the cells that stored the most antigen stained. An increase to a 48-h incubation time resulted in higher background in most sections that could be eliminated by a 2–4 fold further increase in the antibody dilution (Childs and Unabia, 1982a).

We also determined that optimal working dilutions and times were similar in both the unembedded cell cultures and the embedded plastic sections. The percentages of each cell type did not vary following dissociation or embedding. Hence, we concluded that the relative amounts of specific antigens required for detection of a given cell type were not altered appreciably by the processing methods used to date.

The stains at the EM level were performed initially with a 48-h incubation in primary antibody diluted as in the LM stains. The sections were over-labeled with a dense punctate or a cloudy reaction that masked the stain. Therefore, we reduced the time in primary antibody to 4–12 h. The results were cleaner, but some background was noted. Thus, the times were

---

* National Institute Arthritic, Diabetic, Digestive and Kidney Diseases.

reduced further and the minimal time for the detection of stain was noted. Our quantitative measurements of the staining intensity showed that the stain for LHβ was detected after a 15-min incubation in 1:10 000 anti-LHβ (Childs and Unabia, 1981b). It is optimal at 30–120 min. Longer times are required for the other antisera, however the optimal incubation period for most antisera on normal rat pituitaries seems to be 2 h.

B. Application of Biotinylated Second Antibody (Step 3; Fig. 1)

After the plastic sections or cell monolayers have been reacted with diluted primary antibody, they are jet washed in 0·05 M phosphate buffer (Fig. 2) and treated with a 1:400 dilution of affinity purified biotin conjugated anti-rabbit IgG. The solution is available from Vector Laboratories (Burlingame, Calif.). It is stored in 10 μl aliquots at −70°C and is diluted, prior to its use, in 3990 μl of 0·05 M phosphate buffer + 2·5 mg/ml human serum albumin.

The second antibody is applied for *30 min* to semithin sections or cell monolayers. *However, it is applied for only 3 min to the ultrathin sections on nickel grids.*

C. Production and Application of the Avidin-Biotin Complex (Steps 4 and 5; Fig. 1)

The ABC components are available in a kit from Vector Laboratories. The avidin DH and biotinylated peroxidase are stored separately in 25 μl aliquots in the refrigerator (4 °C). Thirty min prior to their use in the stain, 25 μl of each component is added to 4000 μl of 0·05 M phosphate buffer containing 2·5 mg/ml human serum albumin. The complex forms at room temperature for 20 min prior to its use in the stain. *The ABC solution is applied to the cell monolayers or semithin sections for 45–60 min. It is applied to ultrathin sections for 3 min.* The sections or cells are then jet washed and the remaining ABC solution discarded. Phosphate buffer is applied to the sections while the diaminobenzidine-hydrogen peroxide solution is made.

D. Application of the Peroxidase Substrate Solution (Step 6; Fig. 1)

The solution applied to the pituitary cell monolayers or semithin (1 μm) sections contained 5–10 mg of diaminobenzidine tetrahydrochloride in 100 ml of Tris buffer + 100 μl of 10% H_2O_2. This solution was applied for 4–6 min and then removed rapidly by washing in distilled deionized milli-

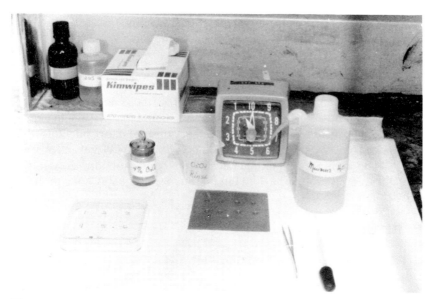

FIG. 5. The OsO_4 step is optional. It will enhance the stain and help counterstain the tissues. The grids are placed on drops of 4% ultrapure aqueous OsO_4 for 8–10 min and covered with the square petri dish lid. They are then jet washed and allowed to dry on filter paper. They are viewed without further counterstaining.

pore filtered water. The reaction is maximal in 5 min. The substrate can be intensified by allowing the sections to dry and then treating them with 1% OsO_4 for 1–2 min (aqueous), ultrapure, EM Sciences), or by the addition of 2·5% nickel ammonium sulfate to the DAB in dissolved acetate buffer (Hancock, 1982).

The solution applied to the ultrathin sections contained 18–22 mg of diaminobenzidine-tetrahydrochloride in 175 ml of 0·05 M Tris (pH 7·6, room temperature) + 150 μl of 30% H_2O_2. It was rotated gently in a 250 ml beaker on a magnetic stirrer and the grids were immersed, attached to forceps, for 3 min (Fig. 5). They were then rapidly removed and washed in distilled-deionized millipore filtered water. The stain was punctate or dot-like on the granules or rough endoplasmic reticulum (RER) (Fig. 6). It could be intensified by a brief (4–6 min) treatment in 4% OsO_4 (aqueous, ultrapure) (Figs. 7–9). The sections are washed in distilled-deionized, millipore filtered water and dried.

1. Counterstains

Counterstains are now being tested for their application to the ultrathin sections. The semithin sections or the cell monolayers were counterstained with Nuclear fast red or Eosin. The sections were then washed, dried and coverslips are mounted with permount.

2. Controls

The controls for this technique were similar to those described for other techniques (Childs, 1982a,b). Tests for endogenous biotin, or avidin binding activity should be conducted (see Boorsma, this volume) and, if needed, appropriate blocking steps performed as in the study by Wood and Warnke (1981). If no staining occurs when the first or second antibodies are omitted, then endogenous biotin or avidin binding sites are probably not a problem.

IV. RESULTS

A. Electron Microscopic Staining Patterns

The electron microscopic ABC stain is shown in the next series of Figures. Figure 6 shows the ABC stain on granules that have not been exposed to

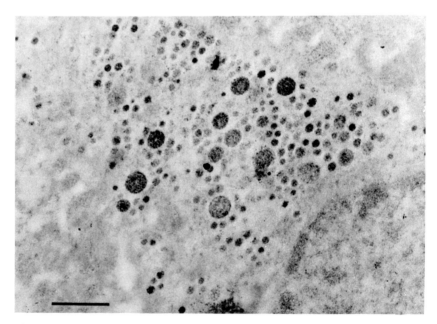

FIG. 6. LH gonadotrope stained with 1:30 000 anti-bLHβ (48-h incubation) and the ABC technique. No OsO$_4$ was used to enhance stain. Note punctate deposits on the granules. Magnification ×24 000; bar = 1 μm.

OsO$_4$ after the DAB reaction. The background is pale and the stained cells difficult to distinguish. Figures 7–9 show gonadotropes stained for LH (Figs. 7, 8) or FSH (Fig. 9). The serial view in Fig. 7 shows an LH cell stained after 1-h incubation in 1:10 000 anti-bLHβ while the view in Fig. 8 shows the stain after 4 h. OsO$_4$ treatment of the DAB darkened the granules, and brought out the tissue density. The granules are stained after a 4-h incubation, at maximal intensity. In Fig. 9, the serial field shows the same cell stained optimally for FSH following a 1-h incubation in a 1:4000 dilution.

The background produced by the ABC stain can be diffuse and filigreed and is illustrated in Fig. 10. This shows an overstained gonadotrope incubated for 48 h in 1:10 000 anti-bLHβ. The background causes a decrease in the staining intensity, in comparison to cells stained after only 1–4 h incubation in the same dilution of antiserum.

The stains shown in Figs 6–10 were reacted with ABC kits produced in 1981. We have since found that newer kits label more precisely. Figure 11 is from a mink pituitary showing the ABC stain for LH on the secretion granules of a gonadotrope. The coarse appearance of the ABC stain is so obvious, that blackening by OsO$_4$ is not necessary, except to help counter-

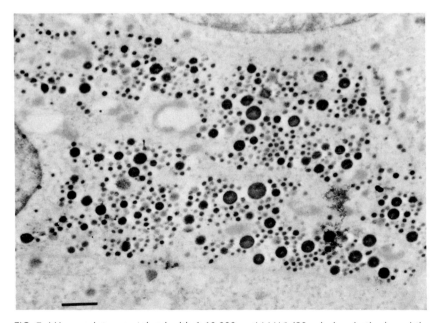

FIG. 7. LH gonadotrope stained with 1:10 000 anti-bLHβ, (30-min incubation), and the ABC technique. OsO$_4$ enhances stain on granules and helps bring out the background. Stain does not fill the granule intensely. Magnification ×15 000; bar = 1 μm.

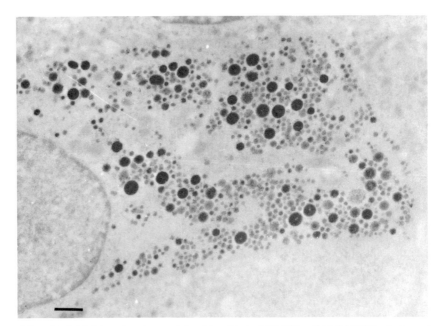

FIG. 8. Serial field to the above stained for 4 h in 1:10 000 anti-bLH (ABC technique + OsO₄). Granule staining is very dense and even has a three-dimensional aspect. Magnification ×12 500; bar = 1 μm.

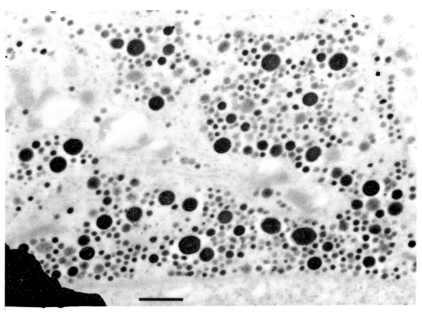

FIG. 9. Serial field to the above stained for 1 h in 1:4000 anti-hFSHβ as above. The gonadotrope stains optimally for FSH as well under these conditions. Magnification ×18 666; bar = 1 μm.

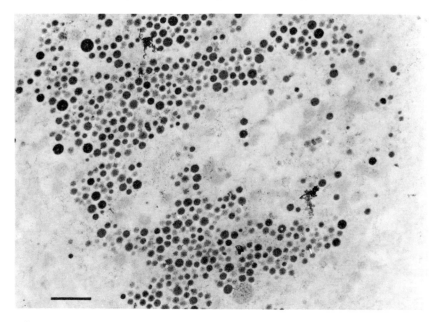

FIG. 10. LH gonadotrope that was stained in 1:10 000 anti-bLHβ for 48 h. The stain is not more intense than that produced at 1–4 h, but it is dirtier. The background resembles a filigreed network over and around the granules and areas adjacent to the cell. Magnification ×17 333; bar = 1 μm.

stain the tissue. Furthermore, a heavy metal counterstain does not appear to mask the specific stain. Therefore, we are now in a position to be able to define more clearly the ultrastructure of the organelles that are staining with lead and uranyl counterstains.

B. Light Microscopic Staining Patterns

Figure 12 is a representative field from the normal rat pituitary showing stain for ACTH on semithin sections of intact pituitaries. Figure 13 shows the stain for LHβ on semithin sections of glutaraldehyde fixed, Araldite-embedded dissociated pituitary cells. The stained cells contain brown–dark brown granules against a pink Eosin-stained background.

Figure 14 is from a fixed monolayer culture cell showing stain for TSHβ in isolated cells. The stain may be diffuse in patches, or it may fill the entire cell. As stated previously, these stains do not require membrane solubilization by detergents, or etching by H_2O_2.

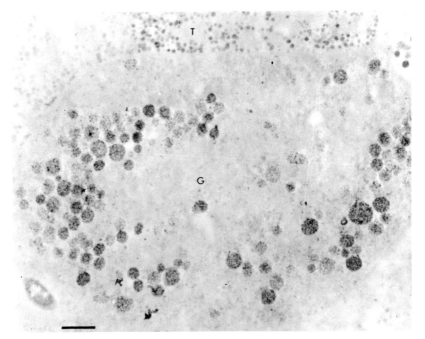

FIG. 11. LH gonadotrope (G) from a mink pituitary stained for 2 h in 1:10 000 anti-bLHβ. Stain is more coarse and punctate with the newest ABC kits, while the background is so low that the unstained areas are almost invisible. T = presumptive thyrotrope. Magnification ×15 000; bar = 1 μm.

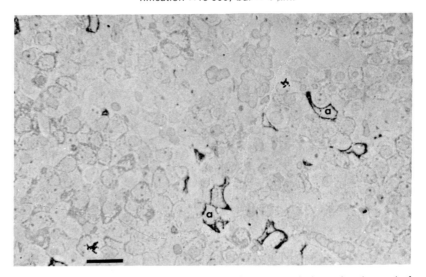

FIG. 12. Light micrograph of semithin section of intact rat pituitary showing stain for ACTH in scattered, stellate cells (a) that contain peripheral storage granules (Moriarty and Halmi, 1972). Stained with 1:20 000 anti-²⁵⁻³⁹ACTH, 12-h incubation. Magnification ×640; bar = 20 μm.

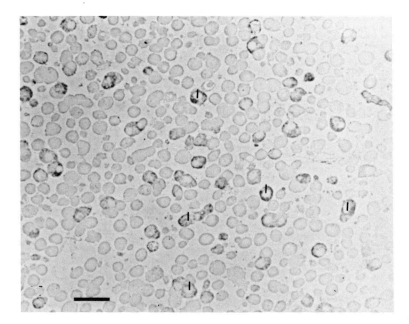

FIG. 13. Semithin section of dissociated pituitary cells that are separated by centrifugal elutriation. This field shows an enriched population of medium sized LH cells (I). Stained with 1:10 000 anti-bLHβ; 12-h incubation. Magnification ×640; bar = 20 μm.

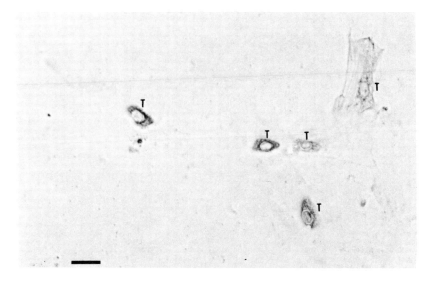

FIG. 14. Pituitary cell monolayer grown for 3 days and then fixed in 2·5% glutaraldehyde and stained with 1:1600 anti-rTSH and the ABC technique. No detergents were used to penetrate cell. Five stained cells (T) appear to be nested in fibroblast sheets. Stain is granular or filamentous in the cytoplasm near the nucleus, 12-h incubation. Magnification ×640; bar = 20 μm.

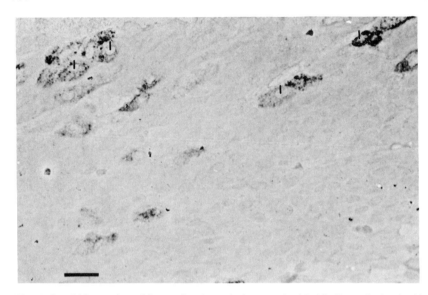

FIG. 15. Semithin section of frozen-fixed rat pituitary embedded in Epon. Stained with 1:50 000 anti-LHβ, 12-h incubation. Most LH gonadotropes (L) are round-ovoid and packed with densely staining granules. Some cells stain less intensely. Magnification ×640; bar = 20 μm.

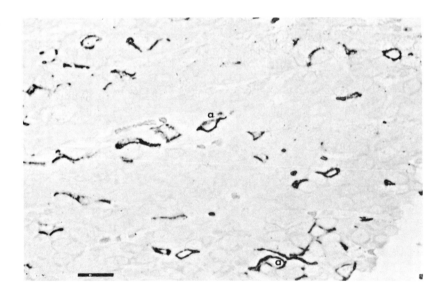

FIG. 16. Semithin section of frozen-fixed rat pituitary embedded in Araldite. Stained with 1:50 000 anti-[1–39] ACTH, 12-h incubation. Stellate ACTH (A) cells are scattered in the field as in Fig. 13 which is from a chemically (glutaraldehyde) fixed pituitary. Magnification ×640; bar = μm.

Stained frozen fixed-plastic embedded semithin sections are illustrated in Figs 15 and 16. These sections require a 2–5 fold increase in the antiserum dilution because there are more antigens retained in the cells.

V. SUMMARY AND CONCLUSIONS

Our experience has shown that the ABC method yields a rapid, efficient stain that conserves both time and solutions. It also has a low background when used properly. Furthermore, the ABC stain offers some advantages over the PAP stain applied previously in our laboratory. These are listed below.

1. It is cleaner and has lower background than most of our stains that use the PAP complex.

2. It can be used at the EM level with 1/10–1/3 the incubation time. Normally, the PAP technique requires a 48-h incubation time in primary antibody diluted >1:5000.

3. The reaction product is coarse and punctate. This factor renders it readily distinguishable from osmiophilic granules and allows the use of a heavy metal counterstain.

4. The stain for FSHβ appears more reliable and intense, especially at the light microscopic level.

5. In general, most primary antisera can be diluted 2–10 fold beyond 1:5000 dilutions if incubation times are prolonged to 48 h. Thus, one may achieve working dilutions similar to those used in the sensitive radioimmunoassays. This conserves antisera and may render a polyclonal antibody more specific, especially if it is preabsorbed with ng or μg quantities of crossreactive antigens.

6. The stains can be applied with the use of the same concentrations of antibody to fixed pituitary cells in monolayer culture. They will penetrate the fixed cells without detergent or H_2O_2 pretreatment.

Thus the ABC immunoperoxidase method has proved to be extremely useful in the efficient localization of pituitary hormones. Future tests of its applicability with gold or ferritin labeled complexes are in progress.

VI. ACKNOWLEDGEMENTS

The author wishes to thank Drs Jim Whitehead and José Perdromo, Vector Laboratories, for our many helpful discussions about the ABC complex and related technique. She is grateful for the technical assistance of Ms Geda Unabia and the secretarial skills of Ms Phyllis Fletcher.

This work was supported by seed funds from UTMB-NIH 507 RR05427, and RO1 HD 15472-01; Dr Childs is the recipient of RCDA HD -00395.

VII. REFERENCES

Childs, G. V. and Unabia, G. (1982). *J. Histochem. Cytochem.* **30**, 713–716.

Childs, G. V. and Unabia, G. (1982). *J. Histochem. Cytochem.* **30**, (in press).

Childs, G. V. (1982). *J. Histochem. Cytochem.* **30**, (in press).

Childs, G. V. (1982). *In* "Electron Microscopy in Biology" (J. Griffith, ed.), Vol.II, pp.107–187. John Wiley and Sons Inc., New York.

Denef, C., Hauteskeete, E., Dewolf, A. and Vandershusen, B. (1978). *Endocrinology* **103**, 724–735.

Dudek, R. W., Childs, G. V. and Boyne, A. F. (1982). *J. Histochem. Cytochem.* **30**, 129–138.

Hancock, M. (1982). *Neurosci. Letters* (in press).

Hsu, S-M., Raine, L., and Fanger, H. (1981). *J. Histochem. Cytochem.* **29**, 577–579.

Hsu, S-M. and Raine, L. (1981). *J. Histochem. Cytochem.* **29**, 1349.

Moriarty, G. C. and Halmi, N. S. (1972). *J. Histochem. Cytochem.* **20**, 590–603.

Moriarty, G. C. (1975). *Endocrinology* **97**, 1215–1225.

Moriarty, G. C. (1976). *J. Histochem. Cytochem.* **24**, 846–863.

Moriarty, G. C. and Tobin, R. B. (1976). *J. Histochem. Cytochem.* **24**, 1131–1139.

Immunological Methods in Scanning Electron Microscopy using Peroxidase

A. L. HARTMAN and P. K. NAKANE

I. INTRODUCTION

A. Historical Background

The theory behind scanning electron microscopy (SEM) was put forth by Knoll in 1935 and the first scanning electron microscope was built by Von Ardenne in 1938. However, it was not until the mid-1960s that scanning electron microscopes became commercially available. Since that time, the scanning electron microscope has become a routine laboratory tool. The images obtained by SEM are considerably different from those of transmission electron microscopy (TEM). Originally, these microscopes were used to obtain high resolution topographical views of the specimen through the use of secondary electrons generated when the incident electron beam

IMMUNOCYTOCHEMISTRY 2
ISBN 0 12 140402 1

strikes the specimen. More recently, detectors for other types of electrons generated when the incident electron beam strikes the specimen have become commercially available. The availability of these new detectors has greatly broadened the practical application of the scanning electron microscope.

When the incident electron beam strikes the specimen, several types of radiation are generated: (1) Auger electrons; (2) secondary electrons; (3) backscattered electrons; (4) X-rays; and (5) cathodoluminescence (Reimer, 1979). Each of these types of radiation can be used to form a different kind of specimen image, each containing unique information on the specimen's composition. In addition, SEM offers several other advantages over TEM: the specimen preparation for SEM is far quicker and easier than TEM; SEM allows the examination of large specimens, thus avoiding the sampling error often encountered with TEM; and SEM allows one to look at both the internal and external composition of the same specimen.

This review is not intended to be a review of scanning electron microscopy as a whole and, therefore, we will not delve into each of the imaging systems. However, a basic concept of secondary and backscattered electrons is necessary to fully understand the rationales employed in the use of scanning electron microscopy for immunohistochemical localization and, therefore, those two types of radiations will be discussed briefly.

B. Secondary Electrons

When the primary electron beam strikes the specimen, the incident electrons interact with the atoms of the specimen. One of these interactions is the inelastic collision of primary electrons with electrons of the specimen's atoms. These inelastic electron-electron interactions are responsible for the liberation of low-energy secondary electrons from the specimen. Because of their low energy (most are less than 15 eV), only those secondary electrons generated in the top 5–10 nm of the specimen are able to exit from the tissue and be collected by the detector. These secondary electrons can be detected at accelerating voltages as low as 1 kV and the number of secondary electrons generated is relatively independent of the atomic number of the specimen. The number of electrons detected, however, is greatly influenced by the topography of the specimen. Therefore, the secondary electron image is formed by secondary electrons which arise from a zone at or very near the surface of the specimen, from an area only slightly larger than the diameter of the primary electron beam, and thus can be used to obtain high resolution surface images (approximately 10 nm for most conventional scanning electron microscopes).

C. Backscattered Electrons

Another type of interaction that occurs when the primary electron beam strikes the specimen is elastic collisions between electrons of the primary beam and the atomic nuclei of the specimen. This type of interaction results in deflection of primary electrons at large angles without the loss of energy associated with secondary backscattered electrons. Because there is little energy loss in this type of primary electron-specimen interaction, backscattered electrons generated deep within the specimen (over several μ below the surface) can exit from the specimen and be detected. Backscattered electrons can normally be detected only at accelerating voltages of 5–7 kV or greater and the number of electrons generated is relatively independent of the topography of the specimen. However, the number of backscattered electrons generated is dependent upon the atomic number of the specimen. Therefore, backscattered electrons can be used to form images of sub-surface structures based upon their atomic number independent of the surface topography. However, because these electrons are emerging from deep within the specimen, the primary electron beam has diffused considerably and, consequently, this is reflected in the resolution which can be achieved (50–200 nm with most conventional scanning electron microscopes).

II. IMMUNOHISTOCHEMISTRY

A. Background

The use of antibodies labeled with a marker for the localization of antigens *in situ* was first introduced by Coons and his coworkers in the 1950s using fluorescein as a marker (Coons, 1958). Although there have been improvements in the isolation of antigens, raising of antibodies, preparation of antibody fragments, and expansion of the types of markers one can use to label the antibody, the basic concept introduced by Coons has remained unchanged: Use of the built-in specificity of antibody-antigen interaction to localize the sites of antigens in tissues and cells *in situ*. The fluorescein marker used by Coons was restricted to the localization of antigens at the light microscopic level. However, with the introduction of an electron dense substrate by Graham and Karnovski (1966) and the peroxidase-labeled antibody method by Nakane and Pierce (1966), it became possible to localize intracellular antigens at the electron microscopic level.

Over the years, a number of markers have been developed to label antibodies for use in ultrastructural localization. Markers for immunohistochemical localization for antigens with scanning electron microscopy have, for the most part, depended upon the physical characteristics of size and shape for their detection, thus restricting their use to the secondary electron mode of the scanning electron microscope. These markers include: viruses (Hämmerling *et al.*, 1975), ferritin (Hattori *et al.*, 1976), hemocyanin (Miller and Teplitz, 1978), latex spheres (Molday *et al.*, 1975), silica particles (Peters *et al.*, 1976) and colloidal gold (Goodman *et al.*, 1979). Because these markers are dependent upon their three-dimensional structure for their recognition, they are limited to localization of antigens on the surface of the specimen. More recently with the advent of low cost, commercially available backscattered electron detectors, the search for new, more versatile markers for use in immunohistochemistry with SEM has begun. Those traditional secondary electron markers which are capable of being detected by backscatter imaging (i.e. colloidal gold) are too large to facilitate their penetration into the intracellular or sub-surface sites of antigen within the specimen and therefore are of limited use in backscattered electron imaging (BSI). Although in the past, enzymes have seldom been used as markers for SEM, Becker and Sogard (1979) and more recently Soligo and deHarven (1981), showed that lead deposited at the intracellular sites of endogenous acid phosphatase can be detected using BSI. In addition, Becker and Debruyn (1976) showed that the diaminobenzidine (DAB) reaction product formed by peroxidase present in leukocytes could be visualized using backscattered imaging following reaction of the DAB reaction product with osmium. Thus, the peroxidase-labelled antibody method which in the past has been widely used for antigen localization by light microscopy and TEM can be applied to antigen localization by SEM as well.

Since its introduction in 1966, a number of modifications of the peroxidase-labeled antibody method have been used in various laboratories (Sternberger *et al.*, 1970; Spicer *et al.*, 1976). We will limit the discussion presented here to the three most commonly used techniques, namely: the direct, the indirect, and the peroxidase-anti-peroxidase (PAP) techniques (see Volume 1 this series).

B. Direct Method

In the direct technique, the antibody molecule or Fab or Fab' fragment of the antibody molecule directed against the antigen of interest is labeled with horseradish peroxidase. The peroxidase-labeled antibody is added to the cells or tissue sections and allowed to react with the antigen. The excess antibody is then washed off and the cells or tissue sections are incubated in the presence of diaminobenzidine and hydrogen peroxide. This results in the deposition of a brown enzymatic reaction product at the site of the enzyme, thus allowing the visualization of the site(s) of antigen.

C. Indirect Method

The indirect method involves one more step than the direct method. The first step is the same: one applies the antibody (or antibody fragment), to the cells or tissue and allows it to react with the antigen. However, in this case the primary antibody is not labeled with peroxidase; therefore, after washing off excess antibody, an anti-antibody (or antibody fragment) labeled with peroxidase is applied and allowed to bind to the primary antibody. Following washing to remove any excess anti-antibody, the site of antibody (i.e. antigen) is localized histochemically as in the direct technique. The indirect method has the advantage that single peroxidase-labeled antibody (e.g. sheep anti-rabbit IgG) can be used to localize several different antigens provided the primary antibodies are from a single species (e.g. rabbit).

D. Peroxidase-anti-peroxidase Method

The peroxidase-anti-peroxidase (PAP) technique involves one more step than the indirect method. With this method, one applies primary antibody and allows it to react with the antigen. The unreacted antibody is washed off and an *excess* of unlabeled anti-antibody is added. By adding the second antibody (anti-antibody) in large excess, one of the two antigen combining sites of the antibody molecule should remain unoccupied. Following washing to remove unreacted anti-antibody molecules, soluble immune complexes of peroxidase-anti-peroxidase (in which the anti-peroxidase was raised in the same species as the primary antibody) are allowed to react with the unoccupied antigen combining site of the second antibody. After washing of any unbound PAP complexes, the site(s) of antigen is visualized histochemically as described above.

The PAP technique has the advantage that no chemical coupling of the peroxidase molecule to the antibody molecule is necessary. However, the PAP method has two major disadvantages. First, because of the large size of the PAP immune complexes, achieving adequate penetration often becomes an insurmountable problem; and second, the primary antibody must be raised in the same species as the anti-peroxidase antibody which renders it useless with certain types of primary antibodies (i.e. human autoimmune antibodies). A typical staining protocol for the direct and indirect methods is given in the Appendices.

III. FIXATION

Perhaps the biggest obstacle which must be overcome for the successful localization of antigens at the ultrastructural level is selection of the proper fixation regimen. In fixing a specimen for immunohistochemistry, one is forced into a compromise between good morphological preservation and good retention of antigenicity. This is brought about by the fact that fixatives which give good morphological preservation in general destroy antigenicity and conversely, fixatives which give good antigenic preservation tend to give poor morphological preservation.

The most commonly used group of fixatives for immunohistochemistry is the aldehydes. Glutaraldehyde, a bifunctional dialdehyde, provides excellent morphological preservation, however, many antigens loose their antigenicity upon fixation with glutaraldehyde. In addition, because of its bifunctional nature, fixation with glutaraldehyde results in extensive cross-linking which greatly retards the penetration of labeled antibodies into tissues and cells.

Formaldehyde, a monoaldehyde, is perhaps the most commonly used fixative for immunohistochemistry. While the ultrastructural preservation obtained with formaldehyde is not as good as that obtained with glutaraldehyde, sufficient antigenicity is usually retained with formaldehyde fixation to allow immunohistochemical localization. In addition, because formaldehyde is a monoaldehyde, the degree of cross-linking is minimal and therefore much better antibody penetration is obtained with formaldehyde fixation. In an effort to improve the morphological preservation while still retaining antigenicity, formaldehyde has been used in combination with other fixatives. Dilute solutions of glutaraldehyde (1·0–0·01%) in combination with formaldehyde (Yokota and Fahimi, 1981) have proved to be useful in this regard, especially with tissues of the central nervous system (Pickel *et al.*, 1975). Picric acid, a protein precipitant, combined with formaldehyde improves morphological preservation while retaining antigenicity in many cases (Stefanini *et al.*, 1967). Another variation on this theme has been the combination of periodate and lysine with formaldehyde, which has also proven to be a useful fixative for immunohistochemistry in many cases (McLean and Nakane, 1974). Unfortunately, there is no good rule of thumb which can be used to select the proper fixation regimen. For each antigen to be localized, a series of fixatives must be screened in order to determine which is best suited for that particular antigen.

IV. PENETRATION

The other major obstacle that must be overcome for the localization of intracellular antigens is that of penetration. If the antibody molecule does not penetrate into the intracellular site(s) of antigen, a false-negative result will occur. In general, it is the membrane structures (plasma membrane, mitochondrial membranes, endoplasmic reticulum and nuclear envelope) which present the biggest obstacles to penetration. There are two main approaches to overcoming this problem: (1) increasing the permeability of the cell or tissues; and (2) decreasing the size of the penetrating molecule. With regard to the former, the specimen can be frozen and thawed, treated with detergents such as saponin (Bohn, 1978) and Triton X-100 (Willingham and Yamada, 1979) or treated with organic solvents such as acetone and alcohol.

Unfortunately, while these methods increase the permeability of the specimen they often adversely affect the morphology or result in increased non-specific background staining. The latter approach can be accomplished by enzymatic digestion of the antibody into Fab′ or Fab fragments (Grey and Kunkel, 1964). This decrease in size of the antibody molecule, due to the removal of the FC portion, leads to increased penetration and at the same time reduces the background staining due to the non-specific sticking of the antibody molecule via the FC region (Nakane, 1975). (This is especially true in the case of central nervous system tissues.) Therefore, whenever possible it is advisable to use antibody fragments rather than whole IgG molecules for the ultrastructural localization of intracellular antigens.

V. TISSUE HANDLING

Because the specimen used in SEM is much thicker than that used in TEM, the electrons from the primary beam cannot pass through it and, thus, if the specimen is not electrically grounded a negative charge builds up in the specimen as it is bombarded by the primary electron beam (charging). This charging causes severe distortion in the secondary electron image (SET) and to a lesser degree, distortion in the backscattered electron image as well. To overcome this charging effect, grounding of the specimen is usually accomplished by coating the specimen with a thin layer of heavy metal such as gold or a layer of carbon. As mentioned above, backscatter imaging is much less sensitive to charging than SEI, therefore in many cases coating of the substrate upon which the specimen is mounted is sufficient to overcome the charging artifacts.

There are currently two methods in use for coating the substrate (i.e. a glass slide or coverslip). The first is the evaporation of indium oxide onto the substrate (Ogura and Laudate, 1980), and the second is the evaporation of carbon onto the substrate (Hartman and Nakane, 1981). The former has the advantage that it leaves the substrate transparent for light microscopic examination; the latter, while being slightly opaque (which does not significantly interfere with light microscopic examination), has the advantage of not interfering with the *in vitro* growth of cells. When mounted on carbon or indium coated substrates frozen sections of fixed tissue or sections of epon embedded tissues require no further grounding. In addition, several types of tissue culture cells, when grown on carbon coated slides or coverslips, are sufficiently grounded to allow SEM examination without further coating.

Thus far, we have examined frozen sections of fresh tissues, frozen sections of fixed tissues, sections of paraffin embedded tissues, sections of epon embedded tissues and preparations of whole cells. Frozen sections of fresh tissues have proven to be unsatisfactory thus far because of the lack of morphological preservation. Frozen sections of fixed tissue can be used although the information obtained from such sections is limited by the relatively poor morphological preservation generally obtained with these sections. To prepare frozen sections of fixed material for SEM, 4–8 μm sections are cut, picked up on carbon-coated slides, and immediately placed in phosphate buffered saline (PBS) (this keeps the collapse of the tissue due to air-drying to a minimum). Following immunohistochemical staining (see Appendix), the sections are reacted with 0·01% osmium tetroxide for 10–15 min at room temperature. (The amount of osmium reacted is much more critical in specimens prepared for SEM than for TEM specimens. If the tissue is overreacted with osmium, the osmium bound to the surrounding cellular components will mask the specific staining making it undetectable. This is especially true for sections over 6 μm in thickness or preparations of whole cells.) After post-fixation in osmium the sections are washed in distilled water, dehydrated in two 10-min changes of acidified 2, 2-dimethoxypropane (Maser and Trimble, 1977), and critical point dried from liquid carbon dioxide.

Paraffin embedded tissue, as has been previously shown by Diehiana *et al.* (1980), can provide excellent morphological preservation provided the specimen has been carefully fixed and embedded. Two to 10 μm thick sections of paraffin embedded material are cut and mounted on carbon coated slides. After the paraffin sections have been allowed to thoroughly dry onto the carbon-coated slides, the paraffin is removed from the section by soaking the slides in toluene, the tissue sections are hydrated in a graded series of ethanols and placed in PBS. These sections are then handled identically to frozen sections of fixed tissues as described above.

Epon embedded material is prepared according to the procedures established for immunohistochemical localization of antigens with TEM (Mazurkiewicz and Nakane, 1972) (see Appendix). One-half to 5 μm thick sections (generally 0·5–1·0 μm prove optimal) are cut using a glass knife, mounted on carbon coated slides and examined by BSI. There are two general methods in which whole cells can be prepared for immunohistochemical localization of antigen with SEM. The first is to start with a suspension of cells. Following fixation the cells are spun onto polylysine-coated slides using a cytocentrifuge (care must be taken not to allow the cells to dry during centrifugation). After washing, the cells are stained immunohistochemically in the same manner as tissue sections. The stained cells are reacted with 0·01% osmium tetroxide for 5–15 min, dehydrated in two 10-min changes of 2,2-dimethoxypropane, and critical point dried from liquid carbon dioxide. Cells prepared in this manner must then be coated with carbon to render them electrically conductive before they can be examined by SEM.

The second approach for the examination of whole cells can be taken with cells which grow as monolayers *in vitro*, or tightly adhere to the surface of the culture cvessel when placed *in vitro* for a short period of time. Cells which behave in this manner can be simply grown on carbon-coated slides (or coverslips), fixed, washed and stained as described above. In this case, following critical point drying, cells which spread and tightly adhere to the substrate (i.e. fibroblasts or endothelial cells) may be examined directly by SEM without further coating by carbon. Cells which adhere less strongly to the substrate and are more rounded (i.e. parietal yolk sac cells, and embryonal carcinoma cells) often require a light coating of carbon to render them sufficiently grounded for SEM examination.

To date, we have not, nor to our knowledge has anyone else, examined the immunohistochemical localization of antigens using the peroxidase-labeled antibody method on tissue fragments using SEM. This type of localization should be possible provided the specific staining is not obscured by the osmium bound to the underlying tissue and cells.

VI. SUMMARY

The methods outlined above provide the means of combining the peroxidase-labeled antibody method with SEM for the localization of intracellular antigens. In combining these two techniques, one takes advantage of the specificity of antigen-antibody interactions of immunohistochemistry and large sample area, speed and ease of specimen preparation of SEM to provide a simple method for obtaining ultrastructural information which has been heretofore achieved only with great difficulty. This methodology provides one with the means of directly comparing the intracellular localization of antigen with the cell surface topography. The use of SEM for localization of intracellular antigens is still in its infancy, and as such it shows much potential.

However, as often the case, there are several obstacles which must be overcome before the full potential can be realized. At present, with currently available instrumentation, the resolution which can be achieved is in the range of 50–200 nm. The resolution of the backscatter imaging will, in all probability, never achieve that obtainable with TEM, however, as instrumentation improves, one can expect the resolution to increase perhaps to the 10 nm range in the near future. Perhaps the biggest obstacle to be overcome is the reaction of surrounding tissue components with osmium which often obscures the staining. There are two ways in which this obstacle may be overcome. First, one could develop a substrate for peroxidase which contains a heavy metal and thereby eliminate the necessity to react the specimen with osmium altogether. Second, one could develop a means of blocking the reaction of the surrounding tissue components with osmium, thereby leaving only the DAB reaction product to react with the osmium. As the improvements of instrumentation and staining technology are made, the burden of bringing to fruition the full potential of the methodology will fall upon those of us who apply it.

VII. ACKNOWLEDGEMENTS

This work was supported in part by NIH grants AI-09109 and CA-15823 and by a gift from R. J. Reynolds Industries, Inc.

VIII. REFERENCES

Ardenne, H. von (1938). *Z. Tech. Phys.* **19**, 407–416.
Becker, R. P. and DeBruyn, P. P. H. (1976). *In* "Proceeding of the Ninth Annual SEM Symposium (O. Jahari, ed.), Vol. V. pp. 171–178. IITRI, Chicago.
Becker, R. P. and Sogard, M. (1979). *In* "Proceeding of the Twelfth Annual SEM Symposium" (O. Johari, ed.), Vol. II. pp. 835–870. IITRI, Chicago.
Bohn, W. (1978). *J. Histochem. Cytochem.* **26**, 293–297.
Coons, A. H. (1958). *In* "General Cytoplasmic Methods" (J. F. Danielli, ed.), pp. 399–422. Academic Press, New York.
Dichiara, J. F., Rowley, P. P. and Ogilvie, R. W. (1980). *In* "Proceeding of the Thirteenth Annual SEM Symposium (O. Johari, ed.), Vol. III. pp. 181–188. IITRI, Chicago.
Goodman, S. L., Hodges, G. M., Trejdosiewicz, L. K. and Livingston, D. C. (1979). *In* "Proceeding of the Twelfth Annual SEM Symposium" (O. Johari, ed.), Vol. III. pp. 619–628. IITRI, Chicago.
Graham, R. C., Jr and Karnovsky, M. J. (1966). *J. Histochem. Cytochem.* **14**, 291–302.
Grey, H. M. and Kunkel, H. G. (1964). *J. Exp. Med.* **120**, 253–266.

Hämmerling, U., Polliack, A., Lampen, N., Sabety, M. and de Harven, E. (1975). *J. Exp. Med.* **141**, 518–523.

Hartman, A. L. and Nakane, P. K. (1981). *In* "Proceeding of the Fourteenth Annual SEM Symposium" (O. Johari, ed.), Vol. II. pp. 33–44. IITRI, Chicago.

Hattori, A., Matsukura, Y., Ito, S., Fugita, T. and Tokunaga, J. (1976). *Arch. Hist. Jap.* **39**, 105–115.

Knoll, M. (1935). *Z. Tech. Phys.* **16**, 467–475.

Maser, H. D. and Trimble, M. D. III (1977). *J. Histochem. Cytochem.* **25**, 247–251.

Mazurkiewicz, J. E. and Nakane, P. K. (1972). *J. Hystochem. Cytochem.* **20**, 969–974.

McLean, I. W. and Nakane, P. K. (1974). *J. Histochem. Cytochem* **22**, 1077–1083.

Miller, M. M. and Teplitz, R. L. (1978). *In* "Proceeding of the Eleventh Annual SEM Symposium" (O. Johari, ed.), Vol. II. pp. 893–898. IITRI, Chicago.

Molday, R. S., Dreyer, W. J., Rembaum, A. and Yen, S. P. S. (1975). *J. Cell Biol.* **64**, 75–88.

Nakane, P. K. (1975). *Ann. N. Y. Acad. Sci.* **254**, 203–211.

Nakane, P. K. and Pierce, G. B. (1966). *J. Histochem. Cytochem.* **14**, 929–931.

Ogura, K. and Laudate, A. (1980). *In* "Proceeding of the Thirteenth Annual SEM Symposium" (O. Johari, ed.), Vol. I. pp. 233–238. IITRI, Chicago.

Peters, K.-R. Gschwender, H. H., Haller, W. and Rutter, G. (1976). *In* "Proceeding of the Ninth Annual SEM Symposium" (O. Johari, ed.), Vol. II. pp. 75–83. IITRI, Chicago.

Pickel, V. M., Joh, T. H. and Reis, O. J. (1975). *Proc. Natn. Acad. Sci. USA* **72**, 659–663.

Reimer, L. (1979). *In* "Proceeding of the Twelfth Annual SEM Symposium" (O. Johari, ed.), Vol. II. pp. 111–124. IITRI, Chicago.

Soligo, D. and de Harven, E. (1981). *J. Histochem. Cytochem.* **29**, 1071–1079.

Spicer, S. S., Phifer, R. F., Garvin, A. J. and Zehr, D. (1976). *In* "First International Symposium on Immunoenzymatic Techniques INSERM Symposium" (G. Feldman, P. Druet, J. Bignon and S. Avrameas, eds.), pp. 59–70. North-Holland Publishing Co., Amsterdam.

Stefanini, M., DeMartino, C. and Zamboni, L. (1967). *Nature* **216**, 173–174.

Sternberger, L. A., Hardy, P. H., Jr, Cuculis, J. J. and Meyer, H. G. (1970). *J. Histochem. Cytochem.* **18**, 315–333.

Willingham, H. C. and Yamada, S. S. (1979). *J. Histochem. Cytochem.* **7**, 947–960.

Yokota, S. and Fahimi, H. D. (1981). *Proc. Natn. Acad. Sci. USA* **78**, 4970–4974.

IX. APPENDICES

A. Preparation of Fab' Fragments by Pepsin Digestion of Rabbit IgG

1. Prepare sodium acetate buffer by adding 5·8 ml of concentrated acetic acid to 800 ml of distilled water and titrating to pH 4·0 with sodium hydroxide. Following titration bring volume to 1000 ml with distilled water.
2. Dissolve IgG in the above buffer at a final concentration of 8 mg/ml. (When not starting with a lyophilized preparation of IgG, this can be accomplished either by passing the IgG over a desalting column or dialyzing it against acetate buffer overnight.)

3. Place the IgG (8 mg/ml in acetate buffer) in a 37 °C water bath and add pepsin to a final concentration of 0·3 mg/ml*. Allow the digestion to proceed for 16 h at 37 °C.
4. Dialyze the digest (including the precipitate) against several changes of 0·3 M Tris-HCl buffer, pH 8·2, for a minimum of 6 h.
5. Add 7 μl of 2-mercaptoethanol (diluted 1:10 in Tris-HCl, pH 8·2) per 8 mg of starting IgG and mix at room temperature for 1 h.
6. Add 1·85 mg of iodoacetic acid per 8 mg of starting IgG, mix until dissolved and let stand at 4 °C for 16 h.
7. Dialyze against 0·01 M sodium phosphate, 0·15 M sodium chloride, pH 7·2 (PBS).
8. Chromatograph on a 2·5 × 30 cm Sephacryl S-200 column (or equivalent) equilibrated with PBS. Run column at a flow rate of 40 ml/h and collect 2 ml fractions.
9. Read the OD_{280} of the fractions and pool the 40 000 MW peak.

B. Conjugation of IgG or Fab' Fragments to Horseradish Peroxidase

1. Dialyze 1 ml of IgG (10 mg/ml) or Fab' (5 mg/ml) for 24 h against several changes of 0·01 M sodium carbonate buffer, pH 9·5.
2. Dissolve 4 mg of Sigma Type VI horseradish peroxidase (RZ > 3)† in 1 ml of distilled water.
3. Add 50 μl of 0·18 M sodium m-periodate (freshly prepared in distilled water) and stir for 20 min at room temperature.
4. Chromatograph the activated peroxidase on a Pharmacia PD-10 column equilibrated wtih 0·001 M sodium acetate buffer, pH 4·0, and collect the peroxidase eluate (reddish brown in color).
5. Add the IgG (10 mg in 1 ml) or Fab' (5 mg/ml) to the activated peroxidase and *immediately* titrate to pH 9·5 with 0·02 M sodium hydroxide. Stir at room temperature for 2 h.
6. Add 100 μl of 0·1 M sodium borohydride (in distilled water) to the mixture and place at 4 °C for 2 h.
7. Dialyze overnight against several changes of PBS.
8. Chromatograph on a 2·5×30 cm Sephacryl S-200 column (or equivalent) equilibrated with PBS at a flow rate of 40 ml/h and collect 2 ml fractions.
9. Read the OD_{280} and OD_{403} of each fraction and pool the 200 000 MW peak if using IgG and the 90 000 MW peak if using Fab'.
10. Add bovine serum albumin to the pooled fractions to a final concentration of 10 mg/ml, aliquot and store frozen.

---

* For species other than rabbit, we currently use the following IgG and pepsin concentrations: rat, 12 mg/ml IgG, 18 mg/ml pepsin; goat, 5 mg/ml IgG, 0·3 mg/ml pepsin; hamster, 5 mg/ml IgG, 0·3 mg/ml pepsin; sheep, 8 mg/ml IgG, 0·8 mg/ml pepsin; human, 8 mg/ml IgG, 0·3 mg/ml pepsin; guinea pig, 8 mg/ml IgG, 0·3 mg/ml pepsin.

† RZ = the ratio of the OD_{403} to the OD_{280} which reflects the amount heme to non-heme protein present. If the RZ value of the peroxidase is < 3, the peroxidase must be chromatographed before using.

C. Direct and Indirect Immunohistochemical Staining of Tissue Sections and Whole Cells for SEM*

1. Prepare a moist chamber (e.g. glass baking dishes lined with moist paper towels secured by tape inverted on a moist paper surface).
2. Wipe off excess PBS from around the tissue with cotton gauze. Using a capillary pipette, apply approximately 20 μl of antibody solution.
3. Thoroughly mix the antibody solution with the residual PBS which remains over the tissue, being careful not to scratch the tissue. place the slide in the moist chamber for 3–24 h—care should be taken to be sure the chamber remains wet and the tissue does not dry.
4. Rinse the antibody off the slides with PBS and wash in PBS: 3 times 10 min. (If using the indirect staining method, repeat steps 2 through 4, applying the peroxidase conjugated anti-antibody.)
5. Incubate the slide in 2% glutaraldehyde in PBS for 30 min.
6. Wash in PBS: 3×10 min.
7. Incubate in $6 \cdot 6 \times 10^{-5}$ M diaminobenzidine (DAB), $0 \cdot 05$ M Tris-HCl, pH $7 \cdot 6$, for 30 min.
8. Incubate in the above DAB solution containing $0 \cdot 005\%$ H_2O_2 for 10 min.
9. Wash in PBS: 3×10 min.
10. Incubate the tissue in $0 \cdot 01\%$ osmium tetroxide, $0 \cdot 1$ M sodium phosphate buffer, pH $7 \cdot 2$, for 5–15 min.
11. Wash in distilled water: 3×10 min.
12. Dehydrate in two changes of acidified 2,2-dimethoxypropane: 10 min each.
13. Critical point dry.
14. Coat with carbon if necessary.

D. Immunohistochemical Staining of Tissue for SEM Examination Following Epon Embedding

1. Six to twelve μM-thick frozen sections of fixed tissue well washed in PBS containing 10% sucrose (PBS-S) are cut, placed on albumin-coated slides, and allowed to dry.
2. Wash in PBS-S: 3×10 min.
3. Make a moist chamber. (e.g. glass baking dishes lined with moist paper towels secured by tape inverted on a moist paper surface.)
4. Wipe excess PBS-S from around the section with gauze. With a capillary pipette, apply approximately 20 μl of antibody solution (this technique is a direct technique using peroxidase-labeled immunoglobulin fragments; if an indirect technique is used, repeat steps 4 through 6 when applying the conjugated antibody which is directed against the first antibody to the section).
5. Mix the antibody solution thoroughly with the residual PBS-S which is still over the tissue, being careful not to scratch the section. Place in the moist chamber for 3 to 24 h. Keep the chamber moist and do not let the section dry.
6. Rinse conjugate off the slides with PBS-S. Wash in PBS-S: 3×10 min.
7. Incubate in a solution of 2% glutaraldehyde in PBS-S for 30 min.

---

* This protocol can be used for frozen sections of fixed tissue, paraffin sections or whole cells.

8. Wash in PBS-S: 3×10 min.
9. Incubate in 6·6×10^{-5} M diaminobenzidene (DAB), 0·05 M Tris-HCl, pH 7·6, solution containing 10% sucrose for 30 min.
10. Incubate in the above DAB solution containing 0·005% H$_2$O$_2$ for 2 to 8 min.
11. Wash in PBS-S: 3×10 min. At this point, the slides may be briefly examined for staining under a light microscope, taking care not to let tissue dry out.
12. Incubate in 2% OsO$_4$–0·1 M sodium phosphate buffer, pH 7·2 for 1 to 2 h.
13. Wash in PBS-S: 3×10 min.
14. Dehydrate in graded ethanols (10 min each) to 100%.
15. Embed by inverting a gelatin capsule of fresh epon-araldite over each section.
16. Polymerize the epon by incubating at 37 °C overnight and at 60 °C for 48 h. The epon block containing the tissue section can then be removed from the slide by briefly heating the slide over a bunsen burner flame and snapping off the capsule.
17. Cut 0·5–2 μm thick sections using a glass knife, mount on carbon or indium-coated slides and examine by SEM using BSI.

Labeling of Cell Surface Antigens for SEM

R. S. MOLDAY

I. INTRODUCTION

Immunomicroscopic labeling techniques have proved to be an extremely valuable means of studying the properties of specific types of cells and their

IMMUNOCYTOCHEMISTRY 2
ISBN 0 12 140402 1

surface membranes. Immunofluorescence microscopy using antibodies tagged with fluorescent dyes (Coon and Kaplan, 1950) and immunotransmission electron microscopy using antibodies conjugated to electron dense complexes (Singer, 1959) have enabled cell biologists and membrane biochemists to detect cellular antigens and study their distribution, dynamic properties and relationship to cellular ultrastructure. Related labeling techniques using lectins as cell surface specific ligands have also proven valuable for localizing specific carbohydrate-containing components, principally glycoproteins, on cell surface membranes.

More recently, immunolabeling techniques have been developed for scanning electron microscopy. Since the first report by Lo Buglio *et al.* (1972) on the use of large polystyrene latex spheres as immunological markers for SEM, a wide variety of markers, modes of detection and labeling procedures have been developed for analysis of antigens and receptors on cell surfaces by SEM (Molday, 1977; Brown and Revel, 1978; Molday and Maher, 1980). In this chapter the preparation and properties of immunological markers and labeling techniques which have been widely used to detect and localize cell surface antigens and receptors by SEM are described. Additional information on electron microscopic markers and labeling techniques can be obtained in this series (Hartman and Nakane; Roth, this volume) and in recent reviews (Brown and Revel, 1978; De Petris, 1978; Horisberger, 1981; Molday 1977; 1981; Sternberger, 1979).

II. CELL SURFACE MARKERS FOR SEM

A. General Properties

Most markers are large macromolecular complexes which can be resolved under the scanning electron microscope with the conventional secondary electron mode of detection. Identification of these markers on cell surfaces is based on their characteristic size and shape. Macromolecular markers which have been used for SEM (Molday and Maher, 1980) range in size from 12 nm in the case of ferritin to over 500 nm for various polymeric latex spheres. Although most markers are essentially spherical in shape, some markers, in particular, bacteriophages and viruses, have more complex morphologies which further aid their recognition on irregular cell surfaces (Kumon, 1976).

Small markers less than 30 nm in size are particularly useful for high resolution mapping of labeled antigens and receptors on cell surfaces. Markers of this size are also required when the accessibility of antigens or receptors on cell surfaces is restricted due to steric hindrance (Horisberger *et al.*, 1978). Small markers, however, are sometimes difficult to resolve and identify clearly on complex, irregular cell surfaces or on cells which have a thick (10–20 nm) heavy metal coating. Macromolecular complexes in the size range of 30–50 nm are easily recognized on most cells and have been most widely used to study the distribution of antigens and receptors on cell surfaces by SEM (Molday, 1977). Large markers over 100 nm in size are suitable for the detection of surface antigens in mixed cell populations (De Harven *et al.*, 1979; Kumon, 1981). Such markers can be readily seen at low magnification, and therefore, large areas of a specimen can be efficiently surveyed under the SEM. Morphological features on cell surfaces are often masked by markers of this size (Gamliel *et al.*, 1981) and therefore, they have limited use in correlating the distribution of antigens with cell surface topography.

Properties other than size and shape have also been utilized to detect labeled antigens and receptors on cell surfaces by SEM. Markers having a high content of heavy metal such as iron or gold have been detected and localized on cell surfaces using X-ray microanalysis with SEM (Molday, 1981; Hoyer *et al.*, 1979). Certain dyes such as fluorescein have been detected as a result of both a high emission of secondary electrons and generation of cathodoluminescent signals (Springer *et al.*, 1974; Soni *et al.*, 1975; Cavellier *et al.*, 1978). Silver granules obtained with autoradiographic procedures have also been used to localize cell surface receptors labeled with tritiated lectins (Suzuki *et al.*, 1979). Backscattered electron imaging has recently been used to visualize fibronectin antigens using immunogold markers (Trejdosiewicz *et al.*, 1981).

In addition to characteristics required for detection, SEM markers must also exhibit properties required for specific labeling of cell surface antigens and receptors. An important parameter is the extent of nonspecific binding of markers to cell surfaces. Ideally, the markers should not bind to cells except through the specific antibodies or ligands. In practice, however, there is usually some nonspecific binding of the markers to cells, the extent of which will depend on the surface characteristics, i.e. charge, polarity, molecular groups, etc. of both the markers and the cells. Conditions used in labeling, i.e. temperature, concentration, type of buffers, time, etc. may also affect the level of nonspecific binding. In general, successful labeling requires that nonspecific binding of the marker or immunomarker conjugate to cells as measured control experiments should be at least an order of magnitude less than that observed in actual test experiments.

Markers must be capable of interacting strongly with antibodies or other ligands. This interaction most often involves covalent bond formation between antibodies and markers. This is accomplished by crosslinking functional groups, such as amino, carboxyl, hydroxyl or aldehyde groups on the surface of markers to the ϵ-amino groups of lysine residues on antibodies or other ligands under mild chemical reaction conditions. In the case of markers which are devoid of surface functional groups, non-covalent hydrophobic and electrostatic forces have been used to form antibody marker conjugates for labeling. In some procedures described in a later section, specific high-affinity binding, i.e. antibody-antigen binding has been used to indirectly label surface antigens.

The stability of markers is also an important consideration. Markers which are aggregated prior to or during labeling: (1) are less readily recognized on cell surfaces; (2) obscure cell surface features, and (3) generally result in a higher degree of nonspecific binding. Likewise, markers which are easily fragmented may be difficult to identify on cell surfaces due to alterations in their characteristic size and shape. The stability of markers during preparation of labeled cells for SEM has not generally been a problem however since fixation of cells with glutaraldehyde also stabilizes the structure of most markers.

B. Specific SEM Markers

A wide variety of biological macromolecular complexes and synthetic polymeric particles have been developed as cell surface markers for SEM (Molday and Maher, 1980). These are listed in Table I. The properties and methods of preparation of the most commonly used markers are described below.

1. Hemocyanin

Hemocyanin is a glycoprotein complex having a cylindrical shape with a diameter of approximately 35 nm and a length of 50 nm. It was initially introduced by Smith and Revel (1972) as a TEM marker for use with replica techniques, but since this time, it has also proved to be a valuable marker for SEM (Weller, 1974; Brown and Revel, 1976). The dimensions of hemocyanin are such that it can be readily resolved under conventional scanning electron microscopes, yet small enough that it does not obscure cell surface features. Its distinctive cylindrical shape aids in the identification of this marker on complex cell surfaces. Functional amino groups of lysine residues can be reacted covalently with glutaraldehyde for conjugation to antibodies (Ostrand-Rosenberg et al., 1979; Geltosky et al., 1980), Staphylococcus aureus protein A (Miller et al., 1981) and lectins (Brown and Revel, 1976). Furthermore, since hemocyanin is glycoprotein which binds concanavalin A, it can be used to label Con A-treated cells for visualization of Con A receptors on cell surfaces (Smith and Revel, 1972; Weller, 1974).

Although most labeling studies have employed hemocyanin isolated from

TABLE I
Visual markers for SEM.

Marker	Shape/size (nm)	Conjugate formation	Principal mode of detection used	References
Hemocyanin	Cylindrical 35 (diameter) × 50 (length)	Covalent via —NH$_2$ groups	SEM — secondary electrons TEM — replica methods	Weller, 1974; Ostrand-Rosenberg et al., 1979
Copolymer microspheres	Spherical 30–340 ,	Covalent via —NH$_2$, —COOH or —OH	SEM — secondary electrons; fluorescent microscopy	Molday et al., 1975; 1976
Polystyrene latex spheres	Spherical 200–1000	Hydrophobic	SEM — secondary electrons	Lo Buglio et al., 1972; Linthicum and Sell, 1975
Gold particles	Spherical or oblong 5–150	Electrostatic	SEM — secondary electrons, backscatter electrons or X-ray TEM — thin sections	Horisberger et al., 1975; 1976; Hoyer et al., 1979; Trejdosiewicz et al., 1981
Silica spheres	Spherical 7–25	Covalent via —NH$_2$ groups	SEM — secondary electrons TEM — replica methods	Peters et al., 1976; 1978
Ferritin	Spherical 12–15	Covalent via —NH$_2$	SEM — secondary electrons TEM — thin sections	Tokunaga et al., 1976
Viruses				
Tobacco mosaic virus	Rod 15×300	Covalent via —NH$_2$	SEM — secondary electrons TEM — thin sections	Hammerling et al., 1975 Nemanic et al., 1975
Bushy stunt virus	Spherical 30	Covalent via —NH$_2$		
Bacteriophage T-4	220 head-tail 85×115 hexagonal head	Covalent via —NH$_2$	SEM — secondary electrons	Kumon, 1976; 1981
Iron copolymer microspheres	Spherical 30–50	Covalent via —NH$_2$	SEM — secondary electrons and X-ray	Molday et al., 1977
Iron dextran microspheres	Spherical 20–40	Covalent via —C$\overset{\text{O}}{=}$ or —NH$_2$	SEM — secondary electrons TEM — thin sections	Molday and MacKenzie, 1982; Baccetti and Burrini, 1977
Peroxidase reaction product	Irregular particles or crystals	Covalent —C$\overset{\text{O}}{=}$ or —NH$_2$	SEM — secondary electrons TEM — thin sections	Bretton et al., 1973; McKeever et al., 1977
Fluorescein		Covalent via —N=C=S	SEM — brightness by secondary electrons or cathodoluminescence Fluorescent microscopy	Springer et al., 1974; Cavellier et al., 1978
^{3}H-(autoradiography)	Irregular silver deposits 200–300	Covalent	SEM — secondary electrons or X-ray TEM — autoradiography	Suzuki et al., 1979

the hemolymph of the marine whelk, *Busycon canaliculatum* (Woods Hole Marine Biological Laboratories, Woods Hole, MA), hemocyanin from other sources including the snail *Levantina hierosalina* and the keyhole limpet, *Megathura crenulata* (Pacific Biomarine Supply Co., Venice, CA) have also served as SEM markers (Ben-Shaul *et al.*, 1977; Carter, 1978).

(a) Procedure for purifying B. canaliculatum hemocyanin (Brown and Revel, 1976)

The hemolymph fluid of the whelk is collected after the shell is cracked and an incision is made through the foot and into the cardiac region. Large particles are removed by centrifuging the fluid at low speed (2000–15 000 g for 10 min). The supernatant is then spun at 57 000 g for 30 min in a Beckman Ti 40 rotor. The blue layer near the bottom of the tube containing the hemocyanin is retained and the pellet consisting of aggregated material is discarded. Residual aggregated hemocyanin can be removed by chromatography on Sepharose 2B or by filtration through a 0·45 μM Millipore filter.

Hemocyanin is stored at 4 °C in phosphate buffered saline (PBS) under sterile conditions or in the presence of 20 mM NaN$_3$ to prevent bacterial contamination. The concentration of hemocyanin in mg/ml can be determined from the absorbance at 280 nm using an extinction coefficient $E_{280\,nm}^{1mg\,ml}$ of 1·51 (Miller *et al.*, 1981).

Hemocyanin is now available commercially as a sterile solution (Polyscience Inc., Warrington, PA) for use as an electron microscopic marker. Lyophilized preparations, however, can not be used since such treatment causes dissociation of this protein complex into small subunits.

2. Functional Copolymer Microspheres

Polymeric microspheres in various sizes and compositions have been developed as SEM markers (Rembaum *et al.*, 1979). Copolymer methacrylate microspheres consisting of 53% (w/w) methyl methacrylate, 30% hydroxyethyl methacrylate, 10% methacrylic acid and 7% ethylene glycol dimethacrylate have been particularly useful (Molday *et al.*, 1975). These microspheres can be easily synthesized in uniform sizes between 30 and 340 nm in diameter. Hydroxyl and carboxyl groups provide a hydrophilic, negative surface charge which prevents aggregation of the spheres in physiological buffer above pH 6 and limits nonspecific binding to most types of cells. Alkyl diamines, such as 1,7 diaminoheptane, can be chemically coupled either to the hydroxyl groups by the cyanogen bromide procedure or to carboxyl groups by the carbodiimide reaction (Molday, 1976). Free amino groups on these derivatized spheres, in turn, can be conjugated to proteins, fluorescent dyes or other reagents.

Copolymer microspheres have a number of advantages for use in immunological cell labeling studies for SEM. They can be easily synthesized by emulsion polymerization in large quantities and stored indefinitely in aqueous solution containing 20 mM NaN_3. When these microspheres are tagged with fluorescent dyes such as fluorescein isothiocyanate or tetramethyl rhodamine isothiocyanate, they can be used as markers for fluorescent microscopy as well as SEM (Maher and Molday, 1979). Microspheres of different sizes can be used to visualize the distribution of different receptors on the same cell (Molday et al., 1976; Molday, 1981) or on different cell types by SEM. Labeling of antigenic sites on neuroblastoma cells with functional copolymeric immunomicrospheres is illustrated in Fig. 1.

The chemical composition of these markers, however, limit their application as general markers for electron microscopy. Since the electron density of methacrylate microspheres is similar to that of most embedding resins they are not visible under the TEM in thin sections. The high negative surface charge from the methacrylic acid and the partial hydrophobic property arising from methyl methacrylate can result in some nonspecific binding to certain types of cells and extracellular matrices in tissues samples.

(a) A simplified procedure for the synthesis of microspheres (approximate diameter 50 nm)

Methacrylate monomers obtained from either Rohm and Haas Co. (Philadelphia, PA) or Polysciences Inc. (Warrington, PA) can be either used directly in the synthesis of the microspheres or first purified by vacuum distillation (Molday et al., 1975). A 5% (w/w) aqueous solution of monomer is prepared by adding 2·65 g methyl methacrylate, 1·50 g hydroxyethyl methacrylate, 0·50 g methacrylic acid, 0·35 g ethylene glycol dimethacrylate, 0·1 g sodium dodecyl sulfate and 0·01 g ammonium persulfate to 95 ml of distilled water in a 250 ml Erlemmeyer flask. The solution is heated to 95 °C with stirring in a water bath for 30–60 min. The opalescent solution which forms is then cooled and filtered through a Whatman No. 1 filter. Residual monomer and sodium dodecyl sulfate is then removed by passing the solution through a 3·5 × 20 cm mixed-bed ion exchange column consisting of equal quantities of Biorad AG 1 × 10 and AG 50W12 (500–100 mesh) resins (Biorad Lab., Richmond, CA) which have been previously washed sequentially with 1N HCl, 1N NaOH and finally distilled water.

The size of these microspheres can be altered by varying the concentration of total monomer in the reaction mixture. A linear relationship between the total monomer concentration and the size of the microspheres as measured by SEM has been observed (Molday et al., 1975; Molday, 1976).

For preparation of immunomicrosphere conjugates, carboxyl groups on these microspheres are derivatized with 1,7 diaminoheptane by the carbo-

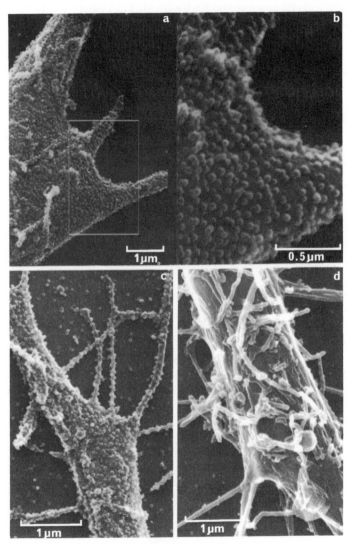

FIG. 1. Scanning electron micrographs of mouse neuroblastoma cells indirectly labeled for surface antigens with copolymeric microspheres (50 nm diameter). Cells on glass coverslips were first treated with rabbit antiserum specific for neuroblastoma cell surface antigens, then washed in PBS and finally labeled with goat antirabbit Ig-microsphere conjugates. A dense uniform distribution of microspheres can be seen on the cell surface (a, b) and on the neurite extensions (c). Control in which the specific rabbit serum is omitted is shown in (d).

diimide procedure (Molday, 1976). A solution of 10 ml microspheres (10–20 mg/ml as determined by dry weight analysis) containing 0·02 M diaminoheptane and 0·05 M N-2-hydroxyethylpiperazine N'-2-ethane sulfonic acid (HEPES) is adjusted to pH 7 and cooled to 4 °C. Fifty mg of 1 ethyl-3-(3 dimethyl aminopropyl) carbodiimide is added and the reaction mixture is stirred for 2 h at 4 °C. The diaminoheptane derivatized microspheres are then extensively dialyzed first against 1 l of 0·1 M NaCl and finally against two changes of 0·01 M sodium phosphate buffer at pH 7 in order to remove excess diaminoheptane. These diaminoheptane-derivatized microspheres can be stored indefinitely at 4 °C in the presence of 20 mM NaN_3 until needed for preparation of antibody-microsphere conjugates.

3. Hydrophobic Latex Spheres

Latex spheres widely used in immunoagglutination assays have also been used as immunological SEM markers. Monodispersed 230 nm diameter polystyrene latex spheres available under the trade name Lytron 612 from Monsanto Corp. (Cincinnati, Ohio) were first used by Lo Buglio *et al.* (1972). Commercial polymethyl methacrylate latex spheres have also been used by Fuchs and Bächi (1975) as immuno-markers for SEM. Both types of spheres lack functional groups on their surface. As a result, antibodies and other surface specific ligands must be adsorbed to the surface of these spheres through noncovalent forces. These weak interactions can result in some dissociation of antibodies during labeling. Furthermore, the hydrophobic surfaces of these spheres can cause aggregation of these markers and some nonspecific binding to cells. These properties have limited the use of polystyrene and polymethyl methacrylate spheres in immunological labeling studies for SEM.

4. Colloidal Gold Particles

Colloidal gold particles, originally developed as electron dense markers for TEM (Faulk and Taylor, 1971), were first employed as SEM markers by Horisberger *et al.* (1975). These particles are easily prepared in a wide range of sizes from 5 nm to over 160 nm by reduction of chloroauric acid (Frens, 1973; Horisberger, 1979). The smallest particles are essentially spherical in shape, whereas the larger particles are oblong in appearance (Goodman *et al.*, 1981).

   Gold particles have many properties which make them versatile microscopic markers. The high emission of secondary electrons from gold enables these markers to be seen under the SEM on cells which have not been coated with heavy metals (Horisberger and Rosset, 1977a). Gold markers can also be detected on cell surfaces by backscatter electron imaging (Trejdo-siewicz *et al.*, 1981) and by X-ray microanalysis (Hoyer *et al.*, 1979). Since gold particles are excellent visual markers for TEM because of their high electron density, they can be used in combined TEM-SEM studies (Horisberger *et al.*, 1978) in which the surface distribution of antigenic sites is correlated with intracellular ultrastructure. Gold particles of different sizes can be used in multiple labeling studies to map the distribution of different components on cell surfaces (Horisberger and Rosset, 1977a; Horisberger and Vonlanthen, 1979). A disadvantage of gold particles over most other markers is their lack of functional surface groups. As a result, proteins must be adsorbed to their surface through noncovalent forces. Not all proteins form stable conjugates with gold and the number of protein molecules bound per gold particle can not be regulated (Goodman *et al.*, 1981).

For SEM studies gold particles in the size range of 30–75 nm in diameter are generally prepared by reduction of cholorauric acid with sodium citrate as described by Frens (1973) and modified by Horisberger (1979).According to their procedure gold particles having a diameter of 32 nm are prepared by adding 3·0 ml of 1% sodium citrate and 0·5 ml of 4% $HAuCl_4$ to 200 ml of boiling distilled water in an Erlenmeyer flask. The reaction mixture is maintained at 100 °C for 30 min with continuous stirring to allow complete reduction of the gold. In this reaction it is essential to use thoroughly clean glassware since impurities can affect the formation of mono-dispersed particles. The size of the particles can be increased by reducing the amount of sodium citrate (Frens, 1973). For example, gold markers having an average diameter of 50 nm can be prepared by the procedure described above if the amount of sodium citrate is reduced to 2·0 ml (Horisberger, 1979).

The size of the gold markers can be estimated from wavelength of the absorption maximum between 520–550 nm (Goodman *et al.*, 1981). More accurate determinations, however, are generally made by electron micro-scopic measurements. Additional information on the preparation of gold particles and their properties are discussed by Roth in this volume and in several recent reviews (Horisberger, 1979; 1981; Goodman *et al.*, 1980).

The application of gold particles as SEM markers is illustrated in Fig. 2 for labeling of antigenic sites on mouse fibroblasts.

5. *Colloidal Silica Spheres*

Colloidal silica spheres were introduced as SEM and TEM markers by Peters *et al.* (1976; 1978). These markers can be obtained from E.I. du Pont de Nemours and Co. Inc. (Willmington, DE) in several sizes under the trade

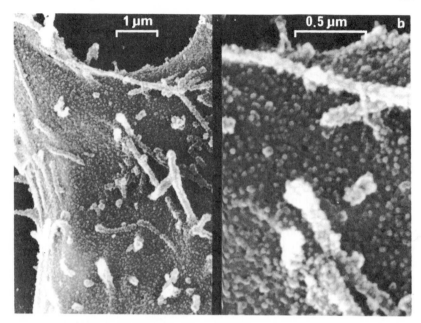

FIG. 2. Scanning electron micrographs of prefixed cells indirectly labeled with gold particles (diameter 32 nm). Mouse fibroblasts were labeled with rabbit antiserum specific for fibroblast cell surface antigens, then washed, and finally labeled with protein A-gold conjugates. Labeled cells were coated with gold-palladium layer prior to examination by SEM. Gold particles are seen to be distributed in a dense, uniform pattern in (a) and (b) at higher magnification.

names Ludox SM 30 (average diameter 7–8 nm), Ludox SM-40 (average diameter 13–14 nm) and Ludox TM (average diameter 22–25 nm). Unlike gold spheres, silica spheres contain functional groups in the form of negatively-charged silanol (Si—OH) groups. These groups can be derivatized with γ-aminopropyl triethoxysilane in order to introduce amino groups required for the preparation of immunoconjugates.

Although these markers appear to be useful for both SEM and TEM, only a few applications of silica spheres as specific cell surface markers have been reported to date (Peters et al., 1976; 1978).

6. Ferritin

Ferritin which has been extensively used as a TEM marker due to its electron dense iron core, can also serve as a useful SEM marker. Under the SEM, ferritin coated with a conductive heavy metal layer appears as particles 15–20 nm in diameter (Tokunaga et al., 1976). The actual size on cell surfaces, however, will vary with the thickness of the heavy metal coating used in the sample preparation. Although ferritin was initiall; seen with scanning electron microscopes having a field emission electron source (Tokunaga *et al.*, 1976; Ito *et al.*, 1978), it can also be seen on cell surfaces with SEM equipped with conventional electron sources. This is illustrated in Fig. 3 for the labeling for surface Thy antigens on rat thymocytes.

Ferritin from horse spleen is available as a highly purified, sterile solution from a number of biochemical suppliers (Sigma Chemical Co., Miles Biochemicals, Calbiochem-Behring Corp) for use in electron microscopy. As in the case of all biological macromolecular markers, ferritin should be stored at 4 °C since freezing and thawing can cause irreversible aggregation.

Ferritin is one of the smallest markers used in labeling studies for SEM. It is particularly useful in the precise localization of antigens on cell surfaces and in correlating this topographical distribution with the cell surface morphology and subcellular ultrastructure as viewed by TEM. Antigenic sites which may be sterically inaccessible to large markers, can often be labeled with ferritin and other markers of this size. The small size of ferritin, however, also has its limitations. Ferritin particles are often difficult to see on rough, irregular cell surfaces or on samples requiring a thick heavy-metal coating. Ferritin which is densely packed over the surface of a cell may appear as a fuzzy coating on the cell rather than distinct particles.

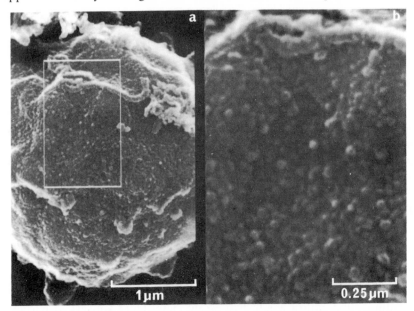

FIG. 3. Rat thymocytes labeled in suspension with a mouse monoclonal antibody against Thy surface antigen followed by goat anti-mouse Ig-ferritin conjugate. Ferritin appears densely packed over the cell surface.

7. Plant Viruses and Bacteriophage

Various plant viruses and bacteriophage with characteristic shapes have been used by several laboratories as morphological SEM markers for cell labeling. Tobacco mosaic virus (TMV) and bacteriophage T-4 have been particularly popular (Kumon et al., 1976; Nemanic et al., 1975; Hammerling et al., 1975). TMV is a long rod with dimensions of approximately 15 × 300 nm. On labeled cells, however, it may appear either straight, curled or bent due to its fragile nature. Some variations in length may also be observed due to fragmentation of this marker during purification or cell labeling procedures. TMV may sometimes resemble cell surface projections such as microvilli, making identification of this marker on certain cells difficult. TMV has been used with a variety of immunological labeling techniques including the indirect sandwich technique (Kumon, 1976), the hybrid antibody technique (Hammerling et al., 1975) and the hapten antibody technique (Nemanic et al., 1975).

TMV can be harvested from infected tobacco leaves and purified by differential and density-gradient centrifugation (Aoki et al., 1971). Kumon (1976) purified TMV for use as an SEM marker by centrifugation of the extract of infected tobacco leaves on a 10–50% sucrose gradient for 2 h at 50 000 g.

Plant viruses with other sizes and shapes can also serve as SEM markers. Small spherical viruses with an approximate diameter of 25–30 nm such as bushystunt virus and ϕX-174 have been developed as visual markers for SEM (Nemanic, 1975; Umeda et al., 1977).

Bacteriophage T-4 is a relatively large marker having an easily recognizable hexagonal head joined to a tail (Kumon et al., 1976; Kumon, 1981). This marker, like TMV, can be seen under the SEM at relatively low magnification. T-4 bacteriophage can be prepared according to the method of Kumon (1981) by inoculating host bacterium E. coli B with the phage. Bacterial lysate is centrifuged at low speed to remove the cell debris. The supernatant is then centrifuged at 11 000 g for 30–40 min. The pellet is resuspended in phosphate buffered saline and centrifugation is repeated to obtain pure T-4 phage.

8. Other SEM Markers

A variety of other markers developed for light and electron microscopy have been adapted for SEM. Fluorescein isothiocyanate routinely used as a visual probe for immunofluorescent labeling studies (De Petris, 1978) has been used in immunological labeling studies for SEM. The relatively high emission of secondary electrons and generation of cathodoluminescence have enabled detection of cell surface antigens labeled with fluorescein antibodies

(Springer *et al.*, 1974; Soni *et al.*, 1975; Cavellier *et al.*, 1978). Relatively low resolution and sensitivity, however, have limited the application of this marker in SEM cell labeling studies.

Autoradiographic techniques on cells labeled with ^{3}H-concanavalin A have been investigated by Suzuki *et al.* (1979). Labeled cells were coated with a photographic emulsion. After exposure and development, silver grains ranging in diameter of 0·2–0·3 μm could be observed over the ^{3}H-concanavalin A-labeled sites by SEM. X-ray analysis as well as backscatter electron imaging under the SEM can also be used to verify the existence of silver grains deposited on cells by such autoradiographic procedures (Hodges and Muir, 1974; 1976).

Horseradish peroxidase coupled with 3,3'-diaminobenzidine (DAB)-hydrogen peroxide reaction has also been used as a SEM marker for cell surface antigens and receptors. Bretton *et al.* (1973) observed small irregular particles on mouse fibroblasts which had been labeled with concanavalin A and horseradish peroxidase and subsequently reacted with DAB-H$_2$O$_2$. Under reaction conditions, used by McKeever and Spicer (1979), horseradish peroxidase-antibody complexes on macrophages yielded long crystals when the cells were treated with benzidine-containing substrates.

Iron-containing polymeric microspheres have also been used as SEM markers. Copolymer methacrylate microspheres containing a colloidal iron oxide core have been conjugated to antibodies and lectins (Molday *et al.*, 1977), as well as toxins (Kronick *et al.*, 1978) and used to label cells. The presence of these markers on cell surfaces has been detected using both secondary electrons and characteristic X-ray signals under the SEM (Kronick *et al.*, 1978; Molday, 1981). Iron dextrans have also been used to indirectly lozalize Con A receptors on rat spermatozoa by SEM (Baccetti and Burrini, 1977). Recently, our laboratory has prepared immuno-specific ferromagnetic iron dextran particles. These reagents have been used to detect antigens on red blood cells and thymocytes by both SEM and TEM (Molday and MacKenzie, 1982) and to separate labeled from unlabeled cells using magnetic fields. Commercial iron dextran particles sold under the trade names of Imferon and Imposil have recently been used by Dutton *et al.* (1979) as TEM markers. Such markers should also find future application as SEM markers.

III. PREPARATION OF IMMUNOMARKER CONJUGATES

A. Covalent Conjugation Methods

Immunomarker conjugates used in routine cell labeling methods are generally prepared by covalently bonding antibodies to markers under mild conditions which do not adversely affect the binding properties of the antibody nor cause aggregation of the markers. Glutaraldehyde has been most commonly used as a bifunctional reagent to couple amino groups of antibodies to amino group of such markers as diaminoheptane-derivatized copolymer microspheres (Molday *et al.*, 1975), ferritin (Neauport-Sautes and Silvestre, 1972; Kishida *et al.*, 1975), hemocyanin (Ostrand-Rosenberg) *et al.*, 1979), bacteriophage T-4 and viruses (Kumon, 1976), amino-derivatized silica spheres (Peters *et al.*, 1976) and horseradish peroxidase (Avrameas, 1969). Other ligands including *Staphylococcus* protein A, lectins, toxins and hormones have also been successfully coupled to these markers using glutaraldehyde.

The glutaraldehyde reaction can be carried out in one or two steps (Otto *et al.*, 1973) to produce stable reaction products. The primary products generated in these reactions are shown below.

One-Step reaction:

$$(1) \text{ Antibody-NH}_2 + \text{H}_2\text{N-marker} \xrightarrow[\substack{\text{0.05\% glutaraldehyde} \\ \text{PBS} \\ \text{1 h 25 °C}}]{} \begin{cases} \text{Antibody-NH} \sim \text{HN-Antibody} \\ \text{Antibody-NH} \sim \text{HN-Marker} \\ \text{Marker-NH} \sim \text{HN-Marker} \end{cases}$$

Two-Step reaction:

$$(1) \text{ Marker-NH}_2 \xrightarrow[\substack{\text{1–5\% glutaraldehyde} \\ \text{PBS} \\ \text{1 h 25 °C}}]{} \text{Marker-NH} \sim\!\!\sim\!\!\sim \text{C} \overset{\displaystyle O}{\underset{\displaystyle H}{\diagup\!\!\diagdown}}$$

$$(2) \begin{array}{l} \text{Antibody-NH}_2 + \\ \text{Market-NH} \sim\!\!\sim \text{C} \overset{\displaystyle O}{\underset{\displaystyle H}{\diagup\!\!\diagdown}} \end{array} \xrightarrow[\substack{\text{PBS} \\ \text{5–12 h 25 °C}}]{} \text{Antibody-NH} \sim \text{HN-Marker}$$

In a typical one step reaction, 0·2 ml of 0·5% glutaraldehyde is slowly added to a 2 ml solution containing 2–4 mg antibody and 10–20 mg marker in 0·01 M sodium phosphate, pH 7 or phosphate buffered saline (PBS). The solution is stirred for 1 h at room temperature, and subsequently quenched by the addition of excess glycine.

In the two step procedure, the markers (5–10 mg/ml) in PBS are first reacted with 1–5% glutaraldehyde for 1–2 h at room temperature. Higher glutaraldehyde concentrations have also been used to further limit crosslinking of markers (Kishida *et al.*, 1975). Excess glutaraldehyde is then removed either by gel filtration chromatography on a Sephadex G-50 column or by dialysis overnight against two 1 l changes of PBS. Although dialysis is slower than column chromatography, it has the advantage that little, if any, dilution of the markers is obtained and, therefore, additional steps involving concentrating the markers can be avoided. In the second step an equal volume of antibody 1–2 mg/ml is added to the glutaraldehyde-activated markers (5–10 mg/ml). The reaction solution is stirred from 6–12 h at 25 °C and finally quenched by the addition of glycine to a final concentration of 0·05 M.

Although the two-step glutaraldehyde procedure is more time consuming and involves extra manipulations, it has the advantage over the one-step procedure in that: (1) intramolecular crosslinking of amino groups which can lead to a reduction in antibody binding activity is avoided, and (2) intermolecular crosslinking leading to the formation of antibody–antibody and marker–marker species is minimized. Several laboratories, in fact, have reported that conjugates prepared by the two step method are more active (Otto *et al.*, 1973; Boorsma and Kalsbeek, 1975; Molday, 1976).

Reactions between aldehydes and amino groups result in the formation of Schiff base linkages which generally must be reduced to a secondary amine by reduction with sodium borohydride. In the case of glutaraldehyde reactions with primary amines on proteins, stable bonds are formed even without reduction. The glutaraldehyde crosslinking reaction has been discussed by Peters and Richards (1977).

A variety of other chemical coupling procedures have been used to conjugate antibodies or lectins to markers containing reactive functional groups. The periodate-borohydride method (Boorsma *et al.*, 1976; Dutton *et al.*, 1979; Molday and MacKenzie, 1982) has proved to be valuable for linking periodate-oxidized sugar residues on some markers, e.g. horseradish peroxidase and iron dextran, to amino groups on antibodies or other proteins. Other procedures include the carbodiimide method (Kishada *et al.*, 1975; Modlay, 1976), toluene 2,4-di-isocyanate method (Singer and Schick, 1961), the benzoquinone method (Ternynack and Avrameas, 1976) and cyanogen bromide method (Molday *et al.*, 1975). These methods have been reviewed by De Petris (1978).

The preparation of highly-active conjugates relies on the use of purified antibodies or other ligands in the coupling procedures. For indirect labeling methods anti-immunoglobulin (anti-Ig) antibodies are generally purified from serum by affinity chromatography on an Ig-Sepharose column. For example, goat anti-rabbit Ig antibody can be purified by passing 5 ml of commercially available goat antirabbit Ig antiserum through a small column containing 2 ml of rabbit Ig Sepharose 4B (5–20 mg Ig per ml of Sepharose 4B) or equivalent immunoadsorbent. The antiserum is washed through the column with PBS until the absorbance at 280 nm is less than 0·1 units. The goat antirabbit Ig antibody is then eluted from the column with 3 M sodium thiocyanate. The sodium thiocyanate is removed by dialysis against PBS.

The fractions containing the goat antirabbit Ig as measured by the absorbance at 280 nm are pooled and dialyzed against PBS.

For use in direct immunological labeling studies monoclonal antibodies obtained from hybridoma cells (Koehler and Milstein, 1975) can be obtained in highly purified form by precipitation of the immunoglobulin from ascites fluid of tumor-bearing mice with 40–50% ammonium sulfate and subsequent chromatography on DEAE cellulose (Mishell and Shiigi, 1980). The concentration of antibody can be determined from the absorbance at 280 nm using an $E_{280}^{1\,mg/ml} = 1\cdot4$.

Staphylococcus protein A which can also be used in indirect labeling (Miller *et al.*, 1981) can be obtained commercially (Pharmacia). This protein, of molecular weight 42 000, has an extinction coefficient ($E_{280}^{1\,mg/ml}$) of 0·15. It has a high affinity for subclasses of IgG from a variety of species including rabbit, mice and human (Goding, 1978).

Lectins which are used as specific markers for cell surface glycoproteins are also available from a variety of biochemical companies. These proteins can be coupled to various markers using the same procedures described above (Nicolson, 1978; Molday, 1981).

B. Non-covalent Adsorption

Polystyrene latex spheres and colloidal gold particles do not contain functional groups on their surface. As a result immunomarker conjugates must be prepared by adsorbing the antibody or other ligand to the surface of these markers through nonspecific adsorption (Lo Buglio *et al.*, 1972; Horisberger, 1979).

In a typical procedure described by Horisberger *et al.* (1976) immunogold markers are prepared by adding a 10 ml solution of antibody (1·5 mg) in 0·005 M NaCl to 100 ml of gold particles with stirring. After 1 min 5 ml of 1% Carbowax 20-M (pre-filtered through 0·45 μM Millipore filters) are added. The solution is then neutralized with 1·25 ml of 0·2 M K_2CO_3 and centrifuged at 27 000 g for 15 min to remove unbound antibody. The pellet is resuspended in 0·05 M Tris buffer pH 7·4 containing 0·15 M NaCl.

Other gold conjugates including protein A-gold conjugates (Roth *et al.*, 1978), lectin-gold conjugates (Horisberger *et al.*, 1976) and toxin-gold conjugates (Schwab and Thoenen, 1978) have been prepared by similar methods. More detailed procedures are described by Roth (see this volume).

Antibodies are adsorbed to polystyrene latex surfaces primarily through hydrophobic interactions. Adsorption procedure involves incubating a suspension of latex spheres with antibody in 0·2 M phosphate buffer at pH 9·2.

The optimal antibody concentration is determined by adding serial dilutions of antibody to the spheres and checking for flocculation of the spheres (Linthicum and Sell, 1975). The highest antibody concentration which does not flocculate the polystyrene markers is generally used to prepare immuno-polystyrene markers for labeling. Antibody-coated polystyrene markers are most stable above pH 8·5 and as a result cell labeling must be carried out at alkaline pH (Lo Buglio *et al.*, 1972; Linthicum and Sell, 1975).

C. Purification and Characterization of Immunomarkers

Immunomarker conjugates must be separated from unbound antibody prior to their utilization in labeling studies. In most cases, this is accomplished by gel filtration chromatography which separates immunomarker conjugates from free antibodies on the basis of differences in size (Kishida *et al.*, 1975). The type of gel matrix used depends on the size of the marker. Generally, the conjugates and unconjugated markers are collected in the void volume of the column, whereas the unconjugated monomeric antibody or small aggregates are eluted in the included volume of the column. Larger aggregated species of antibodies often elute with the conjugate. Therefore, it is desirable to remove such aggregated species prior to conjugate preparation and to use coupling procedures in which such species are not likely to form, e.g. two step glutaraldehyde reaction.

In the case of hemocyanin, ferritin, iron dextran and copolymer microsphere conjugates, Sephacryl S-300, Sepharose 6B (Pharmacia) or Biogel A 1·5 m (Bio Rad Lab) columns have been widely used. These columns are routinely calibrated with unconjugated markers and antibodies. Unconjugated markers are not generally separated from the conjugates. Unconjugated markers and inactive conjugates, however, can be removed from the conjugate preparation by affinity chromatographic techniques if required to reduce the level of nonspecific binding.

Conjugates consisting of large and/or dense markers such as bacteriophage T-4 (Kumon, 1976), copolymer microspheres (Molday *et al.*, 1975) or gold particles (Horisberger and Rosset, 1977; Roth *et al.*, 1978) can be separated from unconjugated antibody by differential or gradient centrifugation. For example immunocopolymer microspheres have been routinely purified by centrifugation through 15% (w/w) sucrose onto a layer of 60% (w/w) sucrose in a SW-27 rotor at 100 000 g for 3–5 h. Immunomicrospheres are collected at the interface between 15% and 60% sucrose and dialyzed against PBS to remove the sucrose.

Purified conjugates are routinely stored at 4 °C in sterile vials or in the presence of antibacterial agents such as 10 mM NaN_3 since freezing and thawing can cause aggregation and inactivation of markers. If NaN_3 is used, it may be necessary to remove this agent prior to labeling since it can affect the distribution of labeled antigens (De Petris, 1978) and morphology of cells as seen under the SEM (Molday *et al.*, 1975).

The final conjugate should be tested in terms of its activity and specificity prior to its use in cell labeling studies. A wide variety of biochemical and immunological assays have been used with the various markers. Such methods as immunoelectrophoresis (Avrameas and Ternynck, 1971; Kishida *et al.*, 1975) and antibody and lectin agglutination assays have been used (Maher and Molday, 1979). These assays, however, are often qualitative in nature. Our laboratory routinely tests immunomarker or lectin marker conjugates by SEM on previously characterized cells. For example, we use glutaraldehyde-fixed human red blood cells to test goat antirabbit Ig or protein A markers. Generally, 10^6 RBC in PBS are first incubated with rabbit antihuman RBC antiserum (Cappel Laboratories, Downington, PA) for 30 min, washed three times by centrifugation in 3 ml PBS and then labeled with various dilutions of the immunoconjugate. The samples are then processed for SEM. A dense packing of the markers over the cell surface for several dilutions of the immunomarkers will indicate that it is highly active and suitable for use with other cells. The specificity is tested at the same time by omitting the specific rabbit antihuman antiserum in control samples. Absence of labeling will indicate that the conjugates do not specifically bind to red blood cells.

Lectin-markers can be directly tested on RBC, thymocytes, or cultured cells which are known to have large quantities of specific lectin receptors (Molday, 1981).

The ratio of immunoglobulin to marker is also important in the analysis of cell labeling. This can be determined by quantifying the amount of Ig molecules using ^{125}I-labeled Ig and the marker concentration by a characteristic property such as adsorbance in the visible wavelength range for ferritin or hemocyanin. It is often desirable to use conjugates having a 1:1 molar ratio in order to limit the effect of multivalent conjugates on the distribution of antigens and receptors (De Petris, 1978).

IV. IMMUNOLOGICAL LABELING METHODS

A. Methods Employing Immunomarker Conjugates

1. Direct Method

Cell surface antigens can be directly labeled in a single step with immunomarkers consisting of the cell surface specific antibody bound to the SEM marker (Fig. 4). Cells are incubated with the conjugate under well defined experimental conditions, i.e. time, temperature, buffer, etc. The concentration of conjugate normally used is that sufficient to saturate accessible antigenic sites on the cell surface. After this incubation the cells are washed in buffer to remove excess, unbound conjugate and prepared for SEM by standard procedures.

Control experiments to measure the extent of nonspecific binding of the conjugates to cell surfaces are carried out in parallel. Typically, cells are incubated with the conjugate in the presence of excess cell surface specific antibody which can effectively compete with the conjugate for cell surface binding sites. A reduction or elimination of binding by the conjugate should be visualized by SEM. Alternatively, cells can be incubated with the conjugate in the presence of inhibitors or antigens which bind to the conjugate and prevent subsequent binding of the conjugate to sites on the cell surface.

The direct labeling method has the advantage that it is rapid and simple.

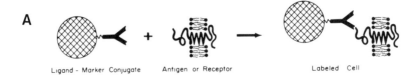

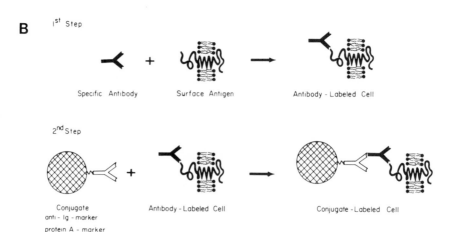

FIG. 4. General scheme for the direct immunological labeling method (A) and the indirect "sandwich" immunological labeling technique (B).

Since cells need be incubated and washed only once, adverse effects on cell surface morphology is minimized. Furthermore, ligand-induced rearrangements of labeled sites can be more easily controlled. This is particularly true when monovalent antibodies are conjugated to markers in a 1:1 molar ratio (De Petris and Raff, 1973; De Petris, 1978). Direct labeling also enables one to localize more precisely labeled sites for high resolution studies since the markers are in closer proximity to the cell surface sites than when indirect methods are used.

The major disadvantages of direct immunological labeling are: (1) the cell suface sites must be sterically accessible to the relatively large SEM markers, and (2) highly purified antibodies are required in sufficient quantities for the preparation of active conjugates. The latter drawback, however, has been overcome by the recent development in the production of monoclonal antibodies from hybridoma cells (Köhler and Milstein, 1975; Mishel and Shiigi, 1980). As a result, the direct labeling method should become more widely used to detect and localize cell surface antigens.

2. Indirect Sandwich Method

The indirect sandwich labeling method involves two labeling steps (Fig. 4). Cells are incubated with the antiserum containing the cell surface specific immunoglobin (Ig) in the first step. The cells are then washed in buffer, and treated with anti-Ig-marker conjugate in the second step. In some studies protein A-marker conjugates which bind to the Fc region of certain classes of IgG molecules of various species (Goding, 1978) have been used in the second step instead of anti-Ig-marker conjugates (Miller *et al.*, 1981; Roth *et al.*, 1978).

In control experiments, nonspecific control serum or its Ig fraction is used in place of the specific antiserum in the first step. Pre-immune antiserum should be used if possible. If a high degree of nonspecific binding of the conjugates to the cells is observed in this control, a second control, in which the control serum is substituted with buffer, should be carried out in order to determine if the observed nonspecific binding is due to nonspecific binding of the conjugate to cells (conjugate would label cells in both controls) or to Ig in the control serum which binds to cells (conjugate would label only cells treated with control serum).

The indirect "sandwich" method has been most widely used in immunological labeling for light and electron microscopy. Advantages of this method include:

1. Antiserum containing anti-Ig antibodies, e.g. goat antirabbit Ig or goat antimouse Ig is available commercially. The anti-Ig can be easily purified by immunoaffinity chromatography;

2. Only small quantities of the cell surface antiserum are needed in labeling studies;

3. Anti-Ig-marker conjugates can be used to localize different cell surface antigens for which specific antiserum from the corresponding species is available;

4. These conjugates can be easily tested for activity on well-established systems, i.e. goat antirabbit Ig-markers can be tested on fixed human red blood cells (see Purification and Characterization of Immunomarkers);

5. Steric inaccessibility of antigen sites is less of a problem since, in the first step, antibodies are used instead of larger conjugates.

A variation of this method is the indirect "bridging" method which requires three labeling steps. In this method cells are first labeled with the primary antiserum containing the cell surface specific antibody, then with anti-immunoglobulin antibody, and finally with excess Ig-marker conjugate. Cells are washed between labeling steps to remove unbound reagents. In this method, bivalent anti-Ig antibodies serve to bridge the Ig-marker to the specific antibodies bound to the cell (Fig. 5). The cell surface specific Ig and the Ig conjugated to the markers must be obtained from the same species, i.e. rabbit Ig if goat anti-rabbit Ig is used as the bridging antibody.

This method has the advantage that purified Ig required in the preparation of the conjugate is available commercially. The disadvantage, however, is that an extra labeling step is introduced which can have additional adverse effects on the cell surface morphology and may cause additional nonspecific binding.

B. Other Indirect Immunological Methods

A variety of specialized immunological labeling methods based solely on antigen-antibody binding have also been introduced for localizing antigenic sites by light and electron microscopy. These are illustrated in Fig. 5.

1. Hapten-sandwich Method

The hapten-sandwich method initially developed for TEM studies (Lamm *et al.*, 1972) was used in SEM studies by Nemanic *et al.* (1975). It involves a three-step procedure in which cells are sequentially treated with hapten-derivatized cell surface specific antibodies, antihapten antibodies and hapten-derivatized SEM markers. Bivalent antihapten antibodies served to bridge the marker to the specific antibody through specific, high affinity binding. After each labeling step the cells must be thoroughly washed in buffer to remove excess labeling reagents. The concentration of antibodies used should be sufficient to saturate all available sites.

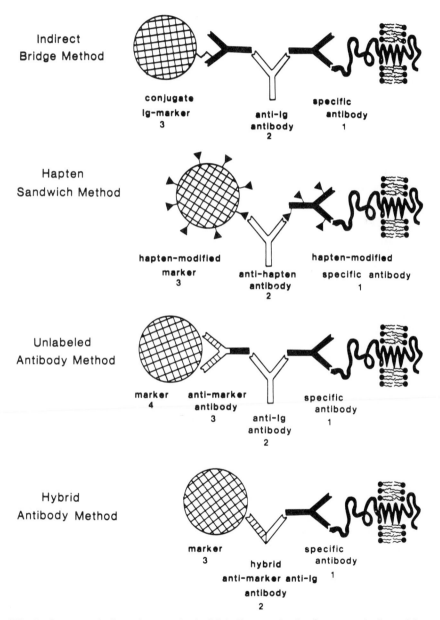

FIG. 5. Common indirect immunological labeling methods. Steps are indicated by numbers.

A variety of small organic compounds which can be linked to proteins can serve as haptens. Nemanic *et al.* (1975) have used mainly *p*-azophenyl-*β*-lactoside. Other haptens, however, such as fluorescein isothiocyanate or tetraethylrhodamine isothiocyanate may be particularly useful since they can be used in combined fluorescent light microscopy and SEM. The hapten-sandwich method has been discussed in detail in several recent papers (Nemanic, 1979; Wofsy, 1979).

2. Unlabeled Antibody Method

The unlabeled antibody method involves four separate labeling steps, but avoids derivatization or conjugation of either the markers or antibodies. In this procedure as introduced for SEM labeling by Gonda *et al.* (1979), cells are sequentially treated with:

    i. The specific cell surface antibody
    ii. Bivalent anti-Ig antibody
    iii. Anti-marker antibody, e.g. antihemocyanin antibody and
    iv. Marker, e.g. hemocyanin.

As for all labeling methods, the cells must be thoroughly washed between labeling steps. The cell surface specific antibody and antihemocyanin antibody must be from the same species. This technique has been used to localize virions and viral proteins on the surface of virus-infected cells (Gonda *et al.*, 1979).

3. Hybrid-Antibody Method

The hybrid-antibody method is a three step procedure in which cells are first labeled with the cell surface specific antibody, then with a $F(ab)_2$ hybrid antibody consisting of anti-Ig and anti-marker fragments and finally the marker. Although in the procedure the markers do not have to be conjugated to antibodies, the hybrid antibodies which bridge the cell surface specific antibody to the marker must be prepared and purified. Such procedures have been discussed in detail by Hämmerling *et al.* (1973). Due to the lengthy procedures required to prepare and purify hybrid antibodies, this labeling method has not been widely used.

4. Controls for Indirect Methods

Controls for these methods generally involve substitution of the specific cell surface antiserum with nonspecific control antiserum. Other controls, however, should also be run to confirm the specificity of binding. Generally one of the intermediate labeling steps is omitted or replaced with nonspecific control immunoglobulin from the same species and having a similar concentration as the corresponding specific immunoglobulin used in the test sample.

In some studies related cell types which are known not to express the antigenic site have been used as controls to test for nonspecific binding (Molday, 1976). Although this is an important control, it is not sufficient by itself since even slight differences in cell surface properties may result in differences in the extent of nonspecific binding of markers to the cells used in the labeling studies.

V. LECTIN LABELING METHODS

Lectins are a class of proteins derived from plant and animal cell extracts which bind reversibly to carbohydrate residues (Sharon and Lis, 1972; Nicolson, 1974). Most lectins are multivalent and agglutinate cells to which they bind. For further details see Leathem and Atkins (this volume).

A. Direct Lectin Methods

Direct labeling methods using lectins covalently bonded or adsorbed to visual markers have been routinely used to localize lectin binding sites on cell surfaces by SEM (Molday *et al.*, 1976; Horisberger and Rosset, 1977a; Tsutsui *et al.*, 1978). This is primarily due to the availability of pure preparations of lectins and the relative ease with which they can be conjugated to markers without significant loss in binding activity.

Generally, cells are treated with the conjugate for 10 min at 25 °C or 60 min at 4 °C then washed to remove unbound conjugate and fixed in glutaraldehyde prior to processing of the samples for SEM. Longer incubation times can be used, but redistribution and internalization of labeled sites can occur (Weller, 1974; Molday *et al.*, 1976; Maher and Molday, 1979). In control experiments, cells are treated with the lectin-marker conjugate in the presence of a large excess (0·01–0·1 M) of the appropriate sugar inhibitor. The direct labeling of con A-receptors on the surface of *Dictyostelium discoideum* cells with con A-microsphere markers is illustrated in Fig. 6.

B. Indirect Lectin Methods

A number of indirect lectin labeling methods have also been developed for microscopic analysis (Fig. 7). The most common is the indirect con A

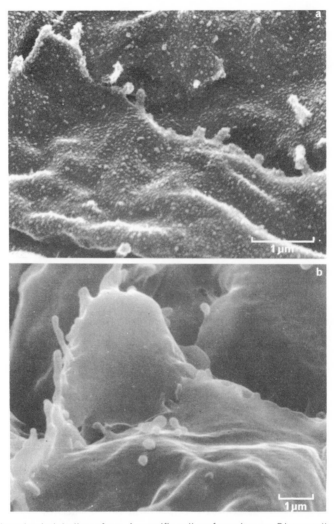

FIG. 6. Direct lectin labeling of con A-specific cell surface sites on *Dictyostelium discoi-deum* cells. Cells were prefixed in 0·25% glutaraldehyde-PBS for 30 min and subse-quently labeled with con A-microsphere conjugates (35 nm diameter) in the absence (a) and presence (b) of α-methyl mannoside inhibitor of con A. In (a) microspheres coat the surface of the cells; in the control (b) no labeling is observed.

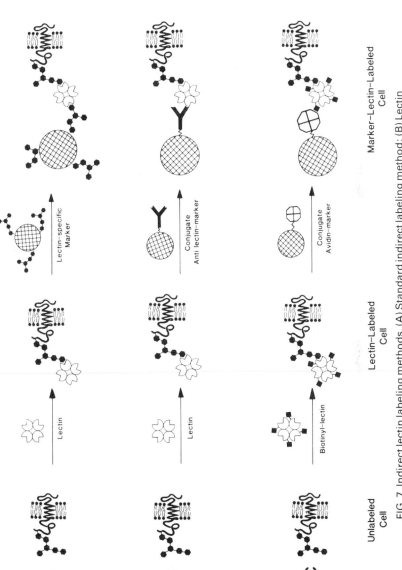

Unlabeled Cell   Lectin–Labeled Cell   Marker–Lectin–Labeled Cell

FIG. 7. Indirect lectin labeling methods. (A) Standard indirect labeling method; (B) Lectin antibody method; (C) Biotin–avidin lectin method.

method used with hemocyanin (Smith and Revel, 1972). In this method, cells are first treated with con A, then washed in buffer and finally treated with hemocyanin. Since con A is multivalent, i.e. tetrameric under physiological buffer conditions, it can bind both to the con A-specific cell surface receptors and to the con A specific residues on hemocyanin. Although this two step indirect method has been used principally with hemocyanin for SEM studies, it can also be used with the markers such as horseradish peroxidase (Bretton et al., 1973) and iron dextran (Baccetti and Burrini, 1977) which also bind con A. A similar indirect method can be used with other lectins and markers derivatized with the corresponding sugar residues (Schrevel et al., 1979). For example, markers derivatized with oligomers of N-acetyl glucosamine can be used to label cells treated with the lectin wheat germ agglutinin.

Indirect methods relying on the high affinity binding of biotin by the protein avidin have also been employed (Bayer et al., 1976). In this method lectins derivatized with biotin are used to label cells in the first step. After washing the cells they are treated with an avidin-marker conjugate in the second step. Biotinylated lectins and ferritin-avidin markers are now commercially available (Vector Laboratories, Burlingame, CA). This technique is also applicable with biotinylated antibodies for labeling antigenic sites (Heitzmann and Richards, 1974; Skutelsky and Bayer, 1979).

Finally, lectin receptors can be labeled using immunological methods. In a two step procedure, cells are first labeled with the lectin and subsequently treated with conjugates consisting of the antilectin antibody coupled to a marker. Alternately, a three-step procedure can be used in which cells are sequentially treated with the lectin, the anti-lectin antibody and the anti-Ig marker or protein A-marker conjugate. Such immunological methods, however, do not offer significant advantages over the direct or other indirect methods.

Controls for indirect lectin labeling generally involve incubation of cells with the lectin in the presence of excess sugar inhibitor in the first step. Omission of the lectin in the first step or substitution of derivatized lectin with underivatized lectin as in the case of the biotin-avidin method can also be used to confirm the specificity of labeling.

VI. CONDITIONS FOR LABELING CELLS

Cells in suspension or grown on solid supports such as glass coverslips can be used in labeling studies. In the latter, small coverslips or pieces of coverslips containing bound cells are washed in phosphate-buffered saline or other suitable physiological buffer. The cells are then immersed in the primary antibody or conjugate. This can be conventionally done by inverting the coverslip onto a drop of the reagent placed on a piece of dental wax. The cells should be completely in contact with the reagent. After the specified time, the coverslip is picked up with forceps and repeatedly dipped into 100 ml beakers of buffer to wash out excess reagents. In multi-step labeling procedures, this labeling procedure is repeated. It should be noted that some cells require Ca^{++} and Mg^{++} to stay bound to solid supports. In such cases it is necessary to include these ions in labeling reagents and buffers used in washing. Precaution should also be taken to prevent air drying of the samples during labeling, washing and subsequent sample manipulations.

Cells in suspension are routinely labeled by adding 100 μl of reagent to 100 μl of 10^6 cells. After the required time, 10–30 fold excess buffer is added and the cells are sedimented by low-speed centrifugation (400–1000 ×g for 10 min). The cells are gently resuspended in 1 ml of buffer and this washing procedure is repeated twice more to ensure complete removal of excess reagents before proceeding to the next labeling step or fixation of cells for SEM. A disadvantage of labeling cells in suspension is the potential agglutination of cells caused by multivalent antibody or lectin reagents.

Cells prefixed in glutaraldehyde or formaldehyde can be used, provided the antigenic binding sites are not destroyed by these fixatives. Prefixation is not a problem if lectin binding sites on cell surfaces are being labeled. Routinely cells are prefixed in 0·1–0·2% glutaraldehyde in PBS for 10–30 min, washed in PBS to remove excess glutaraldehyde and finally treated with PBS containing 0·01–0·05 M glycine or other primary amines to block glutaraldehyde groups remaining on the cell surface. Fixed cells can be labeled either in suspension or after the cells have been adsorbed to poly-lysine-treated coverslips (Mazia *et al.*, 1975). Unfixed cells, however, should not be adsorbed to polylysine-treated coverslips, since alteration in cell surface morphology may occur.

Glutaraldehyde fixation has the advantage that it preserves cell surface morphology during subsequently labeling procedures and prevents redistribution and loss of labeled components from the cell surface by endocytosis or shedding (Molday, 1977; De Petris, 1978). However, pre-fixation with glutaraldehyde often destroys antigenic sites (Ostrand-Rosenberg *et al.*, 1979; Van Ewijk *et al.*, 1980) and also causes autofluorescence of cells which can limit their use in combined fluorescent microscopic and SEM studies. These difficulties are often overcome by using 0·1–4% para-formaldehyde instead of glutaraldehyde as a pre-fixative.

The experimental conditions under which labeling is carried out are important. One generally uses the lowest antibody and conjugate concentrations which will label essentially all accessible cell surface antigens. Non-specific binding as measured in control experiments are minimized under these conditions. This concentration can be determined by labeling cells with serial dilutions of reagents and analyzing the extent of labeling by SEM or other semi-quantitative assays.

The length of time of labeling is also important. Binding of antibodies and lectins to cell surface antigens and receptors is relatively fast at 25 °C. Most sites are labeled within 5 min at 25 °C, although it is more common to label cells for 30–60 min. Redistribution of labeled antigens and receptors into clusters and caps and loss of labeled sites from the surface of unfixed cells through endocytosis, however, can occur over this time period (Raff and De Petris, 1972; Molday *et al.*, 1976; Brown and Revel, 1976).

When labeling is carried out at 4 °C, longer incubation times are often required. Redistribution is often, but not always, prevented, but alteration in cell surface morphology can occur at low temperatures (Lin *et al.*, 1973). Factors which influence the distribution of antigens and receptors are discussed in more detail by De Petris (1978) and Nicolson (1976).

VII. PREPARATION OF SAMPLES FOR SEM

Labeled cells are processed for SEM in the same way as unlabeled specimens (Revel, 1975; Brunk *et al.*, 1980). This involves washing the cells in an isotonic buffer, fixation with glutaraldehyde, post-fixation with osmium tetroxide, dehydration in a graded series of aqueous ethanol, acetone or amyl acetate solutions, critical point drying from freon or more commonly carbon dioxide and evaporative or sputter-coating with gold or gold-palladium. Post-fixation with osmium tetroxide is not required, but it is generally desirable not only for improved preservation, but also for greater contrast due to an increased production of secondary electrons in the SEM. In fact osmium complexing agents such as thiocarbozide and tannic acid have often been employed in post-fixation procedures in order to increase the disposition of osmium in the specimen (Malick *et al.*, 1975; Murakami, 1974). This increases the image contrast as well as the electrical and thermal conductivity of the specimen. In some cases, this procedure eliminates the need to further coat the specimens with heavy metals which otherwise may obscure the definition of small markers on the cell surface.

Preparation procedures are most easily carried out if cells are attached to solid supports. Polylysine coated glass coverslips serve as a convenient support to attached cells which have been labeled in suspension (Mazia *et al.*, 1975). In this procedure, glass coverslips are immersed in an aqueous solution of polylysine (0·1 mg/ml) for 30 min, rinsed in distilled water and air dried. Cells which have been fixed in glutaraldehyde are allowed to settle on the coverslip overnight. Alternatively, a 13 mm diameter polylysine coated coverslip can be placed in a small plastic Millipore filter holder and the cells are then sedimented onto the coverslip by centrifugation at 1000 rpm for 10 min in a table-top clinical centrifuge. The coverslip must be carefully removed from the filter holder to prevent air drying of the specimen. In either method the cell-laden coverslips are rinsed in buffer to remove unattached cells and subsequently post-fixed in osmium tetroxide or indirectly immersed in 50% aqueous ethanol for dehydration.

Routine procedure for the preparation of cells for SEM

1. Cells are washed in isotonic buffer such as phosphate-buffered saline (PBS) and fixed in 1·25% (v/v) glutaraldehyde in PBS for 1 h at room temperature.

2. If cells are in suspension, they are sedimented onto polylysine-coated glass coverslips and rinsed in PBS to remove unattached cells.

3. The cells are then post-fixed in 1% OsO_4 in PBS for 1 h and rinsed in distilled water.

4. Dehydration is carried out in a graded series of aqueous ethanol solutions (60%, 70%, 80%, 90% and 95%) for 5 min each, followed by three changes of 100% ethanol over a period of 1 h.

5. Dehydrated cells are subjected to critical point drying.

6. Specimens are then attached to an appropriate SEM stub with silver conducting paste.

7. A 5–10 nm layer of gold or gold-palladium is applied by the evaporative method using a rotating tilting stage or by the sputter-coating method.

8. Specimens are stored in a vacuum dessicator until visualization under the SEM.

An increase in osmium staining of the cells can be achieved by substituting step 3 with the following osmium-thiocarbozide-osmium (OTO) procedure: Cells are post-fixed in 1% osmium tetroxide for 1 h, rinsed in distilled water, and treated in a freshly prepared and filtered aqueous solution of thiocar-bohydrozide for 30 min. After the cells are thoroughly rinsed in distilled water, they are treated a second time in 1% osmium tetroxide for 1 h, followed by washing with distilled water.

VIII. ANALYSIS OF CELL LABELING

An important aspect of cell surface labeling for SEM as well as for other modes of microscopy is the critical evaluation of the results. Negative results i.e. absence of labeling can be due to (1) the use of inactive primary antibody or inactive immunomarker conjugates, or (2) the absence or steric inaccessibility of the cell surface antigen or receptor to the relatively large immunomarker conjugates.

The binding activity of the primary antibody to the cell surface component should be tested prior to its use in labeling studies for SEM. This can be carried out by any of a variety of established immunological assays including cell agglutination, immunodiffusion or immunoelectrophoresis, immunoprecipitation or radioimmune assays. Corresponding control antibody or antiserum should also be tested for activity by similar assays.

A more common problem is the determination of the activity and specificity of the immunoconjugate. This analysis is most easily done for conjugates in indirect labeling. As previously described, the activity and specificity of goat anti-rabbit Ig or protein A markers can be tested on fixed human red blood cells pretreated with rabbit anti-human red blood cell antiserum. If the immunomarker conjugates are highly active, they will appear densely packed over the cell surface as seen under the SEM. Likewise, lectin markers such as wheat-germ agglutinin and *Ricinus communis* agglutinin markers can be tested on human red blood cells (Molday, 1976). Lymphocytes or a variety of cultured cells can be used to test con A-marker conjugates (Molday, 1981). In these cases, dense labeling patterns as visualized under the SEM will confirm that the conjugates are active. Controls should also be run to verify the specificity of labeling.

If the immunological reagents are known to be active in labeling model cell systems, negative labeling for the cell system of interest may indicate the absence of an antigen on the particular cell or its inaccessibility to the immunological markers due to steric hindrance (Horisberger *et al.*, 1978). In such cases it is desirable to use indirect immunofluorescent labeling or radio-immune assays to determine if antigens are present on the cells. Immunoperoxidase labeling for light or TEM can also be used since horseradish peroxidase is a small protein relative to immunoglobulins and, as a result, this marker does not cause the additional steric interference that large markers can cause (Temmink, 1979).

If studies indicate that the antigen is present on the cell surface and is sterically accessible to antibodies, but not large SEM markers, labeling may be possible with smaller markers such as ferritin or gold particles having diameters less than 20 nm. Horisberger and Rosset (1977) have in fact shown that the extent of labeling of lectin receptors on red blood cells and hepatocytes is dependent on the size of the gold markers used in labeling. For example human red blood cells could be labeled only with con A-gold particles smaller than 17 nm diameter and with soybean agglutinin gold particles smaller than 50 nm. These cells, however, could be labeled with WGA-gold particles of all sizes (Horisberger, 1978). Indirect methods

PLATES

Plate 1.   Mononuclear cell suspension of normal peripheral blood labelled with OKT4 and GAMG30. The preparation is stained for endogenous peroxidase (brown reaction product (p) in the cytoplasm of monocytes and granulocytes) and counterstained with methyl green (green–blue colour of the nuclei). Lymphocytes (l) are identified as peroxidase negative mononuclear cells. Lymphocytes reacting with the monoclonal antibodies have numerous dark granules around their surface membrane. The small amount of unstained cytoplasm of these lymphocytes is difficult to see on this picture (magnification × 1400).

Plates 2, 3, 4.   Mononuclear cell suspension of normal peripheral blood labelled with OKT4 and GAMG30. The preparations are stained for acid alpha-naphthyl acetate esterase (Plate 2), acid phosphatase (Plate 3) and beta-glucuronidase (Plate 4). They are counterstained with methyl green (green colour of the nuclei). The monocytes (m) can be identified by their morphological and cytochemical characteristics. Lymphocytes reacting with the monoclonal antibodies have numerous dark granules around their surface membrane. In the cytoplasm of the lymphocytes three different staining patterns for the enzymes can be distinguished: a dot-like activity (d), a diffuse granular activity (g) or no reaction at all. The reaction product for acid alpha-naphthyl acetate esterase is brown and it is red for acid phosphatase and beta-glucuronidase (magnification × 1140).

Plate 5.   Immunogold staining on the peripheral blood of a T-ALL patient. A mononuclear cell suspension is labelled with OKT6 and GAMG30. The preparation is counterstained with the methyl green pyronin technique. The blast cells can be recognized as large cells with a pyronophilic cytoplasm and nucleolus. They react with the OKT6 monoclonal antibody. The remaining normal lymphocytes (l) in the peripheral blood are OKT6 negative (magnification × 1140).

Plate 6.   Examination of a preparation of immunogold-labelled cells in dark-field microscopy. The patches of gold particles on the surface membrane of the immunogold positive lymphocytes (p) strongly reflect the incident light and appear as bright yellow spots. Immunogold negative lymphocytes (n) and red blood cells (r) can easily be recognized (magnification × 1140).

Plate 7.   Experiment to estimate the minimal stabilizing protein amount. In tube 1, the natural colour of unprotected colloidal gold is seen which changes to blue and gives a precipitate after addition of NaCl to the unprotected colloid as seen in tube 2. Tubes 3 and 11 show colloidal gold mixed with serial dilutions of a protein. Tube 7 is the last with no colour change of the colloidal gold upon addition of NaCl, i.e. the minimal protein amount for stabilization of this volume of colloidal gold is reached. The colloidal gold in tube 8 shows already a colour change to blue which is more pronounced and accompanied by precipitate formation in the following tubes. Therefore, the protein amount added to these tubes is not sufficient to stabilize the colloidal gold against flocculation by NaCl.

Plate 8.   Rat pancreas, paraffin section, double staining with protein A-gold and protein A-silver complexes. Amylase in the cytoplasm of pancreatic acinar cells is visualized with protein A-gold complexes and gives a red colouration in these cells. Insulin in the B-cells of an islet of Langerhans is demonstrated with protein A-silver complexes resulting in a yellow colouration of these cells. The section is slightly counterstained with 0·01% Evans blue.

Plate 9.   Rat kidney, paraffin section, incubation with *Helix pomatia* lectin-gold complexes. Lectin binding sites are red stained and present at the level of the plasma membrane (apical and basal) of distal convoluted epithelial cells. This section was not counterstained.

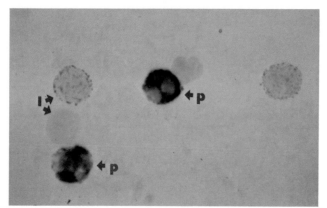

Plate 1

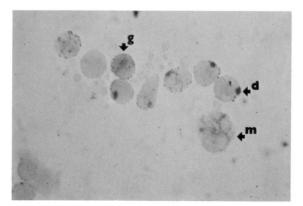

Plate 2

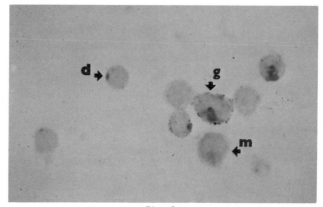

Plate 3

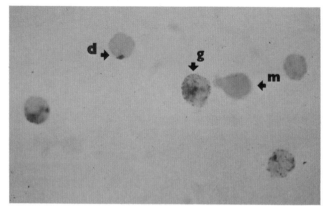

Plate 4

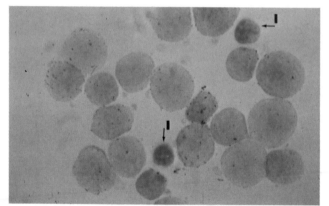

Plate 5

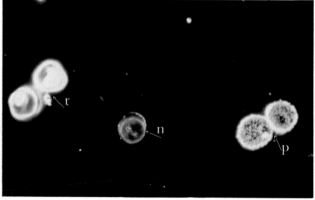

Plate 6

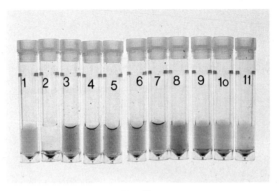

Plate 7

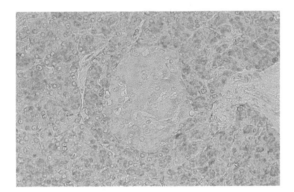

Plate 8

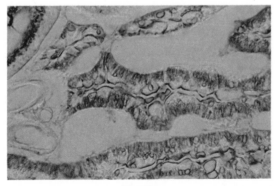

Plate 9

which extend the markers further off the cell surface may also reduce steric interference.

Finally negative labeling as visualized under the SEM may be a result of the conditions used to label cells. If prefixed cells are used, inability to label cells may be due to inactivation of antigenic sites or receptors by the fixation conditions (Van Ewijk *et al.*, 1980). If unfixed cells are used in labeling, cell surface antigens and receptors may redistribute on labeling and be lost from the cell surface through the process of endocytosis or shedding. Correlative studies using immunofluorescence and SEM can be effectively used to study endocytosis of labeled cell surface components (Maher and Molday, 1979). Alternatively, endocytosis can be visualized under the TEM using electron dense immunological markers. The redistribution of antigens and receptors has been the subject of a number of reviews (De Petris, 1978; Nicolson, 1976).

Positive labeling must be evaluated on the basis of controls to test for nonspecific binding. Controls have been discussed. If high levels of nonspecific binding occur which can be attributed to the marker, it may be neccessary to switch to another marker having different surface properties.

IX. CONCLUSIONS

A wide variety of visual markers have been developed for the detection and localization of antigens and receptors on cell surfaces by SEM. Detection of these markers on cell surfaces is generally made on the basis of their characteristic size and shape using secondary electron imaging. Other modes of detection based on generation of a high yield of backscattered electrons, secondary electrons, cathodoluminescence or X-rays, however, have also been reported for some of the SEM markers.

Smaller markers including ferritin, gold particles, silica spheres and co-polymer microspheres are particularly useful in high resolution studies designed for mapping the distribution of cell surface components and correlating this distribution with cell surface morphology. Larger markers including plant viruses, bacteriophage and latex spheres are most suitable for the identification of labeled cells in mixed populations using low magnification.

Electron dense markers such as gold particles, ferritin and iron dextran spheres and fluorescent markers such as fluorescein or rhodamine tagged microspheres are particularly versatile since these visual markers can be used in combined TEM-SEM or fluorescent microscope-SEM studies of labeled cells.

Immunological labeling methods used with SEM markers are identical to the methods developed for immunofluorescent and immunotransmission electron microscopy. The most convenient method is the indirect "sandwich" method using immunomarkers consisting of anti-Ig antibodies or protein A conjugated to the SEM markers. Direct labeling methods in which the markers are directly coupled to the cell surface specific antibodies or their monovalent Fab fragments, however, should prove valuable in future studies. Carbohydrate-containing components on cell surfaces can be visualized using lectin labeling methods in conjunction with visual markers. These methods are similar to immunological labeling methods.

Cell surface labeling techniques for SEM have numerous applications. They can be used to identify and study the surface characteristics of specific cells in mixed cell populations and in tissue specimens under various experimental conditions. The topographical distribution of antigens or receptors on cell surfaces can be studied within the resolution of the markers employed and correlated with cell surface features. Some insight on the relative density of the antigens or receptors on cells can also be obtained although accurate quantification is difficult due to possible steric factors.

Although many of the studies to date have concentrated on the development and improvement of markers and labeling procedures for SEM, application of these techniques in conjunction with related labeling techniques for light and TEM should prove extremely valuable for obtaining further insight into structural and functional characteristics of cell surface antigens and receptors.

X. ACKNOWLEDGEMENT

Research from this laboratory was supported by a grant from the Medical Research Council of Canada. The author also gratefully acknowledges the excellent technical assistance of Don MacKenzie in the preparation of the electron micrographs.

XI. REFERENCES

Aoki, T., Hämmerling, U., de Harven, E., Boyse, E. A. and Old, L. J. (1969). *J. Exp. Med.* **130**, 979–1001.
Avrameas, S. (1969). *Immunochemistry* **6**, 43–52.
Avrameas, S. and Ternynck, T. (1971). *Immunochemistry* **8**, 1175–1179.
Baccetti, B. and Burrini, A. G. (1977). *J. Microscopy* **109**, 203–209.
Bayer, E. A., Wilchek, M. and Skutelsky, E. (1976). *FEBS Lett.* **68**, 240–244.
Ben-Shaul, Y., Ophir, I., Cohen, E. and Moscona, A. (1977). *In* "IITRI/Scanning Electron Microscopy" (O. Johari and R. P. Becker, eds.), Vol. II. pp. 29–35. IIT Research Institute, Chicago.

Boorsma, D. M. and Kalsbeek, G. L. (1975). *J. Histochem. Cytochem.* **23**, 200–207.
Boorsma, D. M. Streefkerk, J. G. and Kors, N. (1976). *J. Histochem. Cytochem.* **24**, 1017–1025.
Bretton, R., Clark, D. A. and Nathanson, L. (1973). *J. Microscopie* **17**, 93–96.
Brown, S. S. and Revel, J. P. (1976). *J. Cell Biol.* **68**, 629–641.
Brown, S. S. and Revel, J. P. (1978). In "Advanced Techniques in Biological Electron Microscopy" (J. K. Koehler, ed.), Vol. II. pp. 65–68. Springer-Verlag, New York.
Brunk, U., Collins, V. P. and Airo, E. (1980). *J. Microscopy* **123**, 121–131.
Carter, D. P. (1978). In "Principles and Techniques of Scanning Electron Microscopy" (M. A. Hayat, ed.), Vol. 6. pp. 317–329. Van Nostrand Rheinhold, New York.
Cavellier, J. F., Berry, J. P. and Lagrue, G. (1978). *Histochemistry* **57**, 313–322.
Coons, A. H. and Kaplan, M. H. (1950). *J. Exp. Med.* **91**, 1–13.
De Harven, E. Pla, D. and Lampen, N. (1979). In "Scanning Electron Microscopy" (O. Johari and R. P. Becker, eds.), Vol. III. pp. 611–618. Scanning Electron Microscopy Inc., O'Hare, Illinois.
De Petris, S. (1978). In "Methods in Membrane Biology" (E. Korn, ed.), Vol. 9, pp.1–201. Plenum Press, New York.
De Petris, S. and Raff, M. C. (1973). *Nature New Biol.* **241**, 257–259.
Dutton, A. H., Tokuyasu, K. T. and Singer, S. J. (1979). *Proc. Natn. Acad. Sci. USA* **76**, 3392–3396.
Faulk, W. P. and Taylor, G. M. (1971). *Immunochemistry* **8**, 1081–1083.
Frens, G. (1973). *Nature Phys. Sci.* **241**, 20–22.
Fuchs, H. and Bächi, T. (1975). *J. Ultrastruc. Res.* **52**, 114–119.
Gamliel, H., Leizerowitz, R., Gurfel, D. and Polliack, A. (1981). *J. Microscopy* **123**, 189–199.
Geltosky, J., Birdwell, C., Weseman, J. and Lerner, R. (1980). *Cell* **21**, 339–345.
Goding, J. W. (1978). *J. Immunol. Meth.* **20**, 241–250.
Gonda, M. A., Gilden, R. V. and Hsu, K. C. (1979). In "Scanning Electron Microscopy" (O. Johari and R. P. Becker, eds.), Vol. III. pp. 583–592, Scanning Electron Microscopy Inc., O'Hare, Ill.
Goodman, S. L., Hodges, G. M. and Livingston, D. C. (1980). In "Scanning Electron Microscopy" (O. Johari, ed.), Vol. II. pp. 133–146. Scanning Electron Microscopy, Inc., O'Hare, Ill.
Goodman, S. L., Hodges, G. M., Trejdosiewicz, L. K. and Livingston, D. C. (1981). *J. Microscopy* **123**, 201–213.
Hämmerling, U., Polliack, A., Lampen, N., Sabety, M. and De Harven, E. (1975). *J. Exp. Med.* **141**, 518–523.
Hämmerling, U., Stackpole, C. W. and Koo, G. (1973). *Methods Cancer Res.* **9**, 255–282.
Heitzmann, H. and Richards, F. M. (1974). *Proc. Natn. Acad. Sci. USA* **71**, 3537–3541.
Hodges, G. M. and Muir, M. D. (1974). *Nature* **247**, 383–385.
Hodges, G. and Muir, M. (1976). In "Principles and Techniques of Scanning Electron Microscopy" (M. A. Hayat, ed.), Van Nostrand Reinhold Co., New York.
Horisberger, M. (1979). *Biol. Cellulare* **36**, 253–258.
Horisberger, M. (1981). In "Scanning Electron Microscopy" (O. Johari, ed.), Vol. II. pp. 9–31. Scanning Electron Microscopy Inc., O'Hare, Ill.
Horisberger, M. and Rosset, J. (1977a). In "Scanning Electron Microscopy" (O.

Johari and R. P. Becker, eds.), Vol. II. pp. 75–81. ITT Research Institute, Chicago, Illinois.
Horisberger, M. and Vonlanthen, M. (1979). *J. Microscopy* **115**, 97–102.
Horisberger, M., Rosset, J. and Bauer, H. (1975). *Experientia* **31**, 1147–1149.
Horisberger, M., Rosset, J. and Bauer, H. (1976). *Arch Microbiol.* **109**, 9–14.
Horisberger, M., Rosset, J. and Vonlanthen, M. (1978b). *Experientia* **34**, 274–276.
Hoyer, L. C., Lee, J. C. and Bucana, C. (1979). *In* "Scanning Electron Microscopy" (O. Johari and R. P. Becker, eds.), Vol. III. pp. 629–636. Scanning Electron Microscopy, Inc., O'Hare, Illinois.
Ito., S., Hattori, A., Ito, S., Ihzumi, T. Sanada, M. and Matsuoka, M. (1978). *Scand. J. Haematol.* **20**, 399–409.
Kent, S. P., Ryan, K. H. and Siegel, A. L. (1978). *J. Histochem. Cytochem.* **26**, 618–21.
Kishida, Y., Olsen, B. R., Berg, R. A. and Prockop, D. J. (1975). *J. Cell Biol.* **64**, 331–339.
Köhler, G. and Milstein, C. (1975). *Nature* **256**, 495–497.
Kronick, P., Campbell, G. and Joseph, K. (1978). *Science* **200**, 1074–1076.
Kumon, H. (1976). *Virology* **74**, 93–103.
Kumon, H. (1981). *Biomed. Res.* **2**, (Suppl.), 41–48.
Kumon, H., Uno, F. and Tawara, J. (1976b). *In* "Scanning Electron Microscopy" (O. Johari, ed.), pp. 85–91. ITT Research Institute, Chicago, Ill.
Lamm, M. E., Koo, G. C., Stackpole, C. W. and Hämmerling, U. (1972). *Proc. Natn. Acad. Sci. USA* **69**, 3732–3736.
Lin, P., Wallach, D. and Tsai, S. (1973). *Proc. Natn. Acad. Sci. USA* **70**, 2492–2496.
Linthicum, D. S. and Sell, S. (1975). *J. Ultrastruc. Res.* **51**, 55–68.
Lo Buglio, A. F., Rinehart, J. J. and Balcerzek, S. P. (1972). *In* "Scanning Electron Microscopy" (O Johari, and I. Corwin, eds.), pp. 313–320. ITT Research Institute, Chicago, Ill.
Lotan, R. (1979). *In* "Scanning Electron Microscopy" (O. Johari and R. P. Becker, eds)., Vol. III. pp. 549–564.
Maher, P. and Molday, R. S. (1979). *J. Supramolec. Struct.* **10**, 61–77.
Malick, L. W. and Wilson, R. B. (1975). *In* "SEM/1975" (O. Johari and I. Corwin, eds.), pp. 259–266. ITT Research Institute, Chicago, Ill.
Mazia, D., Schatten, G. and Sale, W. (1975). *J. Cell Biol.* **66**, 198–200.
McKeever, P. E. and Spicer, S. S. (1979). *In* "Scanning Electron Microscopy" (O. Johari and R. P. Becker, eds.), Vol. III. pp. 601–610. Scanning Electron Microscopy, Inc., O'Hare, Ill.
Miller, M. M., Strader, C. S. Raftery, M. A. and Revel, J. P. (1981). *J. Histochem. Cytochem.* **29**, 1322–1327.
Mishell, B. and Shiigi, S. (1980). Selected Methods in Cellular Immunology. San Francisco, W. Freeman and Co.
Molday, R. S. (1976).*In* "Principles and Techniques of Scanning Electron Microscopy" (M. A. Hayat, ed.), Vol. 5. pp. 53–77. Van Nostrand Reinhold, New York.
Molday, R. S. (1977). *In* "Scanning Electron Microscopy" (O. Johari and R. P. Becker, eds.), Vol. II. pp. 59–74. ITT Research Instutute, Chicago, Ill.
Molday, R. S. (1981). *Biomed. Res.* **2**, (Suppl.), 23–39.
Molday, R. S. and MacKenzie, D. (1982). *J. Immunol. Meth.* **52**, 353–367.
Molday, R. and Maher, P. (1980). *Histochem. J.* **12**, 273–315.

Molday, R. S., Dreyer, W. J., Rembaum, A. and Yen, S. P. S. (1975). *J. Cell Biol.* **64**, 75–88.

Molday, R. S., Jaffe, R. and McMahon, D. (1976). *J. Cell Biol.* **71**, 314–322.

Molday, R. S., Yen, S. P. S. and Rembaum, A. (1977). *Nature* **268**, 437–438.

Murakami, T. (1974). *Arch. Histol. Jap.* **36**, 189–193.

Neauport-Sautes, C. and Silvestre, D. (1972). *Transplantation* **13**, 536–540.

Nemanic, M. K. (1975). *In* "Scanning Electron Microscopy" (O. Johari, and J. Corwin, eds.), pp. 341–349. ITT Research Institute, Chicago, Ill.

Nemanic, M. K. (1979). *In* "Scanning Electron Microscopy" (O. Johari and R. P. Becker, eds.), Vol. III. pp. 537–547. Scanning Electron Microscopy, Inc., O'Hare, Ill.

Nemanic, M. K., Carter, O. P., Pitelka, D. R. and Wofsy, L. (1975). *J. Cell Biol.* **64**, 311–321.

Nicolson, G. (1974). *Int. Rev. Cytol.* **39**, 89–190.

Nicolson, G. L. (1976). *Biochim. Biophys. Acta* **457**, 57–108.

Nicolson, G. L. (1978). *In* "Advanced Techniques in Biological Electron Microscopy (J. K. Koehler, ed.), Vol. II. pp. 1–38. Springer-Verlag, New York.

Ostrand-Rosenberg, S., Edidin, M. and Wetzel, B. (1979). *In* "Scanning Electron Microscopy" (O. Johari and R. P. Becker, eds.), Vol. III. pp. 595–600. Scanning Electron Microscopy, Inc., O'Hare, Ill.

Otto, N., Takamiya, N. and Vogt, A. (1973). *J. Immunol. Meth.* **3**, 137–146.

Peters, K. R., Gschwender, N. H., Haller, W. and Rutter, G. (1976). *In* "Scanning Electron Microscopy" (O. Johari, ed.), Vol. II. pp. 75–84. ITT Research Institute, Chicago, Ill.

Peters, K., Rutter, G., Gschwender, N. H. and Haller, W. (1978). *J. Cell Biol.* **78**, 309–318.

Peters, K. and Richards, F. (1977). *Ann. Rev. Biochem.* **46**, 523–551..

Raff, M. and De Petris, S. (1972). *Fed. Proc.* **32**, 48–54.

Rembaum, A., Yen, S. P. S. and Molday, R. S. (1979). *J. Macromol. Sci. Chem.* **A13**, 603–632.

Revel, J.-P. (1975). *In* "Scanning Electron Microscopy" (O. Johari and J. Corwin, eds.), pp. 687–696. ITT Research Institute, Chicago, Ill.

Roth, J., Bendayan, M. and Orci, L. (1978). *J. Histochem. Cytochem.* **26**, 1074–1081.

Schrevel, J., Kieda, C., Caigneaux, E., Gross, D., Delmatte, F. and Monsiquy, M. (1979). *Biol. Cellulaire* **36**, 259–266.

Schwab, M. E. and Thoenen, H. (1978). *J. Cell Biol.* **77**, 1–13.

Sharon, N. and Lis, H. (1972). *Science* **177**, 949–959.

Singer, S. J. (1959). *Nature* **183**, 1523–1524.

Singer, S. J. and Schick, A. F. (1961). *J. Biochem. Biophys. Cytol.* **9**, 519–537.

Skutelsky, E. and Bayer, E. (1979). *Biol. Cellulaire* **36**, 237–252.

Soni, S. L., Kalnins, V. L. and Haggis, G. H. (1975). *Nature* **255**, 717–719.

Smith, S. B. and Revel, J.-P. (1972). *Devel Biol.* **27**, 434–441.

Springer, E. L., Riggs, J. L. and Hackett, A. J. (1974). *J. Virol.* **14**, 1623–1626.

Sternberger, L. A. (1979). "Immunocytochemistry", 2nd edn., John Wiley, New York.

Suzuki, H., Futaesaku, V. and Mizukira, V. (1979). *Acta Histochem. Cytochem.* **12**, 489.

Temmink, J. H. (1979). *Biol. Cellulaire* **36**, 227–236.

Ternynck, T. and Avrameas, S. (1976). *Ann. Immunol. (Paris)* **127C**, 197–298.

Tokunaga, J., Fujita, T., Hattori, A. and Müller, J. (1976). *In* "Scanning Electron Microscopy" (O. Johari, ed.), Vol. I. pp. 301–310. ITT Research Institute, Chicago, Ill.

Trejdosiewicz, L., Smolira, M. A., Hodges, G. M., Goodman, S. L. and Livingston, A. (1981). *J. Microscopy* **123**, 227–236.

Tsutsui, K., Ichikawa, H., Kumon, H. Uno, F. and Tawara, J. (1978). *J. Electron Microscopy* **27**, 321–3.

Umeda, A. and Amako, K. (1977). *J. Electron Microscopy* **26**, 87–93.

Van Ewijk, W., Coffman, R. C. and Weissman, I. L. (1980). *Histochem. J.* **12**, 349–361.

Weller, N. K. (1974). *J. Cell Biol.* **63**, 699–707.

Wofsy, L. (1979). *In* "Scanning Electron Microscopy" (O. Johari and R. P. Becker, eds.), Vol. III. pp. 565–572. Scanning Electron Microscopy Inc., O'Hare, Ill.

Conjugation Methods and Biotin-avidin Systems

D. M. BOORSMA

I. INTRODUCTION

The immunohistochemical or immunocytochemical demonstration of antigen is achieved by reacting the antigen with its corresponding antibody. This antibody must then be visualized. A wide variety of techniques exists for the visualization of specifically bound antibody all of which make use of labels. These labels are linked to the specific antibody by means of chemical, immunological or other biospecific methods or by combinations of these

IMMUNOCYTOCHEMISTRY 2
ISBN 0 12 140402 1

methods. The linkage of the label to the specific antibody can be performed directly in a chemical manner or in indirect or even multistep procedures.

Labels of different nature have been used throughout the past decades. The main types of labels are: fluorochromes, inert electron dense particles and enzymes. Fluorochromes, of which fluorescein is the most important one, were introduced in 1941 by Coons *et al.* The use of these labels is restricted to the light microscopical level. Inert electron dense particles like ferritin (Singer and Schick, 1961) or colloidal gold (Horisberger and Rosset 1977; Roth *et al.*, 1978) are used exclusively at ultrastructural level (see Roth, this volume). Enzymes were first successfully used as labels in 1966 by Avrameas and Uriel (1966) and by Nakane *et al.* (1966). Enzymes can produce coloured insoluble reaction products which in some cases can be made electron dense and so, when properly chosen, they can be used as markers at both light microscopical and ultrastructural level. This contribution will focus on enzymes as labels for the visualization of specific antibody.

II. METHODS EMPLOYED FOR VISUALISATION OF SPECIFIC ANTIBODY

The methods which can be employed for the visualization of specific antibody using enzymes can be divided in three main types: attachment of enzyme directly to antibodies (A), to *Staphylococcal* protein A (B) or to the biotin-avidin system (C).

A. Attachment of Enzyme Directly to Antibodies

In the first type the enzyme is attached directly to the specific antibody or to a developing antibody (an antibody which is directed against the specific antibody). The linkage between enzyme and antibody is a covalent bond achieved by chemical agents. A variant of this type of visualization makes use of an enzyme-anti-enzyme antibody complex, which is linked to the specific antibody by a so-called bridging antibody. In this technique the enzyme is linked to the antibody by immunological means and not covalently. This variant will not be discussed further in this contribution.

B. Attachment of Enzyme of *Staphylococcal* Protein A

In the second type the enzyme is linked to *Staphylococcal* protein A. Protein A has affinity for the Fc region of a wide variety of IgGs from several species

(Goudswaard *et al.*, 1978; Goding, 1978). Thus it can be reacted with the specific antibody or with the developing antibody. The linkage between enzyme and protein A is a covalent bond achieved by chemical agents.

C. Attachment of Enzyme to the Biotin-avidin System

The third type makes use of the interaction between biotin and avidin. This so-called biotin-avidin system depends on the extremely strong interaction between biotin (a vitamin from the B series) and avidin (a protein from egg white). One of these is attached to the specific antibody or the developing antibody and the other one is attached to the enzyme. Usually biotin is attached to the antibody and avidin is coupled to the enzyme. A variant which seems to gain wide popularity is to attach the biotin to both the antibody and the enzyme and use the avidin as a bridge between these biotinylated proteins.

III. SELECTION OF COMPONENTS

The proteins which are essential in the above methods all have in common one feature: they are detector molecules. In this contribution special attention will be given to the covalent linkage of enzymes to these detector molecules. One should bear in mind that for using the immunohistochemical methods three elements are of great importance, i.e. the choice of the *enzyme*, the *detector molecule* and the *coupling agent*.

A. Enzymes

The suitability of a given enzyme as a marker substance depends on a number of factors. The enzyme should not act on the tissue or cell under investigation. The enzyme must generate a reaction product which is insoluble, which has a clear distinctive colour, and which precipitates directly at the site of production. The enzyme should be stable at room temperature, available in large quantities, preferably commercially, and maintain most of its activity after coupling. Only a few enzymes meet all these requirements and beyond doubt the most important of these is peroxidase isolated from the roots of horseradish (horseradish peroxidase, HRP). Next in importance is the enzyme alkaline phosphatase (APh) from *E. coli* or of calf intestinal origin. Glucose oxidase and lactate dehydrogenase respectively from *Aspergillus niger* and pig muscle and heart are rarely used. Acid phosphatase was the first enzyme to be coupled by Nakane *et al.* (1966) but since then it has scarcely been used.

For HRP there are at least three chromogens which are suitable in immunocytochemical procedures: diaminobenzidin (brown), aminoethyl-carbazole (red) and chloronaphthol (blue). For APh the available chromogens belong, for the greater part, to the azo dyes (Pearse, 1960). The chromogens for the other enzymes are not so easy to handle, therefore they are used rarely in immunocytochemistry.

B. Detector Molecules

Protein A, biotin and avidin can be purchased commercially. Antibodies (IgG), or its fragments (Fab or Fab_2) ideally should be present in the affinity purified form. However, good conjugates can be obtained when the IgG fraction, isolated by ion exchange chromatography or by protein A, from antiserum used as the starting material. Care should be taken that these antibodies or IgG fractions are not contaminated with other proteins, with peptides or with substances containing amino groups, e.g. in buffers. Interference in the coupling reaction of IgG and enzyme would then be likely. These remarks also hold for monoclonal antibodies, which must be in a pure form (Boorsma *et al.*, 1982). Monoclonals from ascites fluid should be separated from albumin by gel chromatography, ion-exchange chromatography or by immunoabsorption. Monoclonals from tissue culture fluid should be isolated by immunoabsorption.

C. Coupling Agents

These agents are generally bifunctional so that one function can react with the enzyme and simultaneously or sequentially the other function can react with the detector molecule, e.g. the antibody, thus forming a bridge between them. The chemical bonds causing this bridge of course must be irreversible and not destroy the biological activity of the enzyme and the antibody. The better the preservation of the biological activities of both components, the better the performance of the conjugates.

IV. COUPLING METHODS FOR ENZYMES AND ANTIBODIES

Methods of coupling can be of different types; there are so-called one-step methods and two-step methods. In the one-step methods, the enzyme, the detector and the coupling agent are mixed. The reaction is allowed to proceed for a defined period of time. Using two-step methods, the first step consists of the activation of the enzyme and/or detector molecule with the coupling agent. In the second step either both activated components are mixed or the activated component is mixed with the other reactant and the coupling reaction is allowed to proceed for a defined period of time.

In general, it can be stated that two-step reactions are easier to control and provide more homogeneous conjugates than one-step reactions. However the complexity of the coupling reaction always leads, after completion of the reaction, to a mixture of reactants, the conjugate being one of them. The appearance of dimers and polymers of both enzyme and detector molecule is a common feature, while the composition of the conjugate is seldom homogeneous. Depending on the coupling method used, the extent to which the reaction has proceeded differs considerably.

A. General Overview

1. *Water Soluble Carbodiimides*

These were the first agents to be used and were applied in one-step procedures. In 1966 Avrameas and Uriel prepared conjugates of HRP with anti-albumin antibody and of HRP with albumin using carbodiimide. Simultaneously Nakane *et al.* (1966) succeeded in coupling acid phosphatase with antibasement membrane antibody using the same agent. Later on, in 1973, Clyne *et al.* applied carbodiimides for the preparation of HRP conjugates. However, they found, like Nakane and Pierce in 1966, that conjugates thus prepared proved to be unstable, losing their biological activity after a couple of days.

2. *p,p'-difluoro-m,m'-dinitrodiphenylsulfone (FNPS)*

FNPS was introduced by Nakane and Pierce (1966) for the preparation of HRP antibody conjugates, in a one-step method. Analysis of the reaction mixture obtained (Nakane and Pierce 1967; Modesto and Pesce, 1971) showed that the yield of the conjugation reaction was very low. The conjugates were polymeric in structure and contained large amounts of polymeric IgG.

3. *Cyanuric Chloride*

This agent was also used in a one-step procedure. It produced active antibody conjugates with HRP, acid phosphatase and glucose oxidase (Avrameas and Lespinats, 1967) but, the yield of the conjugation reaction was low and the HRP conjugate was ineffective for ultrastructural studies (Bouteille and Avrameas, 1967). This suggests a high degree of polymerisation.

4. *Toluene Diisocyanate*

This coupling agent, well known for the production of ferritin antibody complexes (Singer and Schick, 1961), was applied in the study of Clyne *et al.* (1973) for the preparation of HRP labelled antibodies. The method used was a two-step method, the HRP conjugates obtained being of relatively low molecular weight and effective in immunohistochemical detection of antigens. However this method has not found widespread application.

5. *Glutaraldehyde*

This agent is an alpha, omega dialdehyde. Both aldehyde groups are reactive with epsilon amino groups present in lysines of proteins so that almost every protein can be coupled with another protein using glutaraldehyde. Because many enzymes retain their activity after treatment with low concentrations of glutaraldehyde, as do antibodies, this reagent has become very popular for the preparation of antibody enzyme conjugates. Glutaraldehyde can be used both in one-step and in two-step procedures.

Initially when this reagent was introduced (Avrameas, 1969) it was used in a one-step method for the coupling of antibodies to a number of different enzymes like HRP, APh, acid phosphatase, glucose oxidase and tyrosinase. The HRP conjugates formed appeared to be heterogeneous and polymerised (Avrameas, 1969; Avrameas and Ternynck, 1971; Boorsma and Kalsbeek, 1975).

Using a two-step method, glutaraldehyde has been used almost exclusively for the coupling of HRP and antibodies (Avrameas and Ternynck, 1971), and recently by Falini *et al.* (1982), for the coupling of light chains (kappa or lambda) with APh. In both cases, the enzyme is first activated with glutaraldehyde and, after removal of excess coupling agent, the antibody or light chain is added.

With HRP the conjugate obtained is homogeneous but the reaction has a low yield. Because of the mild conditions of preparation this type of conjugate has a high biological activity and is very suitable in immunohistochemical techniques.

6. *Sodium Periodate*

This agent, introduced by Nakane and Kawaoi (1974), is not a true coupling agent because it does not constitute a bridge between two proteins. The coupling reaction takes place in two steps. Periodate can be applied when the enzyme contains a considerable amount of carbohydrate, as carbohydrates are oxidised by periodate (thus is true for HRP). Also glucose oxidase can be coupled to antibodies using periodate (Clark *et al.*, 1982). Controlled oxidation introduces in the carbohydrate moiety a number of aldehyde groups. The enzyme-aldehyde can then react with amino groups in proteins, thus forming a conjugate. For the preparation of HRP antibody conjugates this method is very popular because of its simplicity and the high yield.

7. p-benzoquinone

This bifunctional agent, introduced by Ternynck and Avrameas (1976; 1977) is used in two-step methods. It inserts active groups into enzymes, e.g. HRP, APh, glucose oxidase and β-galactosidase, which can then be reacted with antibodies or Fab fragments. An alternative approach is to activate the antibody or Fab with benzoquinone and subsequently add the enzyme of choice, as addition products are formed mainly via the amino groups. Although it was shown that the conjugates obtained were very suitable for immunocytochemical studies, the method has not been commonly applied. This may be due to the fact that the *p*-benzoquinone batches are not well standardized, giving results with low reproducibility (Avrameas, personal communication, 1980).

8. N-succinimidyl 3-(2-pyridyldithio)propionate (SPDP)

This agent, introduced by Carlson *et al.* (1978), is heterobifunctional and must be applied in two-step methods. Using SPDP, both proteins must separately be substituted with 2-pyridyl disulfide structures which must be reduced in one of the proteins creating thiolgroups. The reaction between the 2-pyridyl disulfide structure and the thiol group is then started by mixing both substituted components. SPDP can theoretically be applied to almost all enzymes used in immunocytochemistry. It seemed possible to use SPDP to prepare defined HRP antibody conjugates with varying properties as to molecular size and antibody/enzyme ratio (Nilsson *et al.*, 1981). Unfortunately the HRP-antibody conjugates were not tested in immunohistochemistry.

B. Discussion on the Most Commonly used Methods

In immunocytochemistry HRP antibody conjugates are used most frequently. In general two methods are applied: the two-step glutaraldehyde method and the periodate method. For the preparation of APh antibody conjugates, the one-step glutaraldehyde method is generally used. Therefore these three reactions will be discussed in detail.

1. *The One-step Glutaraldehyde Method*

This method, mostly used for APh, is not now used for preparation of HRP antibody conjugates. The preparation of APh-antibody conjugates, which can be used in immunocytochemistry, e.g. for double-labeling experiments, has been described by Avrameas (1969) and Engvall and Perlmann (1971). Ford *et al.* (1978) analysed extensively the APh-antibody conjugates prepared by using different (0·08%–0·4%) glutaraldehyde concentrations. They found that glutaraldehyde concentrations of 0·07%–0·17% and glutaraldehyde/protein ratios of 0·5–1·0 μmol glutaraldehyde per mg protein gave conjugates which were suitable for immunocytochemistry. Almost all antibody was polymerised with a substantial amount of APh, however homopolymers were expected to be present.

2. *The Two-Step Glutaraldehyde Method*

This method for coupling HRP and antibodies begins with the activation of HRP by glutaraldehyde. A large excess of this reagent is added to HRP which must be in a very pure form. The purity of HRP is expressed in the purity number (RZ). This RZ (a ratio of the optical density at 403 nm versus 280 nm) must be approximately 3·0. HRP with RZ values below 2·8 is contaminated with non-HRP impurities. As pure HRP contains only a few lysine groups, in which the epsilon amino groups are for the most part blocked by allylisothiocyanate, the monomeric form dominates after reaction with glutaraldehyde, dimerisation only occurs to a limited extent and polymerisation not at all (Boorsma and Streefkerk, 1976a). Non-HRP impurities, present in HRP with lower RZ values, contain more free epsilon amino groups and give, therefore, rise to varying degrees of polymerisation. Gel chromatography of HRP of different RZ, activated with glutaraldehyde, shows that the lower the RZ the more extended the polymerisation (Fig. 1). The activated polymers may well be more reactive towards antibody but they definitely have lower enzyme activities which will result in HRP conjugates of poor quality.

Excess glutaraldehyde must be removed after the activation has been completed. This can be done easily by gel chromatography (e.g. Sephadex G-25 fine or by a different gel, e.g. Ultrogel AcA-44). Using Ultrogel monomeric and dimeric activated HRP moieties can be separated from each other, the excess glutaraldehyde is removed simultaneously. The isolated

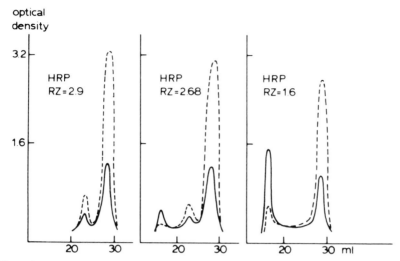

FIG. 1. Gel chromatography on Ultrogel AcA-44 (55 × 1 cm, flow rate 7 ml/cm²/h) of GA-activated HRP; left: HRP, RZ 2·9, middle: HRP, RZ 2·68, right: HRP, RZ 1·6. ———OD 280; ----OD 403.

and activated HRP is then added in eight-fold excess to the antibody preparation. After stopping the reaction, the reaction mixture can be analysed readily, using for example, gel chromatography, as shown in Figs 2 (left) and 3b. These Figs represent elution patterns of a two-step glutaraldehyde prepared HRP antibody conjugate. From this pattern it can be seen that the

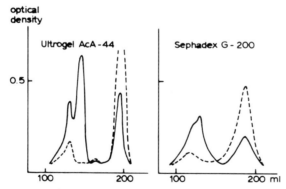

FIG. 2. Gel chromatography on Ultrogel AcA-44 (left) and Sephadex G-200 (right) of HRP conjugate prepared by the two step glutaraldehyde method. Column: 100 × 2 cm, flow rate 3·2 ml/cm²/h.

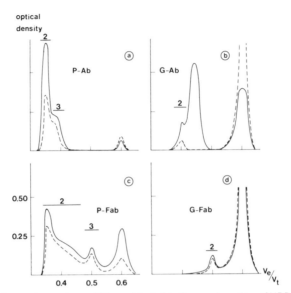

FIG. 3. Gel chromatography on Ultrogel AcA-44 after conjugation of HRP to antibodies (Ab) and Fab fragments of antibodies (Fab) by the periodate (P-) and the two-step glutaraldehyde (G-) methods. Elution patterns: (a) P-conjugation of Ab:P-Ab; (b) G-conjugation of Ab:G-Ab; (c) P-conjugation of Fab':P-Fab; (d) G-conjugation of Fab':G-Fab. The numbers P-Ab-2, P-Ab-3 refer to pools of fractions (conjugates) studied (number 1 refers to the non-chromatographed, "crude" reaction mixtures). These symbols are also used in Fig. 5. Optical density (of protein) at 280 nm (continuous line) and (of HRP) at 403 nm (broken line) plotted against the Ve:Vt ratio (Ve: elution volume; Vt: total volume).

yield of the conjugation reaction is rather disappointing, only about 5% HRP coupled with about 30% antibody, so that HRP antibody conjugate (the first peak, Fig. 2) is only a minor component in the reaction mixture. The bulk of both antibody and HRP has not reacted, these being the second and third peak respectively. The elution volume at which the conjugate elutes strongly indicates that this HRP antibody complex is about 200 000 daltons, which suggests that the complex is composed of one HRP and one antibody. This is confirmed by the optical density ratio of 403 nm to 280 nm, which indicates a molar ratio of 1:1 for HRP to antibody. These data show that this HRP antibody conjugate is both homogeneous and defined. Extensive studies (Boorsma *et al.*, 1976) have shown that both the antibody and the enzyme activity have been well preserved.

It can be expected that the above considerations also apply to the coupling of HRP to Fab fragments of antibodies. Data from the literature (Avrameas and Ternynck, 1971; Boorsma and Streefkerk, 1979) show that HRP-Fab conjugates can be prepared and are defined with a low molecular weight (about 80 000 daltons). The conjugation yield however is low (Fig. 3d), with large amounts of HRP and Fab remaining unreacted. Where the conjugate is prepared from activated HRP which contains also dimeric HRP, it is impossible to separate this dimeric HRP from the HRP-Fab conjugate. A seemingly high yield is obtained after gel chromatography (Avrameas, 1972) but in fact contamination with dimeric HRP occurs. The small molecular dimensions of the HRP-Fab conjugate have distinct advantages in applications where penetration of the conjugate is needed in tissues or cells (Avrameas and Ternynck, 1971).

3. The Periodate Method

This method is very suitable for coupling of HRP to antibodies. Since HRP is covered by a carbohydrate shell which constitutes about 20% of the total enzyme molecule, it is very easy to introduce aldehyde groups onto the outer surface of HRP by controlled oxidation of the glycol groups abundantly present in the carbohydrate moiety using periodate.

This method also requires HRP of high quality (RZ 3·0). HRP of lower RZ has both lower amounts of carbohydrates and many more free amino groups. These facts can, after activation of HRP, cause extensive self coupling by polymerization. Oxidation of HRP with periodate can be performed in bicarbonate solution (Nakane and Kawaoi, 1974) or in distilled water (Wilson and Nakane, 1978). As can be seen from Fig. 4, the introduction of aldehyde groups gives for the most part monomeric HRP, together with some dimers of HRP, but polymerisation of HRP does not occur

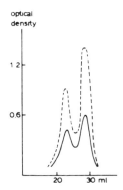

FIG. 4. Gel chromatography on Ultrogel AcA-44 (55 × 1 cm, flow rate 7 ml/cm²/h) of HRP-aldehyde activated with periodate.

(Boorsma and Streefkerk, 1976a). The latter is due to the well documented paucity of free amino groups in HRP. Excess periodate can be removed by dialysis (Wilson and Nakane, 1978) or it can be neutralised by ethylene glycol and subsequent gel filtration (Boorsma and Streefkerk, 1979).

HRP-aldehyde and antibody can then react at high pH (9·0–9·5) and at a relatively high rate due to the high level of activation of HRP. Within two hours both components have reacted almost to completion (Boorsma and Streefkerk, 1976b; 1979). Variation of the ratio of HRP to antibody can give conjugates with different molar ratios, most optimal ratio usually being considered to be 2·2 HRP versus 1 antibody. This will give rise to a conjugate with a molar ratio of 2.

Analysis of such a conjugate by gel chromatography shows (Fig. 3a) that it is largely polymerized, with a molecular weight over 400 000 daltons (Boorsma and Streefkerk, 1976b). A minor fraction of the conjugate is of lower molecular weight (200 000–400 000 daltons). Other studies have revealed that the polymerized conjugate is a heterogeneous mixture of complexes with molecular weights up to several million daltons. This periodate method provides HRP conjugates which retain both enzyme and antibody activities (Boorsma et al., 1976; Boorsma and Streefkerk, 1979), though to a lesser extent than those prepared according to the two-step glutaraldehyde method.

Preparation of Fab-HRP conjugate using the periodate method provides, with high yield, a conjugate of heterogeneous composition. Under the conditions given by Wilson and Nakane (1978), i.e. a molar HRP/Fab ratio of 0·8 in the reaction mixture, the conjugate obtained worked well in immunohistochemistry (Boorsma and Streefkerk, 1979). Analysis with gel chromatography (Fig. 3c) revealed three components: a large fraction of high molecular weight consisting of polymerized conjugate, a minor fraction of conjugate with a molecular weight of 80 000 consisting of one HRP and one Fab, and finally a moiety consisting of a mixture of unreacted HRP and Fab.

V. ISOLATION OF HORSERADISH PEROXIDASE CONJUGATES

From the foregoing considerations it is obvious that conjugation of enzymes with antibody or with Fab fragments, in general, is a complex reaction. Because some of the reactants may interfere with the reaction between the antigen and the labelled antibody it is recommended that the conjugate component should be isolated from the other constituents of the reaction mixture. Three different methods which can be used for the isolation of HRP conjugates will be described.

A. Ammonium Sulphate Precipitation

Using this method, free uncoupled HRP can be removed from antibody and antibody-enzyme complexes. The method is not suitable for the separation of uncoupled and HRP-coupled antibody. In addition Fab-HRP conjugates can not be purified from uncoupled HRP and Fab using this method (Avrameas and Ternynck, 1971; Boorsma and Kalsbeek, 1975).

B. Gel Chromatography

The choice of an appropriate gel enables the isolation of conjugates of very different characteristics. For HRP antibody conjugates, Sephadex G-200, Ultrogel AcA-44 or Sephacryl S-200 are mainly used (Avrameas, 1969; Avrameas and Ternynck, 1971; Boorsma and Kalsbeek, 1975; Boorsma and Streefkerk, 1976b; 1979; Wilson and Nakane, 1978). These gels can also be applied for the isolation of Fab-HRP conjugates (Avrameas, 1972; Boorsma and Streefkerk, 1979). The effectiveness of gels for separation of components with molecular weights close to each other can differ considerably, as illustrated in Fig. 2. In addition, conjugates of antibodies with other enzymes can be isolated choosing the appropriate gels.

C. Affinity Chromatography

Because gel filtration methods are on a small scale and are time consuming, an attempt was made to use affinity methods for purification. Boorsma and Streefkerk (1978) described the isolation of HRP antibody conjugates by using sequential chromatography on protein A-Sepharose and con A-Sepharose. A crude reaction mixture of HRP antibody conjugate, prepared with the two-step glutaraldehyde method, was applied to a protein A-Sepharose column. All IgG molecules, coupled with HRP or uncoupled, adhered to the column whilst all the free HRP passed through. The bound fraction was eluted and applied to a con A-Sepharose column. All HRP-containing moieties adhered to the con A. IgG which was not coupled to HRP passed through. The almost pure HRP antibody fraction could then be eluted from the column. This method of purification is on a large scale and can be performed within a couple of hours. Since the affinity of protein A differs for IgG from different species, the method has its limitations (Boorsma and Streefkerk, 1978). HRP Fab conjugates cannot be purified in this manner, because Fab fragments lack the Fc portion which is essential for binding to protein A.

VI. APPLICATIONS

Enzyme-antibody or enzyme-Fab conjugates can be applied in all fields of immunohistochemistry and immunocytochemistry. As HRP is the enzyme which is used in most cases it is important to review briefly the applicability of the two types of HRP antibody conjugates (i.e. prepared by the two-step glutaraldehyde method and by the periodate method). Although both types of conjugates can equally well be applied, it is generally accepted that different fields have different requirements (Boorsma and Streefkerk, 1979). Moreover both direct and indirect methods can be used for the detection of antigen. The antigen can be present, e.g. in unfixed cryostat sections as deposited immune complexes, as a surface antigen on cells in tissue or in smears or suspensions, and in formalin fixed paraffin embedded tissue. From comparative studies using the direct method (Boorsma and Streefkerk, 1979) it was clear that HRP antibody conjugates, prepared with

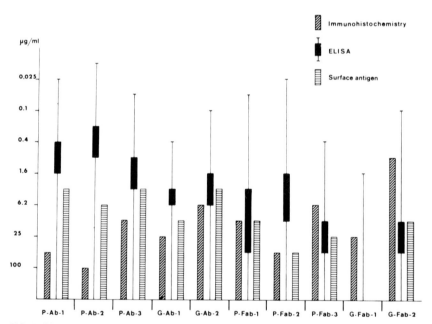

FIG. 5. Diagrammatic representation of test results with the different HRP-conjugates. For nomenclature of conjugates see legend of Fig. 3. Vertical axis: concentration of conjugates in μg/ml. For each conjugate the concentration giving positive reactions for each application is shown as follows: left bar, tissue immunohistochemistry (skin of LE patients); straight line and black bar, direct and indirect ELISA (reaction of human IgG and detection of anti-pencillin antibodies, respectively); right bar, surface antigen detection (Ig on human lymphocytes).

the two-step glutaraldehyde method, were the conjugates of choice for the demonstration of antigen which requires penetration of the conjugate into the tissue section. Antigens exposed on the outer surfaces of cells or tissues can be detected equally well with HRP antibody conjugates prepared with the periodate method (Fig. 5). It is likely that these differences will be less marked when using indirect methods.

VII. COUPLING OF ENZYMES TO *STAPHYLOCOCCAL* PROTEIN A

The affinity of protein A for the Fc portion of a wide range of immuno-globulins, mainly IgGs, from various mammalian species, makes it a powerful tool in immunology (Goudswaard *et al.*, 1978; Goding, 1978). Protein A can be conjugated to enzymes using established coupling methods. It can then be used in immunohistochemistry to detect IgG or to detect antibody to a particular antigen or even developing antibodies.

Enzymes which have been used for coupling to protein A are HRP and APh. Protein A-APh conjugates (Engvall, 1978), though potentially useful, have not yet been used in immunohistochemistry. These conjugates were prepared using glutaraldehyde as coupling agent both in one-step and two-step methods.

Protein A-HRP conjugates were first prepared by Dubois-Dalcq *et al.* (1977) and later on by Celio *et al.* (1979), Trost *et al.* (1980a; 1980b), Falini *et al.* (1980) and by Nygren and Hansson (1981). Most authors used the periodate method to couple HRP to protein A (Nakane and Kawaoi, 1974), or else the modified periodate method (Wilson and Nakane, 1978). Nygren and Hansson (1981) compared three methods of coupling HRP with protein A, i.e. the periodate method, the two-step glutaraldehyde method (Avrameas and Ternynck 1971) and the method using benzoquinone (Ternynck and Avrameas, 1977). From the above studies it appeared that HRP-protein A conjugates prepared with the periodate method were of a relatively high molecular weight, as found from analysis by gel chromatography. The HRP: protein A ratio in the reaction mixture varied in the different studies from 2 to 1. The conjugates obtained were generally excluded in the void volume of the columns used. Conjugates prepared using glutaraldehyde or benzoquinone as coupling agents were of lower molecular weights but required a larger excess of HRP (for their preparation) and the reaction between both components was never complete. Uncoupled HRP and/or protein A remained in the reaction mixture after the reaction had been terminated (Nygren and Hansson, 1981). Unfortunately the latter conjugates were not tested in immunohistochemistry.

The HRP-protein A conjugates, which were prepared with the periodate method, were shown to be suitable in a variety of immunohistochemical situations, i.e. the detection of particular antigens by means of specific antibodies (Dubois-Dalcq *et al.*, 1977; Celio *et al.*, 1979), detection of specific (auto) antibodies to tissue components (Trost *et al.*, 1980a), detection of extracellularly bound immunoglobulins or immune complexes in unfixed cryostat sections of skin tissue (Trost *et al.*, 1980b), and detection of intracellularly located antigens in paraffin-embedded tissue (Falini *et al.*, 1980). Comparative studies of methods using protein A-HRP conjugates with other immunohistochemical methods showed that the protein A conjugates could compete very well with enzyme conjugates used in other methods.

However it must be kept in mind that protein A recognizes, besides the specific antibodies, IgGs which are endogeneously located in the tissue under investigation.

VIII. BIOTIN-AVIDIN METHODS AND THEIR APPLICATIONS

The introduction of the biotin-avidin interaction in immunoenzyme procedures seems to be an important extension in this field (Guesdon *et al.*, 1979). The interaction of biotin with avidin is extremely strong. The affinity constant between both components is in the order of 10^{15} M^{-1} (Bayer and Wilchek, 1978).

As mentioned earlier, the principle, on which the use of the interaction in immunohistochemistry and immunocytochemistry is based, is the attachment of biotin to the specific or the developing antibody and that avidin is attached to the enzyme.

A. Biotin Labelling of Antibodies

Introduction of biotin into antibodies requires activated biotin which is achieved by conversion to biotinyl-N-hydroxysuccinimide (BNHS) (Jasiewicz *et al.*, 1976). BNHS reacts easily with primary amino groups in antibodies. The reaction of BNHS with antibody has been optimized by Guesdon *et al.* (1979), who also formulated optimal BNHS substitutions of antibodies. As a result, both the antigen binding capacity and the avidin binding ability of the substituted antibody are as high as possible.

It is clear that biotin can be introduced in other proteins like enzymes, using the same principles. Reaction circumstances have been studied extensively by Guesdon *et al.* (1979).

B. Linkage of Avidin and Enzyme

Avidin and enzyme can be attached to each other using three main types of binding: covalent coupling of avidin and enzyme; attachment of avidin to biotinylated enzyme via sequential use, and preformation of avidin-biotinylated enzyme complex (ABC).

1. Covalent Coupling of Avidin and Enzyme

In general, the same methods used for enzyme-antibody coupling can be employed for the preparation of avidin-enzyme conjugates. Up to now HRP has been the most commonly used marker enzyme. Avidin-HRP was prepared by Guesdon *et al.* (1979) with the two-step glutaraldehyde method employing a two-fold excess of activated HRP to avidin.

Boorsma (1980) compared the two-step glutaraldehyde method and a number of modifications of the periodate method (Wilson and Nakane, 1978) for the preparation and use of avidin-HRP conjugates. From these studies it became clear that again the coupling efficiency of the two-step glutaraldehyde method was low. The conjugate obtained was of small molecular dimensions. One HRP was conjugated to one avidin which made this conjugate very suitable for immunohistochemistry and immunocyto-chemistry (Guesdon *et al.*, 1979; Boorsma, 1980).

With HRP-aldehyde, prepared by low concentrations of periodate, administered in equimolar amounts to avidin, avidin-HRP conjugates were prepared with a good coupling efficiency. The conjugates consisted partly of polymerized avidin-HRP complexes, but reasonable amounts of monomeric avidin-HRP could also be obtained. The monomeric avidin-HRP prepared with the periodate method was almost equally as suitable as the two step-glutaraldehyde preparation for immunohistochemistry (Boorsma, 1980).

2. Attachment of Avidin to Biotinylated Enzyme

This method is commonly called the bridged avidin-biotin method. The preparation of biotin-labelled enzyme is in fact based on the same principles as are described for biotin-antibody labelling. All enzymes, which are suitable for immunohistochemistry, can be used and easily labelled with biotin. For a number of enzymes the reaction circumstances have been studied by Guesdon *et al.* (1979) with respect to both degree of biotin labelling and retention of enzyme activity.

The bridged avidin-biotin method was found to be somewhat more sensitive in detecting antigen than the method using covalently coupled avidin-enzyme conjugates (Guesdon *et al.*, 1979).

3. *Preformation of Avidin-Biotinylated Enzyme Complex* (ABC)

The ABC will be formed when avidin is incubated at room temperature for 15 min with biotinylated HRP in a molar ratio of about 4:1 (Hsu *et al.*, 1981). ABC is applied to the tissue immediately following the incubation with biotinylated antibody. The method is reported to be even more sensitive than the so-called unlabelled antibody (PAP) procedures (Hsu *et al.*, 1981; Hsu and Raine, 1981).

C. Applications

The biotin-avidin system has been used in various immunohistochemical and immunocytochemical studies. It was used for the detection of intracytoplasmic immunoglobulins in mouse lymphoid cells (Guesdon *et al.*, 1979). Warnke and Levy (1980) and Wood and Warnke (1981) used the interaction for the detection of surface determinants on human and mouse lymphoid cells, applying monoclonal antibodies as the first step. *In-vivo* fixed, extracellularly-located IgG or immune complexes in human skin were equally well detected using the biotin-avidin system as when using HRP labelled antibodies (Boorsma, 1980). Hsu *et al.* (1981) and Hsu and Raine (1981) demonstrated IgG containing plasma cells in human tissue using the ABC method.

However a potential problem arises from the application of the biotin-avidin system because many tissues contain endogenous biotin, which is a widely distributed vitamin. Wood and Warnke (1981) recognized this problem and found that suppression of endogenous biotin activity was achieved readily by incubating the tissue with excess avidin followed by excess biotin preceding the regular immunological incubations.

IX. REFERENCES

Avrameas, S. (1969). *Immunochemistry* **6**, 43–52.
Avrameas, S. (1972). *Histochem. J.* **4**, 321–330.
Avrameas, S. and Lespinats, G. (1967). *C.R. Acad. Sci. Paris* **265**, 1149–1153.
Avrameas, S. and Ternynck, T. (1971). *Immunochemistry* **8**, 1175–1179.
Avrameas, S. and Uriel, J. (1966). *C.R. Acad. Sci. Paris* **262**, 2543–2545.
Bayer, E. A. and Wilchek, M. (1978). *Trends Biochem. Sci.* 257–259.
Boorsma, D. M. (1980). "4th Int. Congress Immunol. Paris", 19.6.05 (Abstr.).
Boorsma, D. M. and Kalsbeek, G. L. (1975). *J. Histochem. Cytochem.* **23**, 200–207.
Boorsma, D. M. and Streefkerk, J. G. (1976a). *Prot. Biol. Fluids* **24**, 795–802.
Boorsma, D. M. and Streefkerk, J. G. (1976b). *J. Histochem. Cytochem.* **24**, 481–486.

Boorsma, D. M. and Streefkerk, J. G. (1978). *In* "Immunofluorescence and Related Staining Techniques" (W. Knapp, K. Holubar and G. Wick, eds.), pp. 225–235. Elsevier/North Holland Biomedical Press, Amsterdam.

Boorsma, D. M. and Streefkerk, J. G. (1979). *J. Immunol. Methods* **30**, 245–255.

Boorsma, D. M., Streefkerk, J. G. and Kors, N. (1976). *J. Histochem. Cytochem.* **24**, 1017–1025.

Boorsma, D. M., Cuello, A. C. and VanLeeuwen, F. W. (1982). *J. Histochem. Cytochem.* **30**, 1211–1216.

Bouteille, M. and Avrameas, S. (1967). *C.R. Acad. Sci. Paris* **265**, 2097–2099.

Carlsson, J., Drevin, H. and Axén, R. (1978). *Biochem. J.* **173**, 723–737.

Celio, M. R., Lutz, H., Binz, H, and Fey, H. (1979). *J. Histochem. Cytochem.* **27**, 691–693.

Clark, C. A., Downs, E. C. and Primus, F. J. (1982). *J. Histochem. Cytochem.* **30**, 27–34.

Clyne, D. H., Norris, S. H., Modesto, R. P., Pesce, A. J. and Pollak, V. E. (1973). *J. Histochem. Cytochem.* **21**, 233–240.

Coons, A. H., Creech, H. J. and Jones, R. N. (1941). *Proc. Soc. Exp. Biol. Med.* **47**, 200–202.

Dubois-Dalcq, M., McFarland, H. and McFarlin, D. (1977). *J. Histochem. Cytochem.* **25**, 1201–1206.

Engvall, E. (1978). *Scand. J. Immunol.* **8** (Suppl. 7), 25–31.

Engvall, E. and Perlmann, P. (1971). *Immunochemistry* **8**, 871–874.

Falini, B., Tabilio, A., Zuccaccia, M. and Martelli, M. F. (1980). *J. Immunol. Methods* **39**, 111–120.

Falini, B., DeSolas, I., Halverson, C., Parker, J. W. and Taylor, C. R. (1982). *J. Histochem. Cytochem.* **30**, 21–26.

Ford, D. J., Radin, R. Pesce, A. J. (1978). *Immunochemistry* **15**, 237–243.

Goding, J. W. (1978). *J. Immunol. Methods* **20**, 241–253.

Goudswaard, J., VanderDonk, J. A., Noordzij, A., VanDam, R. H. and Vaerman, J. P. (1978). *Scand. J. Immunol.* **8**, 21–28.

Guesdon, J. L., Ternynck, T. and Avrameas, S. (1979). *J. Histochem. Cytochem.* **27**, 1131–1139.

Horisberger, M. and Rosset, J. (1977). *J. Histochem. Cytochem.* **25**, 295–305.

Hsu, S. M. and Raine, L. (1981). *J. Histochem. Cytochem.* **29**, 1349–1353.

Hsu, S. M., Raine, L. and Fanger, H. (1981). *J. Histochem. Cytochem.* **29**, 577–580.

Jasiewicz, M. L., Schoenberg, D. R. and Mueller, G. C. (1976). *Exp. Cell Res.* **100**, 213–217.

Modesto, R. R. and Pesce, A. J. (1971). *Biochim. Biophys. Acta* **229**, 384–395.

Nakane, P. K. and Pierce, G. B., Jr (1966). *J. Histochem. Cytochem.* **14**, 929–931.

Nakane, P. K. and Pierce, G. B., Jr (1967). *J. Cell Biol.* **33**, 307–318.

Nakane, P. K. and Kawaoi, A. (1974). *J. Histochem. Cytochem.* **22**, 1084–1091.

Nakane, P. K., Ram, J. S. and Pierce, G. B., Jr (1966). *J. Histochem. Cytochem.* **14**, 789–790.

Nilsson, P., Bergquist, N. R. and Grundy, M. S. (1981). *J. Immunol. Methods* **41**, 81–93.

Nygren, H. and Hansson, H. A. (1981). *J. Histochem. Cytochem.* **29**, 266–270.

Pearse, A. G. E. (1961). "Histochemistry—Theoretical and Applied", Little, Brown and Co, Boston MA.

Roth, J., Bendayan, M. and Orci, L. (1978). *J. Histochem. Cytochem.* **26**, 1074–1081.

Singer, S. J. and Schick, A. F. (1961). *J. Biophys. Biochem. Cytol.* **9**, 519–537.
Ternynck, T. and Avrameas, S. (1976). *Ann. Immunol. (Inst. Pasteur)* **127C**, 197–208.
Ternynck, T. and Avrameas, S. (1977). *Immunochemistry* **14**, 767–774.
Trost, T. H. Weil, H. P., Pullmann, H. and Steigleder, G. K. (1980a). *Klin. Wochenschr.* **58**, 475–478.
Trost, T. H., Weil, H. P., Noack, M., Pullmann, H. and Steigleder, G. K. (1980b). *J. Cutaneous Path.* **7**, 227–235.
Warnke, R. and Levy, R. (1980). *J. Histochem. Cytochem.* **28**, 771–776.
Wilson, M. B. and Nakane, P. K. (1978). *In* "Immunofluorescence and Related Staining Techniques" (W. Knapp, K. Holubar and G. Wick, eds), pp. 215–224. Elsevier/North Holland Biomedical Press, Amsterdam.
Wood, G. S. and Warnke, R. (1981). *J. Histochem. Cytochem.* **29**, 1196–1204.

X. APPENDIX. COUPLING PROCEDURES

A. *Two-Step Glutaraldehyde Method (Avrameas and Ternynck, 1971)*

1. Dissolve 10 mg HRP (RZ = 3) in 0·2 ml of a 0·1 M phosphate buffer, pH 6·8, containing 1·25% glutaraldehyde.
2. After 18 h at room temperature this solution is filtrated on a Sephadex G-25 fine column, equilibrated with 0·15 M NaCl, to remove the excess glutaraldehyde.
3. The fractions containing the activated (brown) HRP are pooled and concentrated to ±10 mg/ml; subsequently 5 mg/ml antibody in 0·15 M NaCl is added.
4. The pH is raised to 9·0–9·5 with sodium carbonate-bicarbonate buffer (pH 9·5).
5. After 24 h at 4 °C 0·1 ml of a 0·2 M lysine-HCl solution is added.
6. After 2 h at 4 °C the solution is dialysed against PBS (pH 7·2).

Instead of step (2) it is possible to isolate the monomeric activated HRP fractions by column chromatography on Ultrogel AcA-44 and to pool the fractions with monomeric activated HRP. In this way activated dimers of HRP are excluded from the conjugation reaction.

A possible step (7) could be removal of uncoupled antibody and HRP, by e.g. gel chromatography.

B. *Periodate Method (Wilson and Nakane, 1978)*

1. Dissolve 4 mg HRP (RZ = 3) in distilled water.
2. Add 0·2 ml freshly prepared solution of 0·1 M NaIO$_4$ and mix gently for 20 min. The colour turns from brown to dark green.
3. The solution is subsequently dialysed against 0·001 M sodium acetate buffer pH 4·4 at 4 °C for 20 h.
4. The pH of the HRP solution is then raised to 9·5 by the addition of 20 μl 0·2 M sodium carbonate-bicarbonate buffer (pH 9·5) and immediately 8 mg antibody is added in 1 ml 0·01 M sodium carbonate-bicarbonate buffer (pH 9·5). Mix gently and let the reaction proceed for 2 h at room temperature.
5. Subsequently add 0·1 ml of a freshly prepared solution of sodium borohydride (4 mg/ml distilled water). Leave this mixture for 2 h at 4 °C.
6. The HRP conjugate is thereafter chromatographed (on e.g. Ultrogel or Sephacryl) or dialysed against PBS.

For minor modifications see: Boorsma and Streefkerk (1979).

Production of Monoclonal Antibodies for Immunocytochemical Use

D. Y. MASON, J. L. CORDELL and K. A. F. PULFORD

I. INTRODUCTION

All immunocytochemical techniques depend upon the successful completion of a series of sequential steps. First, tissue or cell samples are prepared for staining. An antibody, or a sequence of antibodies, is then applied. Finally the antibody label (e.g. a fluorochrome or enzyme) is revealed and examined.

If these steps are considered as links in a chain (and if it is remembered that chains are only as strong as their weakest links) it will be apparent that optimal immunocytochemical labelling can only be achieved if each of these steps is performed as efficiently as possible. The most effective techniques for the preservation of tissue antigenicity and the best antibody sandwich reagents can never compensate for inefficient fluorescence microscopy or sub-optimal enzyme substrates. Similarly all efforts expended in optimising the antibody label will be wasted if tissue has been processed in such a way that antigens are masked or destroyed.

IMMUNOCYTOCHEMISTRY 2
ISBN 0 12 140402 1

In the past 20 years there have been notable advances relating to each of these sequential steps. In particular much more is now known concerning those technical aspects of the preparation and handling of tissues which influence the preservation of antigenic reactivity. Significant advances have also been made in the techniques for labelling antibodies and for constructing multi-layer sandwiches which optimise labelling efficiency. However, in contrast to the advances in these areas, there has until very recently been little progress in one of the crucial stages in the immunocytochemical chain, i.e. in the production of the primary antibodies which enable individual antigens to be recognised. The primary antibodies used by all immunocytochemists until recently were produced by techniques which have been available for many decades, e.g. immunisation with purified antigen, collection of blood samples, isolation of serum etc.

In 1975 Köhler and Milstein described a fundamentally new approach to the production of antibodies. This procedure involved obtaining from an immunised animal not blood but lymphoid cells, and then growing these cells in tissue culture, so that antibody produced by individual lymphoid clones could be harvested. These immune cell clones, which are immortalised by hybridisation with an established tissue culture cell line, produce monoclonal antibodies which are superior in a number of respects to conventional polyclonal antisera. These advantages in the context of immunocytochemistry are listed in Table I.

In the present chapter the techniques used in the authors' laboratories for the production of monoclonal antibodies for immunocytochemical use are described, together with a discussion of the comparative properties of monoclonal and polyclonal antibodies as immunocytochemical reagents.

II. PRODUCTION OF MONOCLONAL ANTIBODIES

The account which follows describes the techniques used in the authors' laboratory when producing monoclonal antibodies for immunocytochemical applications. These methods are identical in principle to techniques used in many other laboratories with the exception that particular emphasis is placed (for reasons explained below) upon the use of immunocytochemical techniques in the initial detection of monoclonal antibodies and in the subsequent monitoring of their production.

A. Principle of the Hybridoma Technique

The principle behind the production of monoclonal antibodies by the cell fusion technique is illustrated schematically in Fig. 1. In essence spleen cells

TABLE I
Properties of monoclonal antibodies compared with polyclonal antisera.

Characteristic	Monoclonal antibodies	Polyclonal antisera
Range of antigens detectable	Potentially very large	Limited to those antigenic constituents which can be purified to homogeneity.
Purity of antibody preparations	Most, if not all, of the antibody produced by a hybridoma cell line is specific for a single antigen.	Only a minor proportion (rarely more than 20%) of the antibody present in an immune serum is specific for the immunising antigen. The remainder consists either of antibodies produced by the animal in the past in response to previous antigenic stimuli, or of antibody against contaminating antigens present in the immunising preparation. It is often difficult even to detect the presence of antibodies of the latter type, let alone to remove them.
Homogeneity of antibody	Monoclonal antibodies are highly homogeneous since each hybridoma cell line produces multiple copies of a single immunoglobulin molecule, all of which possess the same antigen-binding site. In consequence they usually react with only one molecule, and with a single antigenic determinant (epitope) on the molecule.[a]	The antibodies in a polyclonal antiserum which are specific for the immunising antigen are usually highly heterogeneous (in terms of antigen-binding affinity) and are also usually directed against a number of different epitopes on the immunising antigen.
Availability of antibodies	Monoclonal antibodies can be produced in potentially unlimited amounts. In consequence laboratories throughout the world can perform immunocytochemical investigations using identical reagents.	The preparation of satisfactory polyclonal reagents involves considerable expenditure of time and effort, not only in the initial purification of the immunising antigen, but also in subsequent specificity testing and elimination of unwanted antibodies from the antiserum. At the end of these procedures the amount of available antibody is often small and on occasion it is impossible to prepare further antibody of similar quality in other animals (or even on re-bleeding the original animal). These considerations severely restrict the availability of polyclonal antibodies of valuable specificity on a wide scale.

[a] See text (see Section V) for a more extensive discussion of the specificity of monoclonal antibodies compared to polyclonal antisera.

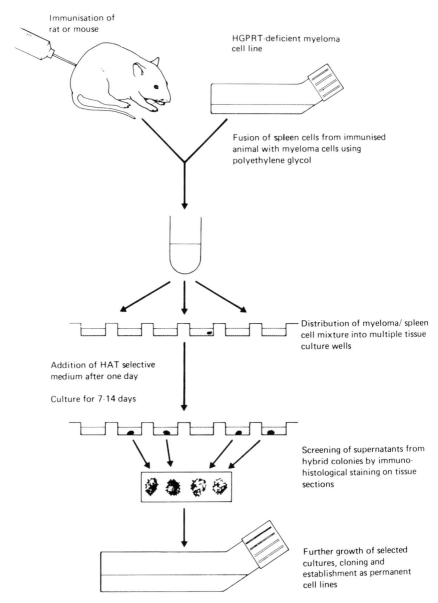

FIG. 1. Schematic illustration of the techniques used in the authors' laboratory when producing monoclonal antibodies for immunocytochemical use.

from an immunised Balb/c mouse are incubated with cells from a myeloma cell line (of murine origin) in the presence of polyethylene glycol. This latter agent promotes the creation of hybrid cells which contain chromosomes from each parent cell.

Cell fusion is a relatively inefficient process (i.e. only a small minority of cells undergo fusion) and it is therefore necessary to give hybrid cells a growth advantage over their neighbours, in order to prevent them being overwhelmed by the vigorously growing myeloma cell line. This is achieved by using a mutant version of the myeloma cell line which lacks an enzyme present on the "salvage" DNA synthesis pathway. The only other pathway for DNA synthesis is the *de novo* or endogenous synthetic pathway and this may be blocked using aminopterin. Under these culture conditions the myeloma cell line will die unless it can acquire an intact salvage pathway by fusion with "wild-type" spleen cells. By this strategy the small numbers of spleen cell/myeloma cell hybrids acquire an absolute growth advantage over the myeloma cell line. Non-fused spleen cells, although they possess a normal salvage pathway for DNA synthesis, do not in practice persist for more than a few days under *in vitro* culture conditions, with the consequence that the only actively proliferating cells which remain after several days culture are hybrids formed between splenic lymphoid cells and the myeloma cell line.

Once spleen cells and the myeloma cells have been exposed to the fusing agent, the mixture is plated out into multiple tissue culture wells so as to increase the chances of isolating individual clones of desired specificity. Cultures which secrete antibody are subjected to further cloning procedures so as to ensure that any cell line which is finally established in culture represents the progeny of a single hybrid cell.

B. Choice of Antigen

Before describing the technical aspects of producing monoclonal antibodies for immunocytochemical use, a brief comment should be made on the choice of antigenic preparation against which the antibodies are to be raised. There are fundamentally two strategies: on the one hand, a recognised antigenic tissue constituent which has been purified to a greater or lesser degree may be used: alternatively, a "blind" approach may be adopted, in which there is no prior knowledge as to the nature (or even existence) of the antigen in the immunising preparation. This latter approach is epitomised by the numerous attempts made in different laboratories to produce monoclonal antibodies reactive with tissue-specific or malignancy-specific antigenic determinants.

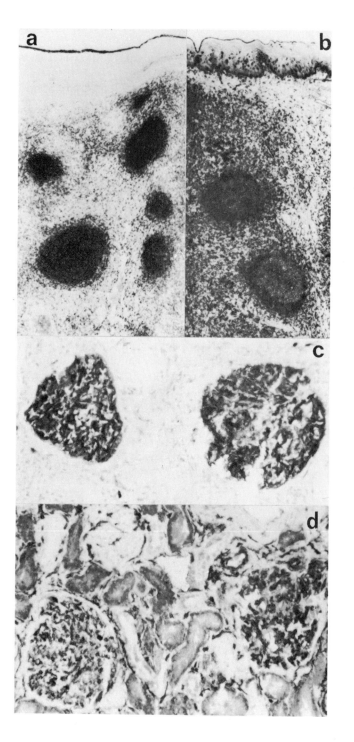

1. Production of Monoclonal Antibodies against purified antigens

This approach is open to the criticism that antibodies against such antigens may already be prepared in the form of polyclonal antisera. However, as discussed at the end of this chapter (see Section V), even optimal polyclonal antisera tend to be inferior, in terms of unwanted background staining, to monoclonal antibodies. Furthermore the production of monoclonal antibodies against a purified antigen may be justified when the antigen in question shows molecular heterogeneity. One example in this context is provided by human immunoglobulin, since satisfactory antibodies recognising either subclass-specific determinants (e.g. those present on IgA1 and IgA2) or "hidden" determinants (e.g. which will allow free light chains to be distinguished from bound light chains) are difficult to prepare. Further examples which would repay study with monoclonal rather than polyclonal antibodies include carcinoembryonic antigen (since this molecule, as conventionally purified, shares some antigenic determinants with molecules on non-epithelial cells such as neutrophils), or neuropeptides (since shared sequences may be found between different molecules).

There is also an argument for preparing monoclonal rather than polyclonal antibodies against already recognised antigenic molecules, since this avoids the complexity of taking the antigen through final purification steps to homogeneity. One example from the authors' laboratory is provided by the human complement (C3b) receptor. Rabbit antisera specific for this constituent can be prepared by immunisation with crude preparations followed by extensive absorption to remove unwanted specificities (Gerdes *et al.*, 1980). The need for absorption could be avoided by immunising a mouse with a similar crude preparation, performing a cell fusion and then selecting a clone secreting monoclonal antibody specific for C3b receptor (Fig. 2) among

---

FIG. 2. Illustration of the way in which immunoperoxidase staining of tissue sections may be used during the primary screening of hybridoma cultures to identify new monoclonal antibodies and to establish their probable specificity. A cell fusion experiment was performed using spleen cells from a mouse previously immunised with a lymphocyte membrane extract enriched for complement (C3b) receptors. Culture supernatants were screened by immunoperoxidase staining of cryostat tonsil sections. One culture was identified which gave strong staining of lymphoid follicles (a), suggesting that it was directed against C3b receptor. Supernatants from other cultures gave superficially similar reactions (b). However, on closer inspection it was evident that these latter antibodies reacted with scattered cells in the T cell areas and also with cells in the tonsillar squamous epithelium. This pattern is typical of antibodies directed against HLA-DR (Ia-like) antigens. Staining of kidney cryostat sections provided additional evidence for the specificities of these two antibodies: the putative anti-C3b receptor reacted only with renal glomeruli (c); whilst the probable anti-HLA-DR antibodies gave a more extensive reaction pattern, in which glomeruli, tubules and interstitial cells were labelled (d) (reproduced with permission from Naiem *et al.*, 1982).

those producing antibodies of unrelated specificity (Gerdes *et al.*, 1982; Naiem *et al.*, 1982).

2. *Production of Monoclonal Antibodies Against Unknown Antigens*

One of the most important consequences of the development of techniques for producing monoclonal antibodies is the possibility of raising antibodies against previously undetected antigens. A substantial number of such new cellular constituents have already been described, including markers associated with different stages of T and B cell maturation, or with different lymphocyte subsets. However it should be noted that the development of such new reagents usually entails much laborious screening in order to eliminate antibodies of unwanted specificity. Furthermore certain antigens are "immunodominant" with the result that after a time successive cell fusions tend to yield repeatedly the same antibodies, rather than those of new specificity. In the case of human lymphoid cells certain antigens such as HLA-DR (Ia-like antigen) or the leucocyte-common molecule show a tendency to dominate the immune response, whilst in the context of T lymphoid subpopulations it appears to be considerably easier to raise monoclonal antibodies against T suppressor cells than against T helper calls.

These factors should be borne in mind by immunocytochemists considering embarking on monoclonal antibody production. It may be added that even if a new monoclonal antibody specific for a previously unknown antigenic molecule is produced by the "blind" approach there may be problems in interpreting its immunocytochemical reactions, since the functions of the target molecule against which it is directed are unknown. In contrast, if the antibody has been raised against a cell constituent the nature and/or function of which is already known (e.g. a hormone receptor etc.), the conceptual framework against which to interpret its immunocytochemical reactions already exists.

C. Technical Details

1. *Immunisation Schedule*

When producing antibodies against *soluble antigens* Balb/c mice are given 2–3 intraperitoneal injections 10 days apart of 50 μg of antigen emulsified with an equal volume of Freund's complete adjuvant. Approximately one week after these immunisations, mice are usually bled (from the retro-orbital plexus or from the tail) and the serum tested by an immunocytochemical technique over a range of dilutions (starting at 1 in 100). If this analysis reveals the presence of antibody (usually detectable at a dilution of at least 1 in a 1000), the mouse is boosted intravenously with 200 μg of antigen in saline 3 days prior to fusion. When difficulty is encountered in performing an intravenous injection, the antigen may be administered by intraperitoneal injection with satisfactory results.

When immunising with *whole cells*, an injection of approximately 5×10^6 cells in serum free medium is given intraperitoneally, followed by a repeat injection after 10 days. The animal does not receive further immunisations until 3 days before a fusion is planned, when 5×10^6 cells are injected intravenously (or, if necessary, intraperitoneally).

2. Preparation for Cell Fusion

A number of preliminary steps should be performed prior to a planned fusion.

(a) Preparation of NS1 cells

The murine myeloma cell line used in the authors' laboratory (and in many other laboratories involved in monoclonal antibody production) is the line known as P3-NS1/1Ag4·1 (usually referred to as NS1). This line is maintained in culture in bicarbonate buffered RPMI 1640 medium supplemented with foetal calf serum, glutamine and antibiotics (see Tables II and III). It grows best at cell densities of between 7×10^4/ml and 1×10^6/ml. In order to prepare NS1 cells for fusion 60 ml of medium should be seeded with these cells at a density of 7×10^4/ml three days before fusion. This should yield ample numbers of healthy rapidly dividing cells by the day of fusion.

(b) Preparation of feeder cell layers

The efficiency of hybridoma growth appears to be enhanced by plating out the cell fusion mixture onto a layer of feeder cells. In the authors' laboratory, feeder cells are prepared by taking the spleen from a normal Balb/c mouse (as for a cell fusion, see below). The cells are then plated out on the day prior to fusion at a concentration of 1×10^6 cells/ml in RPMI medium C (see Table III), dispensing 0·5 ml to each well when using Costar plates, and 50 μl/well when using Microtitre plates. The principal reason for preparing feeder layers 24 h before fusion is to ensure that they are not contaminated. In other laboratories alternative feeder layers have been used, the most common being peritoneal macrophages prepared by washing out the peritoneal cavity of a Balb/c mouse with phosphate buffered saline and distributing the washings in fusion plates as for spleen feeders. The peritoneal cells from one mouse should be sufficient for a single microtitre culture plate, whilst 2·5 times this amount is required for each Costar plate.

TABLE II

Reagents required for monoclonal antibody production.

Reagent	Source	Catalogue Number
RPMI 1640 medium (bicarbonate buffered)	Gibco	041-1875
RPMI 1640 medium (Hepes buffered)	Gibco	041-2400
Foetal calf Serum	Gibco	011-6290
Glutamine (200 mM)	Gibco	043-5030
P3-NS1/1Ag 4·1 murine myeloma cell line	Flow	05-503
Penicillin, streptomycin	Glaxo	M9377
Polyethylene glycol (M.wt. 1500)	BDH	29575
Hypoxanthine, aminopterin, thymidine (50× concentrated)	Gibco	
Pristane	ICN Pharmaceuticals	
Peroxidase-conjugated rabbit anti-mouse Ig	Dako	P161
Diaminobenzidine tetrahydrochloride	Sigma	D5637
Bovine serum albumin (fraction V)	Miles Laboratories	81-003-2
Dimethyl sulphoxide	BDH	10323

(c) Preparation of media

Details of media used for the cell fusion procedure and during subsequent cell culture are given in Table II.

(d) Sterilisation of instruments

The following instruments should be sterilised by autoclaving: fine forceps, fine scissors, blunt scissors, blunt forceps, curved forceps.

2. Cell Fusion Procedure

The immunised animal is killed by cervical dislocation and then liberally soaked in ethanol so as to minimise the risk of contamination from the skin. The spleen is removed aseptically and placed in 5 ml of medium A in a sterile petri dish. Spleen from immunised animals are sometimes surrounded by

TABLE III

Media and solutions.

Tissue culture Media

Medium A: Hepes buffered RPMI 1640 medium containing 10% foetal calf serum, glutamine[a] (20 mM), penicillin 100 U/ml and streptomycin (100 mg/ml)

Medium B: As for medium A, without foetal calf serum

Medium C: Bicarbonate Buffered RPMI 1640 medium containing foetal calf serum, glutamine and antibiotics (as for Medium A)

Medium D: ("HAT" medium) as for medium A, with the addition of hypoxanthine (10^{-4} M), aminopterin (4×10^{-7} M) and thymidine ($1 \cdot 6 \times 10^{-5}$ M). A concentrated stock solution (50×) of these three additives can be obtained commercially; see Table II

Freezing medium: Medium D containing 10% DMSO

Buffers

Tris buffered saline: Dissolve Tris base at 0·5 M in distilled water. Adjust pH to 7·6 with concentrated HCl. Dilute this stock solution 10× in 0·15 M saline to produce Tris buffered saline

Phosphate buffered saline: Dissolve the following ingredients in 1 l of distilled water: 8 g NaCl; 2 g KCl; 11·5 g Na_2HPO_4; 2 g K_2HPO_4. Measure pH and adjust if necessary to 7·2

Miscellaneous solutions

Tris ammonium chloride (for lysing RBC): Add 10 ml of 0·17 M Tris to 90 ml of 0·16 M ammonium chloride and adjust pH to 7·2

Trypan blue: 0·2% in saline

Polyethylene glycol: Weight out 1 g of polyethylene glycol and sterilise by autoclaving. While the solution is still melted add 1 ml of medium B, and then store at room temperature.

Diaminobenzidine/H_2O_2 solution (peroxidase substrate): This solution should be prepared shortly before use. Dissolve diaminobenzidine in Tris buffered saline at a concentration of 0·6 mg/ml. Immediately before use add concentrated H_2O_2 to yield a final concentration of 0·01%

---

[a] Glutamine at this concentration is unstable and fresh glutamine should be added from concentrated stock (see Table II) at least once a week to stored media.

---

fibrous or connective adhesions, particularly when several intraperitoneal injections have been given. These should be carefully cut away and the spleen washed in the surrounding medium. The spleen is then transferred to 5 ml of medium A in a second sterile petri dish and cut into two halves . A cell suspension is prepared by holding the spleen with blunt forceps and gently teasing cells from the capsule into the medium using curved forceps. Cell clumps are dispersed by aspiration in a Pasteur pipette and the cell suspension is then transferred into a 15 ml sterile plastic centrifuge tube. The cells are then spun down at 300×g for 5 min at room temperature.

(a) Cell counting
The cell pellet after centrifugation is resuspended in 5 ml of medium A and an aliquot is removed for counting. For this procedure 0·4 ml of medium A and 0·5 ml of Tris ammonium chloride solution (Table III) are put into a small glass tube. A 0·1 ml aliquot of the spleen cell suspension is added and the mixture is incubated for 8 min at 37 °C. A small volume (e.g. 100 μl) of the above solution is diluted with an equal volume of 0·2% trypan blue and viable cells are counted in a standard haemocytometer. Dead cells will take up the trypan blue dye and appear dark blue or black, whilst living cells will be free of dye. Note that the cell concentration, as counted in the haemocytometer should be multiplied by 20 to give the concentration of the spleen cell suspension.

The same cell counting procedure should then be applied to the NS1 myeloma cells to determine the number of viable cells. The volume of NS1 cell suspension to be added to the spleen cell at the time of fusion is then calculated, based on a desired ratio of one viable NS1 cell for every 10 viable spleen cells. This ratio has been found to be most successful in the authors' laboratory, although it may be noted that other workers have used NS1 spleen cell ratios of 1:5, 1:2 or even 1:1.

(b) Cell fusion
The calculated volume of NS1 cell suspension is added to the spleen cell suspension in a 50 ml plastic centrifuge tube, and the cells are then mixed by gently swirling the tube. The cells are spun down as before and the supernatant discarded. The cell pellet is resuspended in 10 ml of medium B (serum free medium). The cells are spun down as before and as much supernatant as possible is removed. The cell pellet is then disrupted by gently tapping the tube on the bench.

The tube containing the disrupted pellet of cells is now placed in a 37 °C waterbath and polyethylene glycol (Table II) is added slowly from a glass pipette over the course of 1 min, while gently stirring the cell suspension with the pipette tip. This reagent should be made up as a 50% solution and a volume of 1·2 ml is appropriate for 1×10^8 spleen cells. It is important to add the polyethylene glycol at a steady rate over the course of the minute, in order to minimise the risk of cell lysis. At the completion of this period, 2 ml of medium B are added with stirring in the same way, again taking care to keep the rate of addition as constant as possible. Finally 8 ml of medium B are added at a constant rate with gentle stirring over the course of 3 min. After adding medium B small cell clumps will be visible to the naked eye.

However no attempt should be made to break up these clumps by pipetting.

The cells are pelleted by spinning at 300 g for 5 min. The supernatant is then discarded and the cell pellet resuspended very gently in medium C using a pipette, taking care to avoid disrupting cell clumps. Sufficient medium should be added to yield a concentration of spleen cells of approximately 2×10^6/ml.

(c) Plating out the cell suspension following fusion

Cell suspensions are usually plated out in the authors' laboratory into Costar tissue culture plates (Table IV) each of which carry 24 wells. The wells will already contain 0·5 ml of culture medium (from the previously added feeder cells) and a further 0·5 ml of fused cell suspension is added. If the fusion has been performed using 1×10^8 spleen cells it will be possible to plate out the cell suspension in four Costar plates (a total of 96 wells).

An alternative to the use of this type of plate involves distributing the cell suspension into flat bottomed Microtitre plates (Table IV) each of which contains 96 wells. A volume of 50 μl of cell suspension is added to each well, and one fusion will typically involve plating out in six microtitre plates.

Plating out the fusion in Microtitre plates offers the advantage that it increases the chances of obtaining single colonies in individual tissue culture wells. In contrast when distributing the cell fusion suspension into the larger 2 ml wells of Costar plates there is a greater likelihood that multiple colonies will appear in individual wells, leading to a risk of clonal competition, i.e. of

TABLE IV

Disposable items required for tissue culture and immunochemistry.

Item	Source
Tissue culture	
"Cluster" tissue culture plates (24 × 2 ml wells)	Costar
Microtitre tissue culture plates	Nuhc (Gibco)
Tissue culture flasks	Nunc (Gibco)
Pipettes, centrifuge tubes	Falcon
Immunocytochemistry	
Multispot microscope slides	Hendley (Oakwood Hill Industrial Estate, Loughton, Essex, UK)
Pipette tips	Jencons

a non-producing clone overgrowing a clone which is secreting a potentially valuable antibody. Set against this consideration however is the fact that use of Microtitre plates entails having to screen a larger number of tissue culture supernatants (since the cell suspension is distributed into 6 times more tissue culture wells when using Microtitre plates). Screening of tissue culture supernatants by immunohistological or immunocytochemical techniques (see below) is not readily performed on very large numbers of samples and for this reason the use of Costar plates is generally preferred by us.

(d) Culture of cells following fusion

The tissue culture plates into which the spleen cell/NS1 cell suspension has been distributed, are placed in a humidified 37 °C incubator containing an atmosphere supplemented with 5% CO_2. In order to minimise the risk of bacterial or fungal infection we routinely place culture plates into transparent plastic containers which have a few small perforations in their walls to enable equilibration with the atmosphere in the incubator. Such containers may conveniently be prepared from commercially available sandwich boxes.

On the day following fusion the medium in each well is supplemented with an equal volume of medium C, supplemented with double strength HAT (i.e. stock HAT concentrate diluted 25 times; see Table II). The plates are then left undisturbed in the incubator for at least 3 days. Following a successful fusion it should be possible to identify small colonies by inspecting the plates with an inverted microscope after a period of 4–10 days. It is worth noting that colonies often show a tendency to grow towards the periphery of tissue culture wells. Typical colonies, once they are well established, are unmistakable. However confusion is sometimes caused by "pseudo-colonies" which may mistakenly be identified as true hybrid cell clones. These colonies, which probably represent the transient growth of a mixture of spleen cell types, have a more heterogeneous appearance than true colonies, in that they include cells with a variety of morphological appearances, including fibroblast-like cells. In contrast, true colonies consist of a relatively monomorphic collection of medium sized rounded cells.

(e) Primary screening of cell fusion

Cell fusion experiments can usually be screened for antibody production after a period of 7–14 days. Supernatant is removed from all cultures in which hybrid colonies are of sufficient size to be readily visible to the naked eye. When using Costar plates 1 ml of supernatant is removed from each well containing colonies and replaced by an equal volume of fresh medium D.

Details of the methods used for screening fusion experiments are given below (see section II. D).

Once colonies secreting antibody of potential value have been identified the cells are allowed to reach confluence and are then transferred from their original wells to four 2 ml wells on a Costar plate. Following further growth they are transferred to small (25 cm^2) tissue culture flasks. At this stage many workers used feeder spleen cells, but we often find this to be unnecessary, except on the infrequent occasions when a cell line proves difficult to maintain in culture.

Once cells have been transferred to tissue culture flasks their supernatant medium should be retested, to check that antibody is still being secreted. Provided that this is so, the cells may then be cloned by limiting dilution (see below) in order to ensure that the cells being grown in each culture represent the product of single hybrid cell rather than a mixture of cell clones. It is also advisable at this stage to freeze down an aliquot of the uncloned cells (see below for technique). This minimises the risk that valuable clones will be lost subsequently as a result of infection or overgrowth by a non-producing cell line.

(f) Freezing of hybrid cells

Cells for freezing must be in an actively dividing state. This is indicated by the fact that the medium changes from pink to orange/yellow, by the presence of many "doublets" of dividing cells and by the presence of a refractile "halo" around most cells. They are washed once in medium D and then resuspended in freezing medium (see Table III) at a concentration of $2\text{--}5\times10^6/\text{ml}$.

The cell suspension is distributed in 1 ml aliquots into freezing vials and frozen in a constant rate freezing machine (at a rate of 1 °C per min.) or by placing them in the top of a liquid nitrogen store using the adaptor provided for this purpose.

When recovering cells from the frozen state vials should be warmed as rapidly as possible to 37 °C and the cells then washed immediately in an excess of tissue culture medium before suspending them at a density of $1\text{--}2\times10^5/\text{ml}$ in small tissue culture flasks.

(g) Cloning of hybrid cultures

On the day prior to cloning spleen feeder cells should be prepared (see above) and distributed into a number of Microtitre plates. On the day of cloning the hybrid cell culture is checked to ensure that it is dividing rapidly (see above). Cells are then counted and plated out in Microtitre plates at such a density that each well receives (on average) a single cell.

Plates were then incubated as described above. It is wise to check cloning plates microscopically within 4–5 days in order to ensure that wells do not contain more than a single clone. Movement of the plates from the incubator should be carried out with care, since otherwise single clones may be disrupted leading to the appearance of small "daughter" clones, giving the misleading impression that the well contains the product of more than one hybrid cell. When the diameter of a clone is approximately 0·5 that of the well which it occupies its supernatant can be tested for antibody. Positive clones are then transferred from the Microtitre wells to single 2 ml wells on Costar plates. When these wells reach confluence, their contents are transferred to four different wells on a Costar plate and then finally onto 25 cm^2 tissue culture flasks. At this stage it is advisable to freeze down multiple vials of individual clones in order to insure against subsequent loss of the cell line.

(h) Long-term culture and production of ascites
Cloned hybridoma cell lines will usually continue to proliferate and to secrete antibody into the culture supernatant for an indefinite period. In consequence, antibody can be produced by continuously maintaining a small number of cells in culture. In practice, however, it is usually more convenient to grow up a large number of cells, to harvest the tissue culture supernatant, and then to freeze the cells for possible regrowth in the future.

Tissue culture supernatant from a hybridoma will usually contain antibody at a concentration of approximately 5–10 μg per ml. For immunocytochemical labelling this concentration of antibody should be more than sufficient and indeed it may be possible to dilute the supernatant at least 5 fold without loss of staining intensity. Many laboratories however prefer to establish hybridomas as ascitic tumors in Balb/c mice. The titre of antibody obtained in this material is usually 100 to 1000 fold higher than that found in tissue culture supernatant. However it should be noted that not only is there often no strong reason for preparing antibody in the form of ascites (since this reagent will usually be diluted for use, to an antibody concentration equivalent to that found in supernatant) but there may indeed be a positive disadvantage, in that non-specific serum immunoglobulins from the host animal may give rise to unwanted background staining. It also occasionally happens that a hybrid cell line loses its capacity to secrete a desired antibody following its establishment as an ascitic tumour.

Hybridomas from which antibody is being harvested for immunocytochemical staining should therefore only be established as ascitic tumours if there is a clear reason for doing so, e.g. when a large amount of antibody is required, or if it is intended to purify antibody for direct conjugation. The production of ascites involves priming Balb/c mice by an intra-peritoneal injection of 0·5 ml of pristane (tetramethyl pentadecane). A period of at least 10 days should be allowed to elapse following priming before injecting 1×10^6 hybridoma cells intraperitoneally. The effect of the priming appears to be permanent so that cells may be injected at any interval after the initial pristane injection.

Ascitic tumours will develop in the majority of mice within 10–21 days although there is considerable variation from one animal to another in the rapidity with which this occurs. Once ascites begins to develop, the mouse should be observed regularly since it is unlikely to survive for more than a few days. Ascites fluid may be tapped by inserting a large bore disposable needle (which will allow subsequent re-tapping of more ascitic fluid) or the animal may be sacrificed, the peritoneal cavity opened and ascitic fluid aspirated. The ascitic fluid contains numerous tumor cells which should be removed by centrifugation. They may, if necessary, be injected into new pristane-primed mice (in which case they often lead to the accumulation of ascites at a more rapid rate than previously), or they may be frozen for subsequent recovery.

It may be noted that occasionally ascites do not develop following intraperitoneal injection of cells into primed animals. In a few animals a solid tumour will develop in its place. The serum from these animals usually containes a high titre of monoclonal antibody. If necessary the cells from such solid hybridomas may be dissociated and injected into new primed recipients, whereupon they will frequently grow satisfactorily as an ascitic tumour.

D. Assays for Antibody Production

A wide variety of techniques have been described for the detection of antibodies in hybridoma tissue culture supernatants. These include radio-active binding assays, haemagglutination techniques and cytotoxicity procedures. However in the authors' laboratory the majority of cell fusions are screened by immunocytochemical staining on tissue sections (Naiem *et al.*, 1982) or, more rarely, on cell smears. The same techniques are used subsequently to test for continued antibody production by cell lines, both before and after cloning. The major alternative screening technique used in the authors' laboratory (particularly when testing for antibodies reactive with purified soluble antigens) is the ELISA procedure, details of which may be found in many publications.

The use of immunocytochemical methods as the principal procedure for primary screening and for the monitoring of continued antibody production is dictated by two considerations. First, there is a strong argument for testing antibodies during their production by the same technique by which they will subsequently be used. Not infrequently monoclonal antibodies react strongly by one procedure (e.g. radioimmunoassay) but do not give satisfactory results when tested in an unrelated system. Since the authors' laboratory produces monoclonal antibodies principally for detecting antigens in tissue sections or cell smears it is logical to detect these antibodies in the first place by an immunocytochemical technique.

The second argument for monitoring the production of monoclonal antibodies by immunocytochemical techniques is that these procedures are inherently much more informative than are most of the alternative screening methods, such as, radioactive binding assays or haemagglutination procedures. The latter methods usually provide only a single numerical value for each positive supernatant(e.g. radioactive counts bound, haemagglutination titre etc) without any indication of the constituents to which the antibody is binding. In contrast the immunohistological reaction pattern of a monoclonal antibody on a tissue section represents a highly characteristic "fingerprint" which often allows the specificity of a new antibody to be identified at the primary screening stage. This is illustrated in Fig. 2 which shows the way in which a hybridoma secreting a monoclonal antibody against human C3b receptor was initially detected on the basis of its characteristic immunohistological labelling of lymphoid tissue (i.e. staining of B cell follicles and of scattered cells in the interfollicular areas; Fig. 2). The same cell fusion also produced a number of colonies secreting antibodies which labelled B cell follicles, which would not readily have been distinguishable from the anti-complement receptor antibody if tested by a technique such as a radioactive binding assay against lymphoid cells in suspension. On closer inspection however it was apparent that their labelling pattern differed clearly from that of the putative anti-C3b receptor antibody (see Fig. 2), being typical of that given by anti-HLA-DR antibodies. Immunohistological testing of tissue culture supernatants from this fusion on human kidney sections provided further evidence that the first antibody was specific for C3b receptor, since this reagent labelled only glomeruli (see Fig. 2). In contrast the other antibodies gave more extensive labelling (Fig. 2), in keeping with their anti-HLA-DR reactivity.

1. Screening on Tissue Sections

Tissue culture supernatant may be tested against either paraffin embedded or cryostat sections. In making this choice it should be appreciated that many human tissue antigenic constituents do not survive fixation and embedding procedures, so that the chances of detecting antibodies will be maximal if cryostat sections are used. On the other hand, if it is desired to produce monoclonal antibodies suitable for immunohistological analysis of routine surgical biopsy material there is a strong argument for carrying out the initial screening upon sections prepared from this type of tissue.

Paraffin sections are prepared for immunohistological screening by routine procedures. *Cryostat sections* should be cut (at a thickness of approximately 8 μm) from snap frozen tissue which has been stored at -80 °C or below, picked up on gelatin coated slides and then left to dry overnight at room temperature. It is convenient to use multitest slides (Table IV) since this reduces the number of slides required for screening a cell fusion experiment (Fig. 3). After fixation in acetone for 10 min at room temperature the slides are allowed to dry and are then either used immediately or alternatively are wrapped in aluminium foil and stored at -20 °C for future use.

The first stage in the immunohistological staining procedure involves the application of undiluted culture supernatant to tissue sections. When using paraffin sections these should previously have been dewaxed and hydrated by conventional procedures. Cryostat sections which have been stored before use should be allowed to reach room temperature before unwrapping (in order to prevent condensation forming). Tissue culture supernatants may be applied directly to dry cryostat sections without preliminary washing.

Sections are incubated with tissue culture supernatants at room temperature for 60 min in a humidified chamber. Slides are washed in Tris buffered saline (TBS; see Table III) for 5 min and excess moisture is then removed from around each section before adding 100 μl of peroxidase-conjugated anti-mouse Ig (Table II). The optimal working concentration of this reagent is approximately 1:50, and it is advisable to add normal human serum (at a final concentration of 5%) in order to block the cross-reactivity of the antibody against human immunoglobulin.

Slides are incubated for 30 min at room temperature and are then washed in TBS before flooding with the diaminobenzidine/H_2O_2 peroxidase substrate solution (see Table III). After 5–10 min incubation the peroxidase substrate reaction is stopped by washing in tap water and slides are then counterstained with haematoxylin, dehydrated in alcohol and mounted in DPX.

2. Screening on Cell Smears

As an alternative to immunohistological screening supernatants may be tested on air dried cell smears. This technique is of value when screening large numbers of tissue culture supernatants, since cell smears are more rapidly prepared than are tissue sections. Air dried smears have not been used widely in the past in screening for monoclonal antibodies directed against human cellular constituents, the majority of laboratories preferring to use binding assays or indirect immunofluorescent techniques. It is now apparent however that many cellular antigens (both cytoplasmic and surface membrane located) survive drying and fixation (Moir *et al.*, 1983). This fact, coupled with the practical advantages of staining cell smears (i.e. the

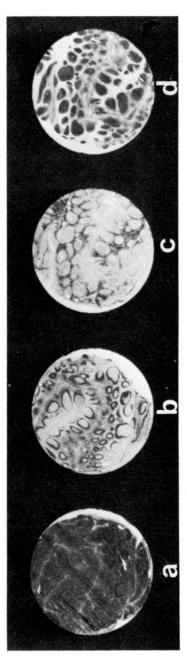

FIG. 3. The immunohistological analysis of multiple cell culture supernatant during the primary screening of hybridoma cultures is facilitated by the use of multi-test slides (see Table IV). In this illustration a slide carrying four cryostat tonsil sections is shown stained with monoclonal antibodies against (a) leucocyte common antigen, (b) IgD, (c) T cells and (d) C3b receptor (the water-repellent masking between each section appears black in this illustration since the slide was backlit for photography). The reaction patterns of the four antibodies are clearly distinguishable, even when inspected without a microscope (reproduced with permission from Naiem, *et al.*, 1982).

possibility of simultaneously visualising intra-cellular and cell surface antigens, and the ability to store slides for long periods for both before and after staining) accounts for the preference in the authors' laboratory for this approach to detecting antibodies reactive with cells extracted from tissue.

The suspension of cells to be used for screening is adjusted to a concentration of 2×10^8 per ml in phosphate buffered saline (PBS; see Table III) which is free of calcium, magnesium and protein. An equal volume of 0·025% glutaraldehyde in PBS is then added dropwise to the cell suspension, the mixture being agitated during the addition of this reagent. We have found this concentration of fixative to preserve a wide range of antigens detectable by monoclonal antibodies.

After 5 min at room temperature fixation is terminated by the addition of a four-fold excess (by volume) of PBS containing 10% bovine serum albumin. Cells are then washed, resuspended in PBS containing 5% bovine serum albumin and passed through a 25 gauge syringe needle. After a final wash the cells are resuspended at a concentration of 5×10^6 cells/ml in PBS containing 10% bovine serum albumin. This mixture is then either frozen in 1 ml aliquots at -20 °C or used immediately to prepare cell smears for screening.

When preparing cell smears the cell suspension is washed in protein-free medium and resuspended at a concentration of 5×10^5 cells/ml. An aliquot of 10 μl of this suspension is placed in each well of a multispot slide and the slides are then allowed to dry overnight at room temperature for use the following day.

Alternative techniques may be used for preparing cell smears for immunocytochemical testing of culture supernatants. Aliquots of unfixed cells in suspension may be dispensed onto multispot slides or they may be cytocentrifuged onto slides. Cell smears prepared by either means are air-dried and stored frozen at -20 °C until required for screening. At this point they are thawed, fixed in acetone at room temperature for 10 min and then air-dried again. The use of cytocentrifuged cells offers the advantage that cell morphology is preserved much better than in preparations produced by allowing drops of cell suspensions to air dry onto slides. However the time required for the preparation of cytocentrifuged preparations means that they are not suitable for the screening of large numbers of supernatants.

Immunocytochemical staining of cell smears, however prepared, is performed by the indirect immunoperoxidase technique described above.

3. Storage of Antibody-containing Supernatants

The majority of monoclonal antibodies present in tissue culture supernatant are stable for long periods when stored at 4 °C (after the addition of 0·02%

sodium azide). For longer-term storage supernatants should be kept at −20 °C or below. Repeated freezing and thawing of supernatants should be avoided.

III. PROBLEMS IN MONOCLONAL ANTIBODY PRODUCTION

A number of problems may be encountered when producing monoclonal antibodies for immunocytochemical use.

A. Infection with Yeast or Bacteria

Any infected cultures should be discarded to avoid the risk of contamination spreading to other culture plates or flasks. Attempts should also be made to identify the source of infection, e.g. by checking the stock bottles of culture medium and foetal calf serum.

B. Fungal Infection

Occasionally an isolated well in a tissue culture plate will be found to contain a fungal colony. It may be possible to abort this type of infection by removing the contents of the contaminated well and swabbing it out with alcohol. However the plate should be inspected at intervals subsequently to make sure the infection has not spread to other wells.

C. Mycoplasma Infection

This organism represents a serious (although not particularly common) infection risk which can threaten the success of monoclonal antibody production. These organisms cannot be visualised without specialised staining techniques; furthermore NS1 cells infected with mycoplasma often appear to grow normally and may undergo fusion with spleen cells with the consequence that mycoplasma infection is not immediately suspected. The most characteristic signs of the presence of mycoplasma are the failure of hybrids to grow following an apparently successful fusion, or the spontaneous death of hybrid colonies following an initial period of active growth.

  If mycoplasma infection is suspected the most effective treatment involves discarding all cell cultures and thoroughly cleaning the incubator and tissue culture work stations.

D. Low Yield of Hybrid Cell Clones

A number of independent factors influence the efficiency of cell fusion (e.g. the responsiveness of the immunised animal to the antigen administered, possible feeder or suppressive influences of non-immune cells from the animal spleen (e.g. splenic macrophages), the inherent "fusability" of the myeloma cell line (which is probably highest when these cells are in an early log growth phase) and culture conditions (e.g. the batch of foetal calf serum used).

In practice there is often little that can be done to influence these imponderable factors, although each laboratory inevitably accumulates a local "folklore" concerning the conditions which favour successful cell fusion. One of the best founded of these beliefs is that the foetal calf serum used for cell fusion and during subsequent cell culture should be carefully selected by testing its ability to support the cloning of NS1 cells by limiting dilution. In the authors' experience different batches of foetal calf serum vary widely in their growth-supporting properties, some of them being positively inhibitory, and screening of this sort is strongly recommended.

E. Death of Hybrid Cell Clones

A proportion of antibody secreting hybrid cell cultures fail to survive after an initial period of growth. This risk is greatest in the earliest stages following fusion and it highlights the importance of freezing aliquots of a valuable cell line at intervals until it is fully established in culture, since this may enable cultures which have died to be re-established from frozen stock.

A number of measures may be of value when a cell line appears to be failing. Increasing the foetal calf serum concentration in the medium to 20% and introducing spleen feeder cells into the culture are frequently beneficial. Cells may also suffer through being present at too low a concentration, in which case they should be spun down and resuspended in a reduced volume of medium. Cultures may also respond to the addition of conditioned medium, prepared by growing NS1 cells or spleen cells at a density of 1×10^5 ml in medium for 24 h. The ailing culture should then be grown in 50:50 mixture of conditioned medium and fresh medium.

Finally it is possible on occasion to rescue an antibody-secreting cell line which is not growing satisfactorily in tissue culture by establishing it as an ascitic tumour in pristane primed mice (see above).

F. Loss of Antibody Production

A proportion of cultures which are found on the initial screening to be secreting antibody will become negative by the time they have been reached sufficient cell numbers to allow cloning. The frequency of this phenomenon is relatively low (of the order of 10%) and may be reduced, as noted above, by plating out fusions in Microtitre rather than in Costar plates, since this reduces the risk of overgrowth by non-producing clones. However even this manoeuvre will not prevent a small proportion of cultures spontaneously losing the capacity to produce antibody, presumably as a reflection of inherent clonal instability.

Loss of antibody secreting function may also occur occasionally at the cloning stage, i.e. the parent culture used for cloning continues to produce antibody but the daughter clones are all negative. This can often be overcome by re-cloning from the parent culture. As noted previously the freezing down of several aliquots of the cells used for cloning represents a valuable insurance against loss during cloning.

Even after cloning there is no guarantee that antibody production by a cell line will continue, although loss of activity at this stage occurs much more rarely than prior to cloning. If this occurs fresh cultures should be established from frozen stock and re-cloning performed.

Although loss of antibody production following cell fusion occurs regularly readers should not overestimate its frequency. In the authors' experience it should be possible to obtain stable cloned lines from at least ⅔ of all cultures which are shown to be positive on initial screening.

IV. ANALYSIS OF SPECIFICITIES OF NEW MONOCLONAL ANTIBODIES

Once a new monoclonal antibody has been raised by the techniques described in the preceding section, it is necessary to analyse its specificity. The ease with which this may be done depends upon the type of antigen which has been used for immunisation (see II. B). If the antibody has been raised against a purified or semi-purified antigen, proof of its specificity is relatively simply obtained since the immunocytochemical distribution pattern of the antigen will already be known and material should be available for inhibition experiments. For example the specificity of a new monoclonal antibody raised against human IgM could be established by showing that it labelled the appropriate number of plasma cells in paraffin embedded samples of human lymphoid tissue, that it stained mantle zone lymphocytes and germinal centre immune complexes in cryostat sections of lymphoid tissue, and that both of these reactions were blocked by purified IgM (but not by other classes of immunoglobulin). If necessary, further evidence for its specificity could be provided by carrying out dual fluorescent labelling of lymphoid tissue using this antibody in conjunction with a well characterised polyclonal anti-μ antiserum. The antibody could aslo be used to prepare an immunoabsorbant to which IgM should bind selectively, and from which it should then be possible to elute the IgM by desorption (e.g at high or low pH).

Many monoclonal antibodies are raised, however, against antigens which cannot be purified in sufficient quantities for such analysis: or they may be raised against hitherto unrecognised antigenic constituents. In these circumstances it may be much more difficult to define with certainty the specificity of the antibody. One widely used technique involves characterising the molecular weight of the target molecule recognised by the antibody, usually by immunoprecipitation of radiolabelled antigen from the material used for immunisation or by "immunoblotting" techniques. The antibody should also be screened as extensively as possible on a wide range of different tissue and cell samples. A full discussion of the technical and theoretical aspects of characterising the specificity of new monoclonal antibodies is outside the scope of this chapter, but information may be found in other publications (McMichael and Fabre, 1982). The value of analysing the molecular characteristics of target antigen lies in the fact that this may provide evidence that a new monoclonal antibody is directed against the same molecule as that recognised by one or more previously described monoclonal antibodies. One example is provided by monoclonal antibodies against common acute lymphoblastic leukaemia antigen (CALLA), since they all bind not only to common acute lymphoblastic leukaemia cells, but also to non-haemopoietic constituents including renal tubules (Fig. 4), glomeruli, bile canailiculi, lymphoid germinal centres, placental syncytiotrophoblast and some intestinal epithelium. It is obviously unlikely that an antibody of unrelated specificity would mimic this pattern, both in terms of tissue stained and detailed cellular labelling pattern (e.g. CALLA is found on proximal but not distal tubules in the kidney).

Immunohistological screening of a new monoclonal antibody on human tissue sections is also essential when attempting to prove that a new monoclonal antibody is of restricted specificity. One example of the need for this type of analysis is provided by antibody Ca1, which detects a malignancy-associated molecule present in human tissue. Initial studies of the reactivity of this antibody against cultured cell lines suggested that it was specific for malignant cells (Ashall et al., 1982). However more extensive immunohistological studies on normal and neoplastic human tissues indicated that the antibody also unequivocally labels normal tissues, e.g. urinary tract epithelium, Fallopian tube epithelium etc (McGee et al., 1982).

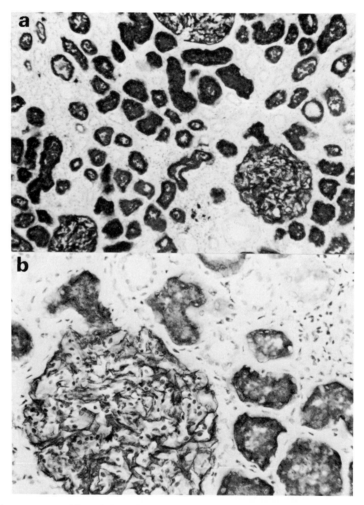

FIG. 4. Immunoperoxide staining of human kidney (cryostat section) with a monoclonal antibody directed against the common acute lymphoblastic leukaemia antigen (antibody J5; Ritz *et al.*, 1980) seen at low (a) and high (b) magnification. Although initially thought to be restricted to haemopoietic stem cells (and to the leukaemias which arise from them) this antigen has since been demonstrated on a wide variety of non-haemopoietic tissues (Metzgar *et al.*, 1981). An immunohistological analysis of this sort would not have been possible using polyclonal antisera against this antigen, because of high levels of non-specific background staining. Note that glomeruli and proximal tubules are strongly stained whilst all other structures are unreactive.

V. COMPARISON OF MONOCLONAL AND POLYCLONAL ANTIBODIES AS IMMUNOCYTOCHEMICAL REAGENTS

Ever since the first monoclonal antibodies were produced the question was raised as to how well they would perform as immunocytochemical reagents when compared to conventional polyclonal antisera. Pessimistic predictions were not infrequently voiced in this context. It was suggested, for example, that monoclonal antibodies would never achieve the labelling intensity obtainable with polyclonal antisera. Further problems envisaged at this stage included a high incidence of non-specific reactions due to the recognition by monoclonal antibodies of similar antigenic determinants on unrelated molecules.

It was thus suggested that monoclonal antibodies would prove inferior (in terms of both labelling intensity and specificity) to polyclonal antisera. It is now possible, however, to see clearly that these predictions were largely unfounded. Whilst it is true that the immunocytochemical characteristics of monoclonal antibodies differ clearly from those of conventional antisera, there is no doubt that in many circumstances monoclonal antibodies are superior reagents. Furthermore some of the unexpected reactions (in terms of specificity) obtained when using monoclonal antibodies for immunocytochemical staining may prove to provide important clues concerning the molecular nature of the tissue antigens being recognised.

In the succeeding section the immunocytochemical characteristics of monoclonal antibodies compared to those of polyclonal antisera are reviewed. This discussion is based partly upon experience in the authors' laboratory, and partly on published accounts from other laboratories. A number of points relevant to this discussion, and to the use of monoclonal antibodies in general for the immunohistological analysis of human tissue samples, are illustrated in Figs 5–10.

A. Relative Strengths of Reaction

Monoclonal antibodies will usually only react with a single determinant on any individual molecule (unless the molecule is multimeric or contains repeating antigenic sequences), whereas polyclonal antibodies frequently recognise a number of different antigenic sites on a target molecule. In consequence it might be predicted that polyclonal antisera will always allow a greater accumulation of Ig molecules on an individual target molecule in the tissue sample, and will hence inevitably lead to greater intensity of immunocytochemical labelling than can be achieved using monoclonal antibodies.

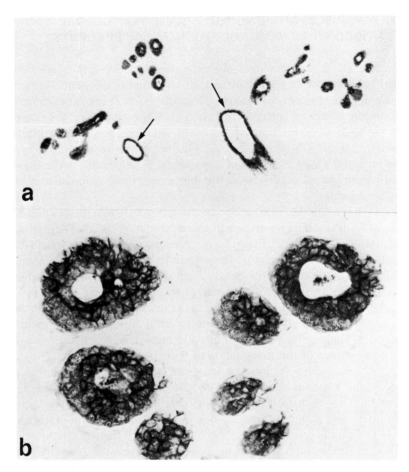

FIG. 5. Immunoperoxidase staining of normal human breast tissue (cryostat section) with a monoclonal antibody which reacts with intermediate filaments present in simple epithelium (antibody LE61; Lane *et al.*, 1982) seen at low (a) and high (b) magnification. Note strong staining of ducts (arrowed) and of glandular structures, contrasting with the non-reactivity of the breast stroma. The absence of background staining in tissue sections is one of the major advantages offered by monoclonal antibodies when used for immunohistological purposes.

Fortunately this theoretical objection does not appear to be supported by practical experience. Although there is considerable variation in the staining intensity obtained with different monoclonal antibodies, the strongest reactions are fully comparable to those obtained using conventional antisera. In the authors' laboratory a direct comparison between monoclonal and poly-

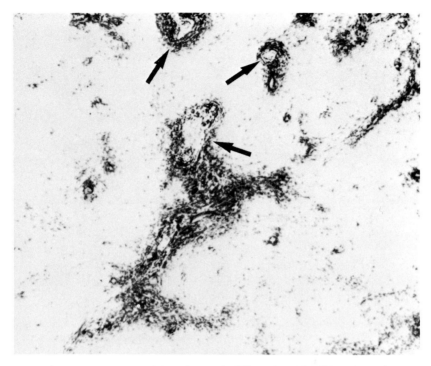

FIG. 6. Immunoperoxidase staining of a poorly differentiated B cell lymphoma (cryostat section) using a monoclonal anti-T cell antibody. Large irregularly shaped clusters of T lymphocytes are seen, particularly in association with vessels (arrowed), contrasting with the unstained lymphoma cells. As in Fig. 5 this Fig. illustrates the absence of background staining obtained when tissue sections are stained with monoclonal antibodies.

clonal reagents has been made for a number of antigens, including IgG, IgM, IgD, λ light chain, F-VIII RAg, and HLA-DR. In each of these instances, monoclonal antibodies gave results as good (in terms of labelling intensity) as those obtained with polyclonal antisera. It should be added that (as referred to below in Section V. B) monoclonal antibodies frequently gave cleaner reactions than the polyclonal antisera.

For every antigen which can be detected by both monoclonal and polyclonal antibodies (and which can therefore be used for a direct comparison of these two types of reagents) there are numerous antigens which can be revealed only with monoclonal antibodies. This fact (which is indeed one of the striking advantages of monoclonal antibodies relative to polyclonal antisera; see Table I) prevents a direct comparison of labelling intensity.

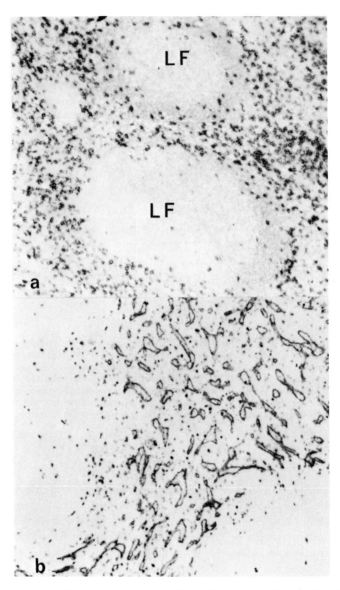

FIG. 7. Immunoperoxidase staining of cryostat sections from (a) human tonsil and (b) spleen using a monoclonal antibody reactive with cytotoxic/suppressor T lymphocytes (Leu 2a). In the tonsil section (a) scattered cells are seen in the interfollicular areas, whereas lymphoid follicles (LF) are almost free of these cells. In the spleen (b) strong staining is seen but the labelled population consists of sinusoidal lining cells. For further details of other unexpected cross reactions of monoclonal antibodies against different cell types see Fig. 4, Table V and main text.

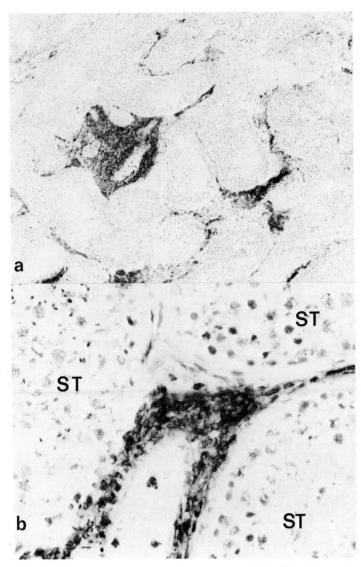

FIG. 8. Immunoperoxidase staining with monoclonal anti-HLA-DR antibody of a testicular biopsy (cryostat section) from a case of acute lymphoblastic leukaemia, seen at low (a) and high (b) magnification. Strongly stained leukaemic blast cells are seen infiltrating between the seminiferous tubules (marked ST in the higher magnification view). This Fig. illustrates the potential value of monoclonal antibodies as reagents for the diagnosis of human malignancy.

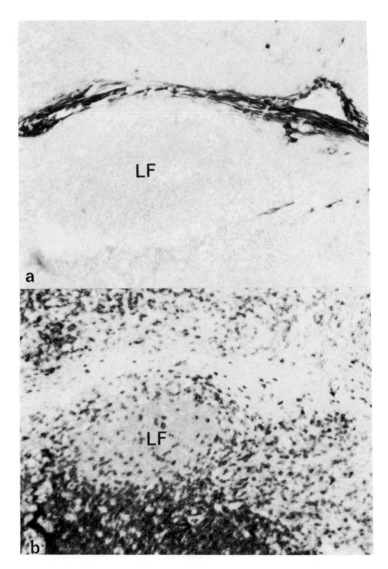

FIG. 9. Immunoperoxidase staining of human tonsil (cryostat section) for carcinoembryonic antigen (CEA), T cells and HLA-DR (Ia-like) antigen. The reactivity for CEA is
shown in low (a) and high (c) magnification and can be seen to be confined to the
superficial layers of crypt epithelium. Note that underlying lymphoid tissue, including a
lymphoid follicle (LF), is devoid of reactivity. In (b) an adjacent section to (a) is seen
stained for T lymphocytes, whilst (d) shows the same area as seen in (c) stained for
HLA-DR. The latter antibody stains lymphoid tissue but its reactivity against epithelial
tissue is restricted to labelling of a minority of cells, often with a linear surface mem-

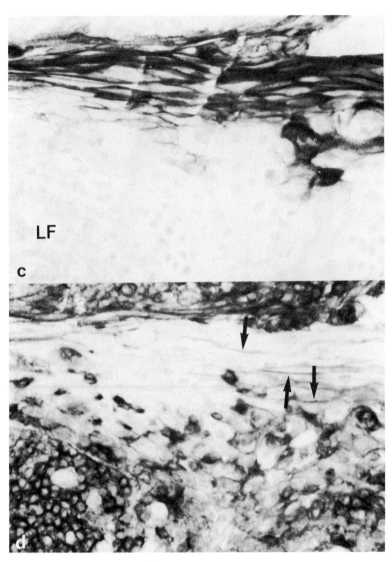

brane pattern (arrowed). Previous immunohistological studies of CEA (based on the use of polyclonal antisera) have been complicated by the antigenic complexity of this constituent: monoclonal antibodies such as the one illustrated in this Fig. offer a means of resolving these problems. HLA-DR antigen has also been the subject of immunocytochemical studies in the past with polyclonal antisera: however almost all reports of the epithelial expression of this antigen have come from the monoclonal antibody era, the absence of non-specific staining associated with the use of these reagents probably facilitating the identification of weak reactions such as those shown in (d).

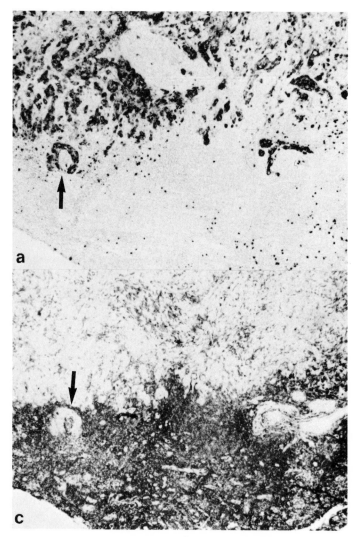

FIG. 10. Immunoperoxidase staining of adjacent cryostat sections of a lymph node infiltrated by metastatic carcinoma. The carcinomatous deposits have been identified in (a) and (b) by an antibody (LE61; Lane *et al.*, 1982) which reacts with epithelial intermediate filaments (see also Fig. 5). The residual lymphoid areas in this biopsy have been revealed with a monoclonal antibody reactive against leucocyte common antigen (c and

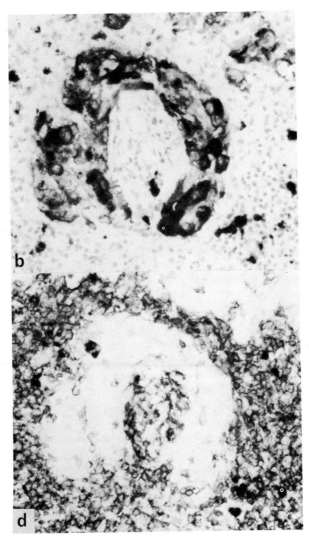

d). Note that a perivascular deposit of carcinoma cells [indicated in (a) and (c) by arrows] is shown in higher magnification in (b) and (d). Scattered myeloid cells are seen (by virtue of their content of endogenous peroxidase) in the sections stained for the epithelial antigen (a, b), but this reactivity does not obscure the specific labelling.

However the strength of labelling for these antigens was usually such that there can be little doubt of the effectiveness of many monoclonal antibodies as primary reagents in immunocytochemical procedures.

It has also been suggested in the past that monoclonal antibodies are unsuitable for immunocytochemical applications because they tend to be of lower affinity than polyclonal antisera. This belief is probably erroneous, although information on this aspect of their reactivity is still limited. Whatever the truth in this regard it is evident from practical results (see above) that there is no evidence to suggest that low affinity represents a significant obstacle to effective immunocytochemical labelling with monoclonal antibodies.

B. Background Staining

Polyclonal antisera contain a mixture of antibodies specific for the immunising antigen (the concentrations of which are of the order of 1 mg/ml) together with an excess of non-specific antibodies directed against unrelated antigens. Since this non-specific immunoglobulin is usually present at a concentration 5–10 times greater than that of the specific antibody, it constitutes a major potential cause of unwanted staining. As a result, the choice of optimal working dilutions and careful attention to washing procedures are essential when using polyclonal antisera.

Monoclonal antibodies in contrast are largely free from this problem of background staining due to non-specific immunoglobulin. This is particularly true when monoclonal antibodies are used in the form of tissue culture supernatant (rather than ascitic fluid) since all of the antibodies secreted into the culture medium should be specific for the target antigen. Being present at low concentration (of the order of 10 μg/ml), the tendency of monoclonal antibody in a tissue culture supernatant to stick nonspecifically to a tissue or cell sample is minimal. Consequently negative control reactions (in which a specific monoclonal antibody is replaced by a monoclonal antibody directed against an antigen absent from the tissue under study) are usually completely free of non-specific labelling. In contrast negative control reactions for polyclonal antisera (involving the use of pre-immune antisera or antisera against unrelated antigens) often give weak nonspecific reactions. Positive labelling has then to be assessed by comparison with these weak "negative" reactions.

This difference between monoclonal and polyclonal antisera is of importance since it is much easier to interpret the significance of a weak staining reaction if it is known that negative control reactions are completely negative (as is the case when using monoclonal antibodies). In contrast, if negative controls frequently reveal weak or scattered areas of non-specific reactivity, the interpretation of low level positive reactions becomes much more difficult.

C. Specificity of Reaction

One of the most important questions to consider when discussing the relative properties of monoclonal and polyclonal antisera concerns the degree to which they are truly specific for the antigen under investigation. This topic may be considered under two headings: first, the possibility that a monoclonal antibody will cross-react with two different molecules; and secondly the risk that a monoclonal antibody will react with two different tissues or cell populations.

1. Cross-reactivity Between Two Different Molecules

The risk that an antibody will react with two different molecules is undoubtedly greatest when polyclonal antisera are used, principally because the non-antigen-specific immunoglobulin present in all conventional antisera may contain antibodies specific for antigens unrelated to those used for immunisation (see Table I). These antibodies are of two types: they may have been elicited by contaminants in the immunising antigen preparation; or they may be antibodies produced by the animal prior to immunisation (and possibly nonspecifically increased in titre as part of an anamnestic response). Monoclonal antibodies in contrast should be free of such unwanted contaminants, especially if culture supernatants are used instead of ascitic fluid or fractions thereof.

It should be realised however that, although monoclonal antibodies should not be contaminated by any antibodies of unrelated specificity, it is quite possible for a single monoclonal antibody to react with two different molecules. This may occur if the two molecules share closely similar or identical antigenic groups, as illustrated in Fig. 11. A similar phenomenon may theoretically also occur when polyclonal antisera are used. However (for reasons explained in the legend to Fig.11) this effect is usually relatively minor, the antibodies against non-shared determinants tending to dilute out the minor population of antibodies directed against shared epitopes (Fig. 11)). In contrast monoclonal antibodies, if they show such cross-reactivity, will tend to exhibit it in a much more marked degree than will polyclonal antisera (Fig. 11).

The frequency with which monoclonal antibodies exhibit intermolecular cross-reactions of this sort remains to be determined. At least one well

CROSS REACTIVITY OF POLYCLONAL ANTIBODIES

Immunising antigen (Ag):

Cross-reacting antigen (CRA):

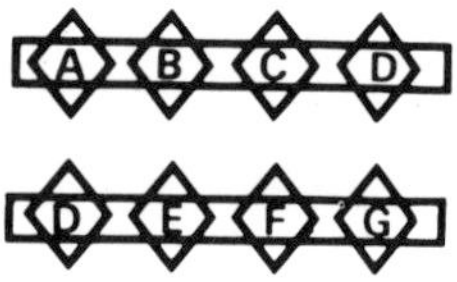

Polyclonal antiserum

   Composition: Anti-A plus Anti-B plus Anti-C plus Anti-D.

   Cross-reactivity against CRA: 25%

   Reactivity following absorption with CRA:

             1) Against CRA   - Nil

             2) Against Ag   - 75% of initial value

CROSS REACTIVITY OF MONOCLONAL ANTIBODIES

Immunising antigen (Ag):

Cross-reacting antigen (CRA):

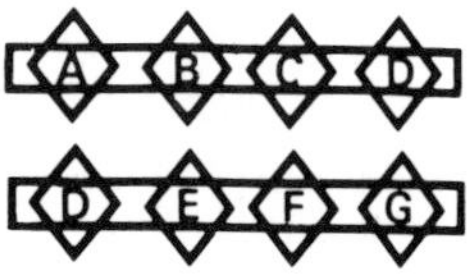

Monoclonal antibodies

   Composition: Anti-A or Anti-B or Anti-C or Anti-D.

   Cross-reactivity against CRA: Nil (anti-A,B or C) or

                                 100% (anti-D)

   Reactivity following absorption (of anti-D) with CRA:

             1) Against CRA - Nil

             2) Against Ag   - Nil

FIG. 11. Schematic comparison of the phenomenon of antigenic cross-reactivity as encountered when polyclonal and monoclonal antibodies are used. For the purposes of this comparison the existence of two hypothetical molecules is proposed: one of these (the immunising antigen) carries four antigenic epitopes (A, B, C and D); the other molecule (the cross-reacting antigen) is structurally distinguishable but shares a single antigenic epitope (D) with the immunising antigen. It is assumed in this model that all epitopes are of equal antigenicity. If polyclonal antibodies are raised against the immunising antigen (upper diagram) equal amounts of antibody will be produced against each of the four epitopes. Antibody against epitope D (constituting a quarter of

attested example exists in the report by Pillemer and Weissman (1981) of a monoclonal antibody which reacts with both Thy-1 antigen and immunoglobulin. This particular cross-reaction appears to reflect the fact that the two molecules share amino acid sequences (and indeed may have arisen from a common precursor). Other instances of shared antigenic epitopes between different molecules may emerge in the future which reflect the sharing of carbohydrate sequences between unrelated glycoproteins (or even between glycoproteins and glycolipids).

2. Cross-reactivity Between Unrelated Cell Types

Given their inherent properties of high specificity it is perhaps surprising to find that there is a steadily growing list of examples of monoclonal antibodies which react with apparently quite unrelated cell types. Some of these examples are listed in Table V. A question raised by such examples of unexpected cellular cross-reactivity is whether they represent the presence of the same molecule in the two cell populations; or whether the monoclonal antibody is reacting with identical (or closely similar) determinants on quite different molecules as discussed above. This question cannot be resolved without relatively complex procedures (e.g. immunoprecipitation of molecules from tissue extracts) and in consequence it is not known which explanation is applicable for most of the instances listed in Table V. However it has been established that the unexpected cross-reactivity of monoclonal antibody J5 (initially thought to be specific for an antigen restricted to leukaemic and early normal haemopoietic cells; Ritz *et al.*, 1980) with renal epithelium (Fig. 4) is probably accounted for by the presence of a similar molecule in both cell types (Metzgar *et al.*, 1981).

---

the antibody produced in response to this antigen) will react against the cross-reacting antigen. However it would be possible to remove this unwanted cross-reactivity by absorption with the cross-reacting antigen, a procedure which would have no effect on the majority of the specific antibody (i.e. antibodies against epitopes A, B and C). In contrast, if monoclonal antibodies are raised against the immunising antigen (lower diagram) four antibodies of quite different specificity would be obtained. One of these (anti-D) would react strongly with the cross-reacting antigen, whilst the other three (anti-A, anti-B and anti-C) would show no reactivity with the cross-reacting antigen. The monoclonal antibody specific for epitope D would show equally strong reactions against both molecules and any attempt to render it specific for the immunising antigen by absorption with the cross-reacting antigen would abolish all its activity. The conclusion from this model is that monoclonal antibodies which exhibit inter-molecular cross-reactivity are likely to manifest this phenomenon to a much greater degree than will polyclonal antibodies. However, it should be possible, by screening a number of monoclonal antibodies against an individual antigen, to select reagents which are mono-specific in their reactivity. For a more extensive discussion of the specificity of monoclonal antibodies readers should consult the informative review by Lane and Koprowski (1982).

TABLE V

Unexpected immunocytochemical reactions of monoclonal antibodies.

Antibody	Principal specificity	"Extra" reactivity	Reference
Na1/34	Cortical thymocytes	Langerhans cells	McMichael *et al.*, 1979; Morris *et al.*, 1983
J5	Haemopoietic stem cells/ acute lymphoblastic leukaemia cells	Renal epithelium	Ritz *et al.*, 1980; Metzgar *et al.*, 1981
OKT4 Leu 3a	Helper/inducer T lymphocytes	Tissue macrophages	Personal observations
OKT8 Leu 2a	Suppressor/cytotoxic T lymphocytes	Splenic macrophages (Fig. 7b)	Personal observations
UCHT1	T lymphocytes	Purkinje cells	Garson *et al.*, 1982
HMFG1	Human mammary epithelium	Smooth muscle	Gatter *et al.*, 1982
Unnamed	*T. cruzi* (causative organism of Chaga's disease)	Neurones	Wood *et al.*, 1982

D. Discrepant Immunocytochemical Reactions of Monoclonal Antibodies of Apparently Identical Specificity

It is generally assumed by immunocytochemists that when two polyclonal antisera reactive with the same molecule are used for immunocytochemical staining, they will give identical labelling reactions. Monoclonal antibodies however are inherently more discriminative reagents, in that they react with only a single epitope on each molecule. There is reason to think that they may provide evidence in the future that many molecules which have been thought of as being homogeneous consist in fact of a "family" of closely related molecules, which may vary in their tissue distribution. One example of this type of newly revealed molecular family is provided by the leucocyte common antigen. A number of laboratories have raised monoclonal antibodies against this constituent of white cells, often as an accidental event in attempting to produce antibodies specific for human white cell subpopulations. Biochemical analysis reveals that many of these antibodies react with a membrane glycoprotein, of molecular weight approximately 200 000. However a monoclonal antibody has been reported by Dalchau and Fabre (1981) which reacts with a subpopulation of the antigen which is largely restricted to human B cells. Furthermore two anti-leucocyte common antibodies recently studied in the authors' laboratory have also been shown to vary in their immunocytochemical reactivity patterns despite the fact that they bind to apparently identical molecules from white cell membrane extracts (Warnke *et al.*, 1983).

An additional possible example of molecular heterogeneity revealed by monoclonal antibodies is to be found in a recent study from our laboratory of the distribution of transferrin receptor in human tissues. Four different monoclonal antibodies reactive with this constituent were studied (Gatter *et al.*, 1983) and one of these differed clearly in its reactivity patterns from the others. Since there was good evidence that all of these antibodies were reacting with the molecule responsible for binding transferrin to cell surface these findings raise the possibility that this molecular structure also shows a degree of antigenic availability.

These findings are disquieting since they suggest that immunocytochemists will have in the future to pay much more attention to defining the molecular basis of the antigenic constituents which they study. However this is an inevitable development given the greater precision brought to the field of immunocytochemistry by the introduction of monoclonal antibodies.

VI. CONCLUSIONS

One of the great attractions of immunocytochemistry to its practitioners lies in the aesthetic appeal of the images which it produces and in the degree to which the observer's imaginative skill is exercised during the interpretation of these images. To this extent immunocytochemistry may be described as an art rather than a science. However in truth immunocytochemistry is a hybrid subject, in which art and science combine — the art lying in the interpretation of results, the science in producing those results. Unfortunately in the past immunocytochemical methods have been less scientifically precise than is desirable, with the result that immunocytochemistry can be seen as one art balancing precariously on the shoulders of another. The introduction of monoclonal antibodies is therefore a major development since it strengthens the foundation upon which immunocytochemistry rests, and promises also to greatly expand the number of scientific problems to which immunocytochemical analysis will be applicable.

VII. ACKNOWLEDGEMENTS

We are grateful to those laboratories who have supplied us with samples of monoclonal antibodies referred to in this chapter. The work on which this chapter is based was supported by grants from the Leukaemia Research Fund.

VIII. REFERENCES

Ashall, F., Bramwell, M. E. and Harris, H. (1982). *Lancet* **2**, 1.

Dalchau, R. and Fabre, J. W. (1981). *J. Exp. Med.* **153**, 753.

Garson, J. A., Beverley, P. C. L., Coakham, H. B. and Harper, E. I. (1982). *Nature* **298**, 375.

Gatter, K. C., Brown, G., Trowbridge, I. S., Woolston, R.-E. and Mason, D. Y. (1983). *J. Clin. Path.* **36**, 539.

Gerdes, J., Klatt, U. and Stein, H. (1980). *Immunology* **39**, 75.

Gerdes, J., Naiem, M., Mason, D. Y. and Stein, H. (1982). *Immunology* **45**, 645.

Köhler, G. and Milstein, C. (1975). *Nature* **256**, 495.

Lane, E. B. (1982). *J. Cell Biol.* **92**, 180.

Lane, D. and Koprowski, H. (1982). *Nature* **296**, 200.

McGee, J. O. D., Woods, J. C., Ashall, F., Bramwell, M. E. and Harris, H. (1982). *Lancet* **2**, 7.

McMichael, A. J., Pilch, J. R., Galfre, G., Mason, D. Y., Fabre, J. W. and Milstein, C. (1979). *Europ. J. Immunol.* **9**, 205.

McMichael, A. J. and Fabre, J. W. (eds.) (1982). Monoclonal Antibodies in Clinical Medicine, Academic Press, London.

Mason, D. Y., Naiem, M., Abdulaziz, Z., Nash, J. R. G., Gatter, K. C. and Stein, H. (1982). *In* "Monoclonal Antibodies in Clinical Medicine" (A. J. McMichael, and J. W. Fabre, eds.), Academic Press, London.

Metzgar, R. S., Borowitz, M. J., Jones, N. H. and Dawell, B. L. (1981). *J. Exp. Med.* **154**, 1249.

Moir, D. J., Ghosh, A. K., Abdulaziz, Z., Knight, P. M. and Mason, D. Y. (1983). *Br. J. Haemat.* (in press).

Naiem, M., Gerdes, J., Abdulaziz, Z., Sunderland, C. A., Allington, M. J., Stein, H. and Mason, D. Y. (1982). *J. Immunol. Methods* **50**, 145.

Morris, H. B., Gatter, K. C., Stein, H. and Mason, D. Y. (1983). *Br. J. Obstet. Gynaecol.* (in press).

Pillemer, E. and Weissman, I. L. (1981). *J. Exp. Med.* **153**, 1068.

Ritz, J., Pesando, J. M., Notis-McConarty, J., Lazarus, H. and Schlossman, S. F. (1980). *Nature* **283**, 583.

Warnke, R. A., Gatter, K. C. and Mason, D. Y. (1983). Submitted for publication.

Wood, J. N., Hudson, L., Jessell, T. M. and Yamamoti, M. (1982). *Nature* **296**, 34.

The Colloidal Gold Marker System for Light and Electron Microscopic Cytochemistry

J. ROTH

IMMUNOCYTOCHEMISTRY 2
ISBN 0 12 140402 1

I. INTRODUCTION

The first comprehensive electron microscopic investigation into the nature of colloidal solutions of gold was performed by Thiessen (1942) and the results of this study proved definitely the particulate nature of colloidal gold. This was confirmation of the brilliant observations on the metallic nature of gold in highly dispersed hydrosols as expressed, but not proved, by Faraday (1857) almost a century before. Furthermore, by investigating the morphology of interaction of various substances with particles of colloidal gold, Thiessen successfully visualized the protective colloid adsorbed onto the surface of gold particles. The protective colloid was seen by him as a surface coat which, as calculated from its thickness, corresponded to a few layers of molecules.

As early as 1939, Kausche and Ruska investigated the morphology of adsorption of proteins onto colloidal gold. Their electron micrographs show tobacco-mosaic viruses tagged with gold particles. However, it took more than 20 years for colloidal gold to be used as a particulate tracer in electron microscopic studies (Feldherr and Marshal, 1962). The modern era of the application of colloidal gold started in 1971 with the introduction of "an immunocolloid method for the electron microscope" by Faulk and Taylor. They used a rabbit anti-*Salmonella* antiserum as a protective colloid for adsorption to colloidal gold particles and succeeded in a specific labelling of the surface of bacteria by incubating them with the immunoglobulin-gold complex. Faulk and Taylor (1971) also reported the preparation of complexes of colloidal gold with antisera to collagen, PHA, ovalbumin, human IgG, BSA, blood groups A, B or D, human light chains and rhinoviruses. The latter immunocolloid was used for the detection of rhinoviruses coupled to red blood cells (Faulk *et al.*, 1971).

Later, the direct labelling technique as described by Faulk and Taylor (1971) was modified by Romano and colleagues (1974; 1975) who used a gold labelled horse anti-human IgG to localize antigen bound human IgG anti-D and anti-A on red blood cell ghosts in an indirect labelling technique. Horisberger and collaborators were the first to prepare a lectin-gold complex (Bauer *et al.*, 1974) and the main methodological contribution from this group was the introduction of colloidal gold as a marker for scanning electron microscopy (Horisberger *et al.*, 1975). Lectin-gold complexes were also used for direct labelling of cell surface antigens and subsequent observation by transmission (Wagner and Wagner, 1976) or freeze-etch electron microscopy (Wagner *et al.*, 1976).

Indirect labelling techniques applying glycoprotein-gold complexes for demonstration of cell surface lectin binding sites were worked out by Geoghegan and Ackerman (1977). These authors made the very important observation that the adsorption of a protein to colloidal gold is pH dependent. Roth and Wagner (1977a) reported for the first time that lectin-gold complexes are useful reagents not only for cell surface labelling, but also for studies on internalization, and of double labelling of different binding sites by the combined use of colloial gold and peroxidase (Roth and Wagner, 1977a,b). Double labelling was also achieved by the use of ferritin and colloidal gold (Wagner and Wagner, 1977) or of colloidal gold of different sizes (Roth and Binder, 1978; Horisberger *et al.*, 1978).

Up to now, a whole variety of ligands such as immunoglobulins, lectins, toxins, protein A and avidin have been used for complex formation with colloidal gold and employed in pre-embedding labelling of living or fixed cells. An important extension of the application of protein-gold complexes as cytochemical reagents became possible through the observation that such complexes show only a very-low degree of nonspecific interaction on thin sections from resin embedded tissues or frozen materials (Horisberger and Rosset, 1977; Roth *et al.*, 1978; Garaud *et al.*, 1980; Bendayan, 1981a; Geuze *et al.*, 1981a; Brands *et al.*, 1980). This provided the possibility of labelling thin sections and allowed the localization of a variety of constituents in different cellular compartments. In addition, it should be mentioned that the two-dimensional distribution of the cell surface label can be studied not only in freeze-etch replicas but also in a less laborious way by the preparation of surface shadow replicas from cell cultures (Tolson *et al.*, 1981).

Finally, colloidal gold is not only a useful marker for transmission, scanning and freeze-etch electron microscopy but also a marker which can be applied for light microscopy as first reported by Geoghegan *et al.* (1978), and later by other investigators (Horisberger and VonLanthen 1979b; Roth *et al.*, 1980; Gu *et al.*, 1981; deMey *et al.*, 1981a,b; Roth, 1982c).

From this short historical introduction it appears that particles of colloidal gold constitute an alternative marker system which can be used for cytochemistry and immunocytochemistry at the level of light and electron microscopy. The aim of this chapter is to give detailed information about the theory and practice of preparation of colloidal gold, the conditions for protein-colloidal gold complex manufacture and finally, the application of such complexes for staining of cells, tissues and sections of biological material. Other relevant reviews on colloidal gold as a marker have appeared and can be consulted for further information (Horisberger, 1981; Goodman *et al.*, 1981; Roth, 1982b).

II. COLLOIDAL GOLD

The general conditions under which colloidal gold can be formed, and several methods for its preparation will be given. There are two principal methods for the preparation of colloids; the *dispersion* method and the *condensation* method. The simplest dispersion method is mechanical grinding. Dispersion can also be produced by electric deflagration, by irradiation with ultrasonic waves, or by chemical means. But none of these techniques produces a colloid which is of use for our purposes. In the condensation method, the colloid is formed from micromolecular units, the so called nuclei which grow into particles of varying sizes depending on the specific conditions employed. The process of condensation may be regarded as a process of crystallization since in many cases the colloidal particles have a crystalline structure. In practice, the most important way to make colloids by condensation is by chemical means. In this method the particle size depends on the rate of formation of nuclei (or crystallization centres) and the rate of crystal growth.

The most popular group of chemical reactions by which colloidal gold can be formed is reduction, and many of the colloids prepared in this way have found application as cytochemical markers. Colloidal gold has been prepared from tetrachloroauric acid by the use of a wide spectrum of reducing agents such as white phosphorus (Faraday, 1857; Zsigmondy, 1905; Zsigmondy and Thiessen, 1925), formaldehyde (Zsigmondy, 1898), ethanol (Vanino, 1905), carbon monoxide (Donau, 1905), hydroxylamine or hydrazine (Gutbier, 1903a,b), hydrogen peroxide (Dörinckel, 1905), ascorbic acid (Stathis and Fabrikanos, 1958), sodium citrate (Zsigmondy and Thiessen, 1925; Frens, 1973) and even an aqueous extract from Dutch cigars (Janek, 1927).

A. General Considerations in the Preparation of Colloidal Gold

1. Glassware

The nature of the glassware surface is an important factor in initiating the reduction process and in determining the reproducibility of the preparations. Small quantities of contaminants on the vessel wall can interfere with the formation of the colloid and can cause variation in particle size or cloudiness of the colloid. Therefore, the glassware must be scrupulously cleaned, rinsed in distilled water, and siliconized. Even in 1857, Faraday wrote

> All the vessels used in these preparations must be very clean . . . . Glass supposed to be clean and even a new bottle is quite able to change the character of a given gold fluid.

This statement is as valid today as in the past.

2. *Reagents*

All solutions must be prepared from double-distilled and filtered (Millipore filter, 0.45 μm pore size) water since the presence of organic substances, dust particles etc. interferes with the formation of the colloid.

Tetrachloroauric acid [H(AuCl$_4$).4 H$_2$O, Merck] is a crystalline substance which is highly hydrophilic. Therefore, one should prepare a 1% aqueous stock solution from the entire sealed ampule. In our experience, this solution can be stored for several months at room temperature in a well-closed vial.

A saturated solution of white phosphorus (Merck) in ether is prepared with diethyl ether of the highest purity. The sticks of phosphorus are cut into small pieces under water, are then dried for a *short* time (a few seconds!) on filter paper and *rapidly* transferred into the ether. With gentle agitation, saturation takes a few hours. The ether-saturated phosphorus can be stored in a *well-closed*, brown vial. It is important to take into account the safety regulations for handling and storing flammable and explosive substances.

Potassium carbonate (K$_2$CO$_3$, water free, Merck) is prepared as a 0·2 M aqueous solution. This solution is not very stable and must be freshly prepared every 4 weeks.

Trisodium citrate (C$_6$H$_5$ Na$_3$O$_7$.2H$_2$O, Merck) is made as a 1% aqueous solution and is stable on storage.

The ascorbic acid (Merck) solution (0·7% in distilled water) is always prepared immediately before use.

Polyethylene glycol (molecular weight 20 000, Merck) or Carbowax-20 M (Fluka) are prepared as 1% aqueous solutions.

B. Recipes to Prepare Colloidal Gold

1. *Reduction with Phosphorus According to Zsigmondy (1905)*

For this purpose 100 ml of 0·01% aqueous tetrachloroauric acid is adjusted to pH 7·2 with 0·2 M K$_2$CO$_3$ and afterwards heated to boiling. As soon as boiling starts, 0·5 ml ether-saturated phosphorus is added rapidly and the mixture shaken. Completion of the reduction is indicated by the appearance of a reddish-orange colour. The colloid consists of 3 nm gold particles with narrow variation in particle size.

2. *Reduction with Phosphorus According to Zsigmondy (1905) and Zsigmondy and Thiessen (1925)*

One hundred and twenty ml of distilled water are mixed with 2·5 ml of 0·6% aqueous tetrachloroauric acid and the solution is neutralized with 0·2

M K_2CO_3. Afterwards, 1 ml of an ether solution of phosphorus is added. The ether solution of phosphorus is prepared by mixing one part of ether-saturated phosphorus with four parts of ether. The mixture is shaken for 15 min at room temperature. During this time a brownish red colour develops. Finally, the solution is heated until the typical wine red colour of colloidal gold appears. The heating also effects evaporation of the ether. Excess amounts of phosphorus can be oxidized by passing air through the colloid. The colloid obtained consists of gold particles with a diameter between 5 and 12 nm.

3. Reduction with Ascorbic Acid According to Stathis and Fabrikanos (1958)

One milliliter of 1% aqueous tetrachloroauric acid is mixed with 1·5 ml of 0·2 M K_2CO_3 and 25 ml of distilled water at 4 °C. To this solution, 1 ml of 0·7% aqueous ascorbic acid is added with stirring. The colour immediately becomes purple/red. The volume is then made up to 100 ml with distilled water and the solution is heated until the colour of the colloid becomes red. The particle size in this colloid varies between 8 and 13 nm.

4. Reduction with Trisodium Citrate According to Frens (1973)

This procedure yields monodisperse colloids, and depending on the amount of sodium citrate added to a constant amount of tetrachloroauric acid, monodisperse sols with particle diameters varying from 15 nm to 150 nm can be obtained. The following protocol is to prepare colloidal gold with a particle diameter of approximately 15 nm. One hundred milliliters of 0·01% tetrachloroauric acid are heated to boiling, and 4 ml of 1% trisodium citrate are rapidly added. The reduction process is practically complete after 5 min of gentle boiling and this is indicated by the appearance of a reddish-orange colour.

5. Reduction with Ultrasonics According to Baigent and Müller (1980)

To 50 ml of distilled water, 0·1 ml of 1% aqueous tetrachloroauric acid is added and the solution is neutralized with 0·2 M K_2CO_3. Afterwards, 0·5 ml ethyl alcohol is added and sonication is carried out at 20 Kc and 125 W by immersing a flat ended probe. The particle size in the colloid varies between 6 and 10 nm.

6. Reduction with Sodium Borohydride (Tschopp et al., 1982)

Colloidal gold with particle diameters between 2 and 5 nm is obtained. One hundred and fifty µl of a 4% $HAuCl_4$ solution and 200 µl of 0·2 M K_2CO_3 were added to 40 ml double-distilled water that had been precooled to 4 °C. Under rapid stirring, 400 μl aliquots (normally 3–5) of a freshly prepared sodium borohydride solution (0·5 mg/ml) were rapidly added until no further colour change from bluish-purple to reddish-orange was observed. The gold solution was then stirred for an additional 5 min.

7. Preparation of Radioactive Colloidal Gold (Kent and Allen, 1981)

The procedure to obtain colloidal gold is identical to the techniques of both Frens (1973) and Zsigmondy and Thiessen (1925). The additional step for both recipes is the addition of 40 μl of ^{195}Au containing approximately 1×10^6 counts per min to the solution of tetrachloroauric acid before reduction.

C. Properties of Colloidal Gold

The colour of colloidal gold in transmitted light is usually red if the particles are spherical and smaller than 80 μm. Colloidal gold which is composed of bigger particles or of distinctly non-spherical particles appears blue in transmitted light. A blue colour can also be found under conditions of gold particle agglomeration. Red solutions of colloidal gold display a single peak of absorption in the visible spectrum ranging between 520 and 540 nm. The position and shape of the peak depends on the mean size of the particles and moves to a longer wavelength with increasing mean particle diameter.

According to Zsigmondy and Thiessen (1925), particles of colloidal gold may be composed of tiny subunits, the so-called primary particles of gold. Later investigations performed by Scherrer (1920) with X-ray analysis showed that colloidal gold particles consist of crystals similar to those of solid gold with primary units probably consisting of minute octahedra. Such particles are approximately spherical but relatively big particles are no longer isodimensional. From the foregoing it must be assumed that the surface of gold particles should resemble that of a growing crystal which has numerous steps and corners. Experimental evidence for the presence of surface irregularities came from studies about the absorption of other substances to colloidal gold (Taylor, 1926). It seems that the corners and edges are most active in adsorption followed by the crystallographic planes.

Another important surface property of particles of colloidal gold is their electrical charge. Particles of colloidal gold move to the anode and, therefore, are negatively charged. The origin of the electrical charge in the case of metal colloids may be either adsorption of ions or dissociation. According to

Pauli (1949), the negative charge of gold particles is caused by dissociation of complex gold compounds formed on the surface of the particles. It is assumed that the aurocomplex, $H(AuCl_2)$, on the surface of the gold particles which dissociates into H^+ and $AuCl_2^-$ is responsible for the charge. To the contrary, Zsigmondy (1924) and Thiessen (1924) assumed that the preferential adsorption of hydroxyl ions from water or alkali by the surface of the gold particles accounts for their negative charge. Whatever theory is right, a more important factor than the question about the origin of the electrical charge on the gold particles is that its presence has several implications for practical work related in cytochemistry.

It is an old observation that the addition of electrolytes to red solutions of unprotected colloidal gold in concentrations above a certain limiting value causes an immediate colour change to blue (Faraday, 1857; Zsigmondy, 1898). This event is due to agglomeration (flocculation) of the single particles in secondary aggregates which ultimately settle out as a fine blue-black precipitate (Zsigmondy, 1898; Scherrer and Staub, 1931). The electrolyte-induced changes in the electrochemical environment which cause coagulation are of a complex nature as discussed in detail by Pauli (1949).

The stability of colloidal gold in water is maintained by electrostatic repulsion. If electrolytes are added to colloidal gold, the ion layers around the gold particles are compressed and allow the particles to approach more closely. If a critical distance is reached, cohesion of the particles occurs and results in flocculation. In 1901, Zsigmondy made the observation that the electrolyte-induced coagulation of colloidal gold can be prevented by prior addition of solutions of various proteins. This observation was the basis for the current use of colloidal gold coated with a variety of biological macromolecules for cytochemical purposes.

III. COMPLEX FORMATION OF COLLOIDAL GOLD WITH BIOLOGICAL SUBSTANCES

A. General Considerations about Adsorption of Proteins to Colloidal Gold

In the preceding section it was pointed out that a protein solution can protect colloidal gold against the action of electrolytes. The addition of a salt solution to colloidal gold protected by protein no longer results in a colour change from red to blue which is an indication of particle flocculation. Such stabilization (i.e. resistance to electrolyte-induced flocculation) of colloidal gold is due to the adsorption of protein to the surface of the gold particles (Weisser, 1933; Jirgenson and Straumanis, 1962). Protein adsorption to gold particles is a highly complex and still incompletely understood phenomenon (Horisberger, 1981; Goodman *et al.*, 1979; 1980). It is generally assumed that protein adsorption is due to electrostatic interaction between the negatively charged surface of gold particles and positively charged groups of the protein. The protein, apparently, is attracted into the action radius of van der Waals-London attractive forces and firmly bound to the gold particle surface.

A number of physicochemical factors influence the adsorption process and the most comprehensive study of the conditions for protein adsorption to colloidal gold comes from the work of Geoghegan and Ackerman (1977). They found that low concentrations of NaCl ($0 \cdot 1$ M) prevented formation of a useful complex since the zeta potential of the colloidal gold was decreased and adsorption could not occur. However, stable complexes could be formed with proteins dialyzed against 5 mM NaCl as already shown by Romano *et al.* (1974; 1975) and by Horisberger *et al.* (1975).

Another parameter of great practical importance is the pH value of the colloidal gold, since it could be clearly demonstrated that adsorption of proteins to colloidal gold is pH dependent. The failure of earlier investigators to prepare stable immunoglobulin-gold complexes (Romano *et al.*, 1974), or lectin-gold complexes (Horisberger and Rosset, 1976), can now be explained by the choice of inappropriate pH conditions for complex formation. It appears from these studies (Geoghegan and Ackerman, 1977; Goodman *et al.*, 1979, 1980) that, as a general rule, strong adsorption of macromolecules and stable complex formation with gold particles occurs at values close to or basic to the isoelectric point of a given protein. At these pH values the zwitterion form of the protein is dominant and the interfacial tension is maximal. Furthermore, it is the condition under which proteins might more readily adsorb to the hydrophobic surface of gold particles.

Horisberger and Rosset (1976, 1977) reported that colloidal gold could not be stabilized with wheat-germ lectin. They assumed that the molecular weight of the lectin was too low and postulated that the molecular weight of a substance is important for complex formation. Later, Geoghegan and Ackerman (1977) explained this as due to an inappropriate pH of the colloidal gold. Wheat-germ lectin has an isoelectric point range of $7 \cdot 9$–$9 \cdot 4$. At pH values of colloidal gold acidic to the isoelectric point of a protein, flocculation of colloidal gold occurs rapidly and it is probable that such an event occurred under the conditions of the experiments of Horisberger and Rosset. However, difficulties have been experienced in the adsorption of wheat-germ lectin and *Lens culinaris* lectin even when appropriate pH conditions were chosen (Roth and Binder, 1978; Goodman *et al.*, 1979). It seems that the particle size is of some importance since only gold particles smaller than 40 nm could be stabilized with these low-molecular weight substances (Roth and Binder, 1978). This observation is in accordance with the data of Frens (1972) who showed that the stability of colloidal gold depends on particle size; colloids with large particles are less stable against electrolyte coagulation than colloids with small particles.

Concerning the nature of the adsorptive forces it was already mentioned that they are considered to be mainly van der Waals-London forces. However, the observations of Horisberger and Rosset (1977) that neutral polysaccharides such as yeast mannan and polyethylene glycol bind to colloidal gold indicate the involvement of other factors such as electrodynamic attractive forces and adsorption due to the surface roughness of colloidal gold particles.

B. Preparation of Protein Solutions and Colloidal Gold for Complex Formation

It was already mentioned earlier that even small amounts of electrolytes added to colloidal gold will decrease the zeta potential and as a consequence will interfere with the adsorption of macromolecules. Faulk and Taylor (1971) dialyzed antisera against 0·2 M ethylene glycol to remove serum electrolytes before complex formation with colloidal gold. Wagner and Wagner (1976; 1977) used the same protocol with *Helix pomatia* lectin. Romano *et al.* (1974) dialyzed horse anti-human IgG against 5 mM NaCl (pH 7·0) and this procedure was found to be useful for many other proteins (Horisberger *et al.*, 1975; Geoghegan and Ackerman, 1977). Goodman *et al.* (1981) recommend extensive dialysis against 1 mM Tris-HCl buffer (pH 7·4) and afterwards filtration through a 0·2 μm membrane filter.

Finally, it should be mentioned that low-density lipoprotein particles (Handley *et al.*, 1981) were brought into 0·05 M EDTA solution and this condition allowed for complex formation with colloidal gold. However, the method of choice is extensive dialysis of the protein solutions against distilled water in which many proteins fortunately remain soluble. In the preparation of immunoglobulins for complex formation, further treatment is necessary (Romano *et al.*, 1974; Geoghegan and Ackerman, 1977). In order to remove aggregates which can form upon storage at low temperature or in solutions of concentration of protein greater than 2 mg ml^{-1}, the immunoglobulin solutions should be centrifuged immediately before use at 105 000 ×g for 1 h.

In order to provide optimal conditions for complex formation with proteins, the pH of the colloidal gold must be adjusted to values depending on the isoelectric point of the protein. Such pH adjustment can be done simply by addition of 0·2 M K_2CO_3 to raise the pH or by addition of 0·1 N acetic acid or 0·1 N HCl to lower the pH in the colloidal gold. The pH must then measured with an electrode for complete accuracy. Unstabilized colloidal gold plugs the pores of the electrode, but this can be prevented by adding a few drops of 1% aqueous polyethylene glycol (molecular weight 20 000) to an aliquot of colloidal gold to stabilize it before the insertion of the pH electrode (Geoghegan and Ackerman, 1977). Another approach for pH adjustment is dialysis of colloidal gold against an appropriate buffer (Goodman *et al.*, 1979). Colloidal particles of gold from 22 nm to 55 nm diameter can be dialyzed against 7 to 10 mM buffers without evidence for flocculation. Citrate-phosphate buffer (pH 3 to 5·8), tris-HCl buffer (pH 5·8 to 8·3) and borate-sodium hydroxide buffer (pH 8·5 to 10·3) at 7 mM concentration were found to be efficient in maintaining the pH upon addition of protein.

C. Estimation of the Minimal Amount of a Substance Needed for Stabilization of Colloidal Gold

In his fundamental investigations on the protective action of various substances on colloidal gold, Zsigmondy (1901) noted that the protective power was different from substance to substance for a given colloid. As a measure for the relative protective power he introduced the term "gold number". The gold number was defined as the number of mg of a protein or another substance added to 10 ml of colloidal gold which just failed to prevent the colour change from red to blue upon addition of 1 ml of 10% NaCl.

This principle was applied by Horisberger *et al.* (1975) and Roth and Binder (1978) to estimate the minimal amount of a protein which fully stabilized a certain volume of colloidal gold against flocculation with NaCl. In other words, under appropriately chosen pH conditions, this amount allows formation of fully stabilized colloidal gold. Horisberger and coworkers (1975) advise the following protocol in which 5 ml of colloidal gold was mixed with 1 ml of serial dilutions of the protein. After 1 min, 1 ml of 10% NaCl solution was added. The absorbance was measured after 5 min at 525 to 540 nm. Geoghegan and Ackerman (1977) determined the optical density at 580 mm and adjusted the pH of the colloidal gold always to or slightly above the isoelectric point of the protein to be adsorbed.

From a series of estimations, a curve was generated, and the point where the curve first appeared asymptotic with the *x*-axis (protein amount) was taken as the minimum quantity of protein needed to stabilize the colloidal gold. Roth and Binder (1978) mixed 0·5 ml of colloidal gold with 0·1 ml of a serially diluted protein solution. After 1 min, 0·1 ml of 10% aqueous NaCl solution was added and the stabilization effect was judged visually by the colour of the colloidal gold (Plate 7, see Plate section, between pp. 148–149).

The lowest protein amount which prevented a colour change from red to blue after addition of NaCl was considered to be sufficiently stabilizing.

D. General Protocol for the Complex Formation of Proteins with Colloidal Gold

1. Preparation of the Crude Complex

The following basic information is needed before one can commence preparation of protein-gold complexes: (1) the appropriate size of gold particles needed in the experiments; (2) the isoelectric point or isoelectric point range of the protein; and (3) the minimal (or optimal) stabilizing protein amount. The colloidal gold can then be prepared and its pH is adjusted to or above the isoelectric point of the protein. Unprotected colloidal gold can be stored under sterile conditions for months but we always prefer to use a freshly prepared colloid for complex formation. The protein is either dissolved in distilled water if available in salt free, lyophilized form or dialysed against distilled water. If problems of protein solubility under such conditions are encountered, dialysis is performed against 2 to 10 mM buffer with properly adjusted pH.

The mixing of colloidal gold and protein is performed either directly in thoroughly cleaned centrifuge tubes or in clean, siliconized glassware depending on the desired volume. Most investigators, including ourselves, add the colloidal gold rapidly to the protein solution. The protein solution is used in a 10% excess of the minimal stabilizing amount. On the other hand, Geoghegan and Ackerman (1977) and Goodman *et al.* (1979; 1980; 1981) add the protein dropwise to the stirred colloidal gold. This may, however, introduce some problems with relatively large particles since occasionally partial or complete flocculation of the colloidal gold has been observed (Horisberger, 1981). In exceptional cases dropwise addition of the protein to the colloid may be imperative as reported for ovomucoid (Geoghegan and Ackerman, 1977). After 1–2 min, a 1% aqueous polyethylene glycol solution (polyethylene glycol 20 000 molecular weight or Carbowax-20 M) is added. Usually 1 ml is mixed with 20 ml crude protein-gold complex but the amount does not seem to be of critical importance. The polyethylene glycol is thought to act as a further "stabilizing" agent which lowers the rate of aggregate formation (Horisberger *et al.*, 1975; Horisberger and Rosset, 1977). Romano *et al.* (1974; 1975) have used bovine serum albumin as a further stabilizing agent and have added NaCl (final concentration 1%) to the crude preparations. Addition of NaCl is thought to "remove" (flocculate) unstabilized or incompletely stabilized gold particles.

2. Purification of the Crude Complex

Purification, i.e. removal of free, uncomplexed protein and of not fully stabilized gold particles, is achieved by ultracentrifugation in a fixed angle rotor. Depending on the particle size of the colloid the centrifugation conditions are as follows: 105 000 ×g for 1·5 to 2 h for complexes formed with 3 nm gold particles; 60 000 ×g for 45 to 60 min for complexes with 15 nm gold particles; 30 000 ×g for 60 min, 30 min or 20 min for complexes formed with 20 nm, 30 nm or 50 nm gold particles respectively. The centrifugation results in the formation of a loose, intensely red coloured sediment in the bottom of the centrifuge tube. In addition, a dark spot of densely packed material is formed on the tube wall slightly above the loose sediment in the bottom of the tube. This material consists of precipitated aggregated complexes or not fully stabilized particles and has to be discarded. The colourless supernatant which possibly contains free protein is carefully aspirated and discarded. The sediment of protein-gold complexes is resuspended with an appropriate buffer containing 0·2 mg ml^{-1} polyethylene glycol (molecular weight 20 000) or Carbowax-20 M. The centrifugation is repeated twice to ensure removal of free protein.

Colloidal gold prepared with ascorbic acid (Stathis and Fabrikanos, 1958) or with diluted ether solution of white phosphorus (Zsigmondy, 1905; Zsigmondy and Thiessen, 1925) varies considerably in particle size. Slot and Geuze (1981) have fractionated such polydisperse colloids complexed with *Staphylococcal* protein A by glycerol or sucrose gradient centrifugation into homogenous subfractions. As a first step, they performed ultracentrifugation as described above. The sedimented complexes were then layered over a 10–30% continuous glycerol or sucrose gradient (volume 10·5 ml, length 8 cm) in PBS. The gradient was centrifuged in a SW 41 Beckman rotor at 41 000 rpm for 45 min in the case of gold prepared with phosphorus or at 20 000 rpm for 30 min in the case of gold made with the ascorbic acid method. From about 1 cm below the surface, successive fractions of about 1 ml were collected and dialysed aganst PBS. In this way, homogenously sized protein A-gold complexes between 4·5 and 15 nm in diameter can be obtained. A simpler way to obtain homogenous subfractions is gel column filtration with Sephacryl (Pharmacia). Tschopp and colleagues (personal communication) sized F(ab')$_2$–gold complexes into homogenous fractions by this procedure.

Depending on the size and molecular weight of the substance to be used for complex formation, the centrifugation conditions must be varied as best illustrated for low-density lipoprotein. Handley *et al.* (1981) performed centrifugation at 20 000 ×g for 20 min in a swing out rotor against a 35% sucrose cushion which ensured that the excess low-density lipoprotein remained in the supernatant. Finally, the complexes were dialysed against PBS.

E. Special Recipes

1. Immunoglobulin-gold Complexes

Antisera, IgG-fractions of antisera or affinity purified antibodies contain a mixture of antibodies having a wide range of isoelectric points. Therefore it is difficult to decide which pH is optimal for their adsorption to colloidal gold and consequently several protocols have been described. Romano et al. (1974) used affinity purified horse anti-human IgG dialysed against 5 mM NaCl at pH 7·0. Horisberger et al. (1975) dialysed an anti-Candida utilis antiserum in the same way. Geoghegan and Ackerman (1977) performed dialysis of an IgG fraction of rabbit anti-goat IgG against triple distilled water. Goodman et al. (1981) used affinity-purified sheep anti-rabbit immunoglobulin after dialysis against 7 mM Tris-HCl buffer at pH 8·2. De Mey et al. (1981b) worked with 2 mM borax HCl buffer (pH 9·0) for dialysis of affinity-purified goat anti-rabbit IgG. These investigators found that 2 mM borax HCL buffer at pH 9·0 gave very satisfactory results with affinity-purified antibodies from goat, rabbit and mouse and seemed to be the method of choice. It was also observed that the solubility of the antibodies was increased under such alkaline conditions. The same conditions proved to be applicable for work with monoclonal antibodies (de Mey et al., 1981a).

The following standard procedure is proposed. Immunoglobulin solutions (1 mg ml^{-1}) are dialysed against 2 mM borax HCl buffer at pH 9 and kept in this low molarity buffer for as short a time as possible. Immediately before complex formation, possible protein aggregates are sedimented by centrifugation at 100 000 ×g for 1 h at 4 °C. The pH of the colloidal gold is adjusted to 9 with 0·2 M K_2CO_3 just before use. A 10% excess of the optimally stabilizing protein amount is mixed with the colloidal gold and after 2 min, bovine serum albumin (in distilled water adjusted to pH 9·0 with NaOH and microfiltered) is added to yield a final concentration of 1%. This crude preparation is filtered with 0·22 μm Millipore filter. After centrifugation, the sedimented immunoglobulin-gold complexes are resuspended in 20 mM Tris buffered saline (pH 8·2) containing 1% bovine serum albumin. The centrifugation is repeated twice and the complexes were resuspended finally in Tris buffered saline containing BSA and NaN_3. The same procedure is used with monoclonal antibodies but the pH of the protein and colloidal gold is adjusted to the isoelectric point of the monoclonal antibodies. Estimation of the isoelectric point is done by isoelectric focusing under non-denaturing conditions.

2. F(ab')₂–gold Complexes

The procedure was described by Ackerman *et al.* (1980a) who used F(ab')$_2$ from an IgG fraction of a rabbit anti-cholera toxin serum. The F(ab')$_2$ preparation was dialyzed against 5 mM phosphate buffer. Before complex formation with colloidal gold, F(ab')$_2$ was dissolved in triple-distilled water. Colloidal gold prepared according to Frens (1973) was adjusted to pH 7·2 with 0·2 M K_2CO_3. To 200 ml of colloidal gold, 3·6 mg of F(ab')$_2$ in 5 ml of triple-distilled water were added dropwise with gentle stirring. After 1 min, 2 ml of 1% aqueous polyethylene glycol (molecular weight 20 000) was added and centrifugation was first performed at low speed to remove any large aggregates followed by high speed centrifugation to sediment the F(ab')$_2$–gold complexes. These complexes were resuspended with 10 ml phosphate buffer (pH 7·4) containing 0·2 mg ml^{-1} polyethylene glycol and 4% polyvinylpyrrolidone (molecular weight 10 000).

3. Protein A-gold Complexes

Protein A from *Staphylococcus aureus* bound to colloidal gold represents a general second step reagent in the localization of antigen-bound antibodies (Romano and Romano, 1977; Roth *et al.*, 1978). A detailed description of the preparation of protein A-gold complex can be found in the first volume of this series (Roth, 1982b). To summarise, protein A is dissolved in water and colloidal gold (pH 5·9–6·2) was added. For stabilization of 10 ml colloidal gold the following amount of protein A is needed: approximately 60 μg for 3 nm gold prepared with ether-phosphorus, approximately 50 μg for polydisperse colloidal gold prepared with ascorbic acid and approximately 30 μg for 15 nm gold particles (citrate method). The sizing of protein A-gold complexes prepared from polydisperse colloids will be described in section III.D.2.

4. Lectin-gold Complexes

Lectins have been extensively used as histochemical reagents coupled to a variety of markers (for review, see Roth 1978) and this is well illustrated (Leathem and Atkins, see this volume). Furthermore, lectin-gold complexes have been prepared in several laboratories (Horisberger *et al.*, 1975; 1978; Horisberger and Rosset, 1977; Wagner and Wagner, 1976; 1977; Roth and Wagner, 1977a,b; Roth and Binder, 1978) but at that time the optimal pH conditions for complex formation were not taken into account. In recent investigations, Roth (1982a; 1983a,b) has considered the different isoelectric points (Table I) of the various lectins and established optimal conditions

TABLE I

Data for pH adjustment of colloidal gold and proteins for complex formation.

Proteins	pH
Immunoglobulins (IgG fractions, affinity-purified antibodies, monoclonal antibodies)	9·0 (7·6; 8·2)
F(ab')$_2$	7·2
Protein A	5·9–6·2
Ricinus communis lectin I	8·0
Ricinus communis lectin II	8·0
Peanut lectin	6·3
Helix pomatia lectin	7·4
Soybean lectin	6·1
Lens culinaris lectin	6·9
Lotus tetragonolobus lectin	6·3
Ulex europeus lectin I	6·3
Bandeirae simplicifolia lectin	6·2
Mannan from *Candida utilis* or *Saccharomyces cerevisia*	7
Horseradish peroxidase	7·2–8·0
Ovomucoid	4·8
Ceruloplasmin	7·0
Asialofetuin	6·0–6·5
Galactosyl bovine serum albumin	6·0–6·5
Bovine serum albumin	5·2–5·5
Peptide-bovine serum albumin conjugates	4·0–4·5
Insulin-bovine serum albumin conjugates	5·3
Cholera toxin	6·9
Tetanus toxin	6·9
DNAase	6·0
RNAase	9·0–9·2
Low-density lipoprotein	5·5
α_2-macroglobulin	6·0
Avidin (unmodified, egg white)	~10·0–10·6
Avidin (tetramethylrhodamine isothiocyanate conjugated, egg white)	
Avidin (*Streptavidin*)	6·4–6·6

for complex formation. The lectins were dissolved in distilled water immediately before use and adsorbed to 15 nm gold particles. The following amounts of protein were needed to stabilize 10 ml of colloidal gold: *Ricinus communis* lectin I, 130 μg; *Ricinus communis* lectin II, 130 μg; peanut lectin, 130 μg; Helix pomatia lectin, 65 μg; soybean lectin, 65 μg; *Lens culinaris* lectin, 130 μg; *Lotus tetragonolobus* lectin, 130 μg; *Ulex europeus* lectin, 250 μg; and *Bandeireae simplicifolia* isolectin B$_4$, 250 μg. In Table I the data for the pH adjustment of the colloidal gold are given. For pH adjustment 0·2 M K$_2$CO$_3$ or 0·1 M HCl or acetic acid was added to the colloidal gold.

Indirect techniques using glycoprotein-gold complexes (see below) for the detection of cell-bound native Concanavalin A or wheat-germ lectin have been worked out by Geoghegan and Ackerman (1977).

Finally, it should be mentioned that Horisberger and Rosset (1977) and Horisberger *et al.*, (1978) used wheat-germ lectin and *Ricinus communis* lectin I cross-linked to bovine serum albumin for adsorption to colloidal gold. The pH of the colloidal gold was 7 (phosphorus gold) or 5·13 (citrate gold). Cross-linking was done by adding 0·05 ml of 0·25% glutaraldehyde to a mixture of lectin (1 mg) and bovine serum albumin (4 mg) dissolved in 0·25 ml 5 mM NaCl neutralized to pH 7 with 0·2 M K_2CO_3. After a conjugation time of 2 h at 25 °C, 12·2 ml 5 mM NaCl were added to the mixture. The crude conjugate was filtered through 0·45 μm Millipore filter and used immediately for adsorption to colloidal gold.

5. Glycoprotein-gold Complexes

Such complexes can be used as second step reagents in the visualization of native, non-labelled lectins (Horisberger and Rosset, 1977; Geoghegan and Ackerman, 1977; Roth, 1983a,b) or as reagents for localization of glycoprotein binding cell surface receptors (Horisberger and Von Lanthen, 1978; Kolb *et al.*, 1981).

Mannan from *Candida utilis* or *Saccharomyces cerevisiae* was dissolved in 5 mM NaCl (pH 7) and mixed with gold at pH 7 (Horisberger and Rosset, 1977) and used for the visualization of Concanavalin A. As an alternative, horseradish peroxidase was used. The glycoprotein enzyme was dissolved in distilled water and adsorbed to colloidal gold adjusted to pH 7·2 (Geoghegan and Ackerman, 1977) or to pH 8·0 (Roth, 1983a,b). Ten ml of 15 nm gold particles (pH 8·0) could be stablized with 65 μg horseradish peroxidase (Fluka, purissimum). Ovomucoid-gold complexes (Geoghegan and Ackerman, 1977; Roth, 1983a,b) for binding to wheat-germ lectin were prepared as follows. Colloidal gold (15 nm) was adjusted to pH 4·8 by addition of 0·1 N HCl. Ovomucoid was dissolved in distilled water and 16 μg were used to stabilize 10 ml colloidal gold.

Asialoceruloplasmin-gold complex (Horisberger and Von Lanthen, 1978) was prepared from ceruloplasmin which was dissolved in 5 mM NaCl (pH 7·0). After centrifugation at 100 000 ×g for 15 min, the optimal stabilizing amount of ceruloplasmin was brought together with colloidal gold. Carbowax-20 M (1% solution) was added after 1 min and the mixture was immediately neutralized with 0·2 M K_2CO_3. After centrifugation, the sediment from a 100 ml crude preparation was resuspended to a volume of 2 ml with 0·02 M Tris buffered 0·15 M saline (pH 7·4). In order to prepare a desialated complex incubation with *Vibrio cholerae* neuraminidase (50 U) was performed for 1 h at room temperature. Neuraminidase was eliminated by two centrifugation cycles, and the complex resuspended finally in Tris buffered saline (pH 7·4) containing 0·5 mg ml^{-1} Carbowax-20 M and 10 mmol ml^{-1} CaCl$_2$.

The procedure for preparing asialofetuin-gold complexes (Kolb-Bachofen *et al.*, 1981) or galactosyl bovine serum albumin-gold complexes (Kolb-Bachofen, 1981) with 17 nm gold particles according to Frens (1973) was recently described. Colloidal gold was adjusted to pH 6·0–6·5 and 130 μg of the glycoproteins were sufficient to stabilize 10 ml colloid. Centrifugation was done at 32 000 ×g for 30 min and the complexes were finally resuspended with phosphate buffered isotonic saline containing 0·02% Carbowax-20 M.

6. *Complex Formation with Peptide-bovine Serum Albumin Conjugates*

The principle of use of conjugates of low molecular weight substances with bovine serum albumin for complex formation with colloidal gold (Horisberger and Rosset, 1977) was adapted for a variety of peptides (Larsson, 1979; Ackerman and Wolken, 1980; 1981).

A variety of synthetic and natural peptides such as synthetic ACTH$_{1-24}$, ACTH$_{1-28}$, β–MSH, β-endorphin, caerulein, human gastrin$_{6-13}$, human gastrin$_{2-17}$, natural porcine ACTH$_{1-39}$ and human growth hormone (between 50 and 200 nmol peptide) and bovine serum albumin (60 nmol) in 250 μl 5 mM NaCl (pH 7·0) were cross-linked with 50 μl 0.25% glutaraldehyde for 2 h at room temperature. Then, the volume was brought to 13 ml with 5 mM NaCl and the pH adjusted to 4·0–4·5. The crude conjugate was filtered (0·45 μm Millipore filter) and mixed with 100 ml of colloidal gold (particle size 18 nm or 30 nm). After addition of 5 ml of Carbowax-20 M, the solution was neutralized and centrifuged. The sedimented complexes were resuspended to 4 ml with 0·05 M Tris HCl buffer (pH 7·9) containing 5 mg ml^{-1} of each Carbowax-20 M and NaN$_3$. A ten-fold dilution was used as the working solution.

Insulin was conjugated to bovine serum albumin by the following procedure. Two mg of porcine insulin and 5·2 mg bovine serum albumin were dissolved in 0·5 ml 0·01 N NaOH and the pH was adjusted to 7·0 with 0·01 N HCl. Glutaraldehyde was added (0·1 ml of 0·25% solution) and conjugation took 2 h at room temperature. Afterwards, 24·5 ml of 5 mM NaCl were added and the crude conjugate was filtered (0·45 μm Millipore filter). Colloidal gold (18–20 nm) was adjusted to pH 5·3 and 66 ml of colloidal gold were added to 25 ml of freshly prepared conjugate. Addition of 6 ml of 1% polyethylene glycol was followed by centrifugation and resuspension of the sedimented complexes in 6 ml of 0·1 M phosphate buffer (pH 7·6) containing 4% polyvinylpyrrolidone and 0·2 mg ml^{-1} polyethylene glycol.

7. Toxin-gold Complexes

Cholera toxin (Montesano *et al.*, 1982) and tetanus toxin (Montesano *et al.*, 1982; Schwab and Thoenen, 1978) were brought into 5 mм NaCl by passage through Sephadex G-25 equilibrated and eluted with 5 mм NaCl. Colloidal gold (15 nm) was adjusted to pH 6·9 with 0·2 м K_2CO_3. The stabilizing amount of cholera toxin and tetanus toxin for 10 ml of colloidal gold was 1·6 mg and 2·7 mg, respectively.

8. Enzyme-gold Complexes

In Volume 3 of this series a whole chapter will be devoted to the preparation and application of enzyme-gold complexes as introduced by Bendayan (1981a). Therefore, only the principal aspects of this procedure will be mentioned here.

Colloidal gold (approximately 15 nm) was adjusted to pH 6·0 for adsorption of DNAase and to pH 9·0–9·2 for complex formation with RNAase. The minimal stabilizing enzyme amount for 10 ml colloidal gold was 0.05 mg DNAase or 0·12 mg RNAase. After mixing and centrifugation, the DNAase-gold complexes prepared with 10 ml colloidal gold were resuspended to a volume of 3 ml with PBS containing 0·2 mg ml^{-1} polyethylene glycol. For RNAase-gold complexes the pH of the PBS was 7·5 and for DNAase-gold complexes it was 6·0.

9. Low-density Lipoprotein-gold Complex

Colloidal gold (19 nm) was used at pH 5·5. Low-density lipoprotein was always freshly prepared from human plasma (Havel *et al.*, 1955) and used immediately after extensive dialysis against 0·05 м EDTA (pH 5·5) for complex formation as described by Handley *et al.*, (1981). To 0.5 ml of low-density lipoprotein containing 1·5 μg protein, 5 ml of colloidal gold were added with rapid mixing. Centrifugation at 9000 ×g for 20 min against a 35% sucrose cushion ensured separation of free protein from the low-density lipoprotein-gold complex which sedimented into the sucrose cushion. Dialysis of the complex was performed against an isotonic buffer. The complex was used within 24 h.

10. α_2-macroglobulin-gold Complex

The procedure was described by Dickson *et al.* (1981). After extensive dialysis of α_2-macroglobulin against distilled, deionized water at pH 6·0, the protein was mixed with colloidal gold whose pH was at 6·0. A volume of

50 ml of colloidal gold and 10 ml of α_2-macroglobulin containing 12 mg protein were mixed, 1·5 ml of 1% polyethylene glycol were added and this was followed by centrifugation (20 000 ×g for 1 h). After several centrifugation cycles, the α_2-macroglobulin-gold complex was resuspended with phosphate buffered isotonic saline (pH 7·4) containing 1·5 mM CaCl$_2$ and 0·01% polyethylene glycol.

11. Avidin-gold Complex

The outstanding advantage of the biotin-avidin interaction is the exceptional high rate of association (10^8 M^{-1} sec^{-1}) and the high stability of the complexes (dissociation rate 10^{15} M^{-1}) (Green, 1974). Therefore, as reported by Boorsma in a separate chapter of this book, this system has been proven to be very useful for light microscopic studies. A main disadvantage of avidin from egg white, with respect to complex formation with colloidal gold is its extremely high isoelectric point pH 10. This causes not only serious problems of nonspecific background staining in some systems (Guesdon *et al.*, 1979) but also problems in the complex formation with colloidal gold. At pH values above 10, colloidal gold tends to aggregate spontaneously in our experience. Colloidal gold (15 nm) brought to pH 10·6 and mixed with avidin always gave highly unstable complexes in our laboratory and these flocculated completely within about 1 h as indicated by a colour change to blue and precipitation. An alternative to egg white avidin seems to be close now since Papermaster and Ward (personal communication) have isolated a bacterial avidin with an isoelectric point of 6·4 and already used it successfully for complex formation and staining experiments at the electron microscopic level.

Nevertheless, Hopkins and coworkers (Hopkins *et al.*, 1979; Tolson *et al.*, 1981) have reported results with avidin-gold complexes used to localize biotinylated epidermal growth factor. Their protocol for avidin-gold complex formation goes as follows. To 1 ml of colloidal gold, 0·1 N NaOH is added in volumes between 10–200 μl, and then 10 μl of 1 mg ml^{-1} avidin in distilled water is added to each aliquot. This is followed by 100 μl 1% NaCl and centrifugation for 1 h. The minimal amount of NaOH which did not cause flocculation in the preparation was considered to be the optimum. Avidin-gold complexes prepared by this procedure were stored in Tris-glycine buffer at pH 11 with addition of 1% polyethylene glycol.

Horisberger and Von Lanthen (1979) used an avidin from egg white which was labelled with tetramethylrhodamine isothiocyanate. Through the coupling procedure amino groups of avidin were blocked and consequently a change of the isoelectric point resulted. The rhodamine-conjugated avidin, after dissolution in 5 mM NaCl (pH 7·0), was mixed with colloidal gold prepared according to Stathis and Fabrikanos (1958). Fifty ml colloidal gold were stabilized with 0·225 mg rhodamine-conjugated avidin. After 1 min, Carbowax was added and the mixture neutralised with 0·2 M K_2CO_3. The complexes were sedimented by centrifugation and resuspended in 0·02 M Tris-HCl buffered 0·15 M NaCl (pH 7·4) containing 0·5 mg ml^{-1} Carbowax-20 M and 1 mM $CaCl_2$ and $MnCl_2$.

F. Storage of the Complexes

Protein-gold complexes cannot be stored frozen since this results in excessive aggregate formation and in some cases in complete loss of bioactivity (Faulk and Taylor, 1971). This can be prevented by mixing the complexes in a 50% glycerol solution so that storage at −18 °C becomes possible (Slot and Geuze, 1981). Usually, the complexes are stored at 4 °C with addition of a bacteriostaticum (NaN$_3$, o.a.). Goodman *et al.* (1979; 1981) and Geoghegan *et al.* (1980) advocated sterile filtration through a 0·2 µm polycarbonate membrane or a 0·22 µm Millipore filter which was pretreated with PBS containing 0·4 mg polyethylene glycol per ml and 1 mg bovine serum albumin per ml in order to minimize protein adsorption.

G. Bioactivity and Stability of the Complexes

It seems that a protein adsorbed on colloidal gold has similar characteristics to the non-adsorbed protein and keeps its binding capacity or enzymatic activity for a long time. The only exception reported so far is beef liver catalase which was found to be completely inactivated after adsorption to colloidal gold (Horisberger and Rosset, 1977). Immunoglobulins (antisera, IgG fractions or monoclonal antibodies) retained their reactivity for several months when stored at 4 °C (Faulk and Taylor, 1971; Romano *et al.*, 1974; de Mey *et al.*, 1981a). The protein A-gold complex prepared from 15 nm gold particles stayed active for more than a year (unpublished observations). Horseradish peroxidase retained its enzymatic activity for at least 14 months (Geoghegan and Ackerman, 1977). Similar observations were made for avidin-gold complexes (Tolson *et al.*, 1981), toxin-gold complexes (Schwab and Thoenen, 1978); Montesano *et al.*, 1982) and lectin-gold complexes (Horisberger and Rosset, 1977; Roth, 1983a,b).

In our experience it appears that the bioactivity of lectins or protein A bound to colloidal gold prepared with the phosphorus method generally does not last as long as colloidal gold prepared by the citrate method. This could be due to the presence of trace amounts of ether or phosphoric acid. Ether can be evaporated by prolonged boiling and by passing a stream of air through the colloid, phosphoric acid can be oxidized. Further investigations are needed to clarify the effect of such treatment on the bioactivity of the complexes. Effective procedures for assessment of the bioactivity of the complexes are provided by agglutination tests or indirect radioassays. Agglutination tests were first applied by Faulk and Taylor (1971) with *Salmonella* as appropriate indicator cells. This type of approach has been adapted since then and proved to be a reliable test for monitoring the activity of complexes (Goodman *et al.*, 1979; 1981). Another convenient means for assessment of the bioactivity of complexes is provided by radio-binding assay (Goodman *et al.*, 1979).

Since the forces involved in complex formation are non-covalent in nature, a most critical question concerns the stability of such complexes. It is generally assumed that proteins are irreversibly adsorbed onto colloidal gold (Horisberger *et al.*, 1975). Evidence to support the assumption that proteins are tightly bound to particles of colloidal gold comes from several experiments. Schwab and Thoenen (1978) have shown the strength of binding of tetanus toxin to colloidal gold. They incubated ^{125}I-tetanus toxin-gold complexes with rat serum and found after 1 h at 37 °C a release of 4% of the radioactivity and after 14 h, 9% of the initial radioactivity released in the supernatant. The possible exchange of previously bound protein was studied by Goodman *et al.* (1980; 1981). The release of protein from colloidal gold was measured in the presence of excess amounts of competing proteins and was found to be reasonably low, especially in the presence of polyethylene glycol. Repeated freezing and thawing of complexes caused only relatively little dissociation (Goodman *et al.*, 1981). Drastic changes in the pH values of the environment (exposure to pH 4 or pH 9) did not destabilize low-density lipoprotein-gold complexes nor did exposure to 600 mOsmol NaCl cause noticeable complex dissociation (Handley *et al.*, 1981). Kolb-Bachofen *et al.* (1981) found no indications for destabilization of glycoprotein-gold complexes after storage for 3 weeks at 5 °C.

In summary, there is evidence that protein-gold complexes retain both bioactivity and stability for reasonable periods of time. However, depending on the macromolecules adsorbed to colloidal gold, release into the buffer solutions can occur. Therefore, the complexes should be used within a short time after preparation or centrifuged again before use.

H. Conclusions

Colloidal gold can be prepared easily and all that is needed is simple equipment and an open mind about straightforward chemical reactions. The preparation is also inexpensive, i.e. from 1 g tetrachloroauric acid, 10 l of colloidal gold can be produced. The formation of complexes between colloidal gold and biological macromolecules is as rapid a procedure as the preparation of colloidal gold by itself. Only small amounts of biological macromolecules are needed. The purification of the complexes is easily achieved and rapid. The marker colloidal gold can be detected in both the light and electron microscope without any further treatment and this allows for precise localization and high resolution.

IV. APPLICATIONS IN LIGHT MICROSCOPY

The natural colour of colloidal gold in transmitted light is red but may appear more reddish-orange or dark red depending on the preparative conditions. This colour remains after complex formation with biological macro-molecules. Structures on cells or in tissues to which protein-gold complexes have been bound appear red when viewed in the light microscope with bright field illumination. No "revealing" agents are necessary as with enzyme-labelled probes to produce this colour. The labelling procedure with pro-tein-gold complexes yields a permanent, non-bleaching staining. Sections or cells can be dehydrated, mounted in commonly-used embedding media and stored to be re-examined.

A. Localization of Cell Surface Components

1. Procedure for Labelling Cells

The cells grown in monolayers or obtained as suspensions may be labelled either unfixed or prefixed. The incubation of unfixed cells is commonly used to prevent any loss of antigenicity upon the action of the fixative. Incuba-tions carried out at 4 °C almost completely prevent lateral movement of cell surface antigens. Labelling of living cells at room temperature or at 37 °C promotes lateral redistribution into patches and allows for cap formation as well as for internalization.

When cells were incubated at 4 °C or after mild prefixation a ring-like pattern of staining appeared. In instances when a low density of cell surface antigens makes it difficult to detect a positive reaction, conditions which allow only for patch formation but not for capping or internalization might be preferable. Such conditions can be easily achieved by addition of NaN_3 (0·2%) to the incubation media and performing labelling at 37 °C, since patching is a metabolically-independent ligand-induced redistribution unlike capping and endocytosis. The focally arranged cell surface labelling can be easily appreciated in the form of "granules".

The general procedure for labelling of unfixed cells is as follows

Cells in suspension or in monolayer are washed with an isotonic buffer solution or maintained in the culture medium provided that it does not contain substances which could interfere with the binding of the specific ligands. Unfortunately, serum constituents are often competitive. However, the media should contain protein especially if multiple centrifugations or reincubation experiments are to be performed. In general, bovine serum albumin in concentrations of 0·1–0·5% does not interfere with the binding of various ligands (Taylor *et al.*, 1971; de Petris and Raff, 1972; Cohen and Gilbertsen, 1975) and the binding of lectins is not impaired (Amherdt and Roth, unpublished observations). On the other hand, addition of bovine serum albumin to the incubation medium lowers, in many instances, the degree of nonspecific binding.

The cells are incubated with the native or gold-labelled protein for 20–30 min (room temperature or 37 °C) or 30–60 min (4 °C) with occasional agitation. The incubation mixture is diluted with washing buffer and cells are centrifuged at approximately 300 ×g for 3–5 min. After removal of the supernatant, the pellet is resuspended in washing buffer and two centrifugation cycles follow. If the cells are grown in a monolayer, they are simply rinsed with the buffer solution.

In the one-step method (primary reagent adsorbed to colloidal gold), this is followed by fixation in 0·01–0·1% glutaraldehyde in PBS for 10 min or by simple air drying on coverslips, and counterstaining is done with 1% methylgreen in distilled water for 3 min. Finally, cells are dehydrated in graded ethanol and xylene and mounted in a common embedding medium.

In the two-step method (primary reagent non-labelled), the washed cell pellet is resuspended with the gold labelled secondary antibodies or the cell monolayer covered with this solution and incubated for 30–60 min with occasional agitation. At the end of the incubation period, rinsing, fixation, staining and mounting is performed as described above.

Staining of prefixed cells is done principally in the same way with the following modifications.

Choose an appropriate fixative which in the most cases will be glutaraldehyde or formaldeyde in an isotonic buffer. Immobilization of cell surface sites can be achieved within a few minutes with 0·5–1% glutaraldehyde. Formaldehyde (1–2%) fixation should last longer (30–60 min) to ensure immobilization of cell surface components.

After fixation with aldehydes, free aldehyde groups must be blocked since they are reactive with ϵ-amino groups and could introudce nonspecific binding of antibodies, lectins, etc. Blocking of reactive aldehyde groups can be done with 0.1–0.5 M NH_4Cl in PBS, or 0.1 M glycine or lysine in PBS for 30–60 min, or borohydride ($NaBH_4$, 0.5 mg ml^{-1}) for 10 min.

Incubation steps and washing procedures are as described above.

Combination staining for a variety of enzymes by histochemical methods can be subsequently performed as described by de Waele *et al.* (1982a,b).

The staining for surface antigens is performed on unfixed cells with monoclonal antibodies and gold-labelled secondary antibodies as a two-step method (see above).

Cell smears are fixed with 4% formaldehyde in absolute ethanol for 2 min, rinsed in distilled water and air dried.

Histochemical reactions according to standard protocols are performed to reveal peroxidase, α-naphthyl acetate esterase, acid phosphatase and β-glucuronidase.

2. Microscopic Observation of the Specimens

Positively reacting cells can be seen clearly in a normal bright field light microscope as red coloured structures. The observation is facilitated with transverse light illumination (Roth, unpublished). De Mey and coworkers (unpublished) have found that polarized light epi-illumination microscopy is more sensitive than bright field illumination. The polarized epi-illumination system can be easily adapted to most epi-fluorescence microscopes. De Mey and co-workers propose the use of a mercury-vapour lamp and planapochromat immersion-objectives with a large numerical aperture in combination with the epi-illumination equipment. The staining resulting from the immunoglobulin-gold complex appeared as a strong yellow-gold colour.

3. Applications in Enumeration of B and T Lymphocytes

Geoghegan *et al.* (1978) visualized surface immunoglobulin D and M on human blood lymphocytes in a two-step technique with rabbit anti-goat

IgG-gold complexes and compared the data with those obtained by direct immunofluorescence. Similar percentages of labelled cells were found with both techniques; i.e. 10% IgD positive cells with immunocolloid staining versus 9·9% with immunofluorescence and 8·5% versus 10·7% for IgM bearing cells. The same approach was used by de Waele *et al.* (1981a,b) and de Mey *et al.* (1981a,b) to enumerate lymphocytes and their subclasses with monoclonal antibodies which were either directly bound to colloidal gold or were visualized with gold labelled anti-species antibodies. These authors used normal human AB serum in the incubation media to prevent binding of the specific antibodies to Fc receptors and, to exclude, therefore, the possibility of a false-positive result. When they compared the sensitivity of the immunoglobulin-gold staining with immunofluorescence almost identical results were found. All groups of investigators agree that this staining method could become a routine technique in clinical laboratories. In their opinion, it provides an alternative to immunofluorescence since no fluorescent microscopes are needed and the preparations are stable and may be re-examined at any time.

B. Localization of Antigens and Glycoconjugates in Tissues and within Cells

1. Fixation and Permeabilization of Cells

The procedure has been described by de Mey *et al.* (1981a,b; 1982).

Cells were grown on glass coverslips.

Mammalian cells were fixed and permeabilized for 10 min in a mixture of 1% Triton X-100 and 0·5% glutaraldehyde in a convenient buffer. They were then washed in buffer and treated with 0·5% Triton X-100 in buffer for 30 min. Plant endosperm cells were treated with 0·5% glutaraldehyde in 0·1 M phosphate buffer (pH 6·9) containing 0·1–0·2% Triton X-100 for 2–5 min followed by 1% glutaraldehyde for 10 min. After washing in buffer, further permeabilization with 0·5% Triton X-100 in buffer followed for 10 min.

Free reactive aldehyde groups were blocked by treatment with borohydride ($NaBH_4$; 0·5 mg ml^{-1}) for 10 min.

After washing with buffer, cells were processed for staining as described above (Section IV.A.1).

2. Fixation and Embedding of Tissues for Paraffin Sections and Semi-thin Resin Sections

For the localization of antigens, indirect techniques using immunoglobulin-gold complexes (Gu *et al.*, 1981) or protein A-gold complex (Roth, 1982b) were applied. Cellular and extracellular glycoconjugates were visualised by means of lectins directly adsorbed on gold particles or by glycoprotein-gold complexes in an indirect technique (Roth, 1983a,b).

Fixation for the localization of various polypeptide hormones introduced no special problems with respect to retention of antigenicity. Fresh tissue pieces were frozen in Arcton and freeze-dried overnight at −40 °C followed by fixation in benzoquinone vapour (60 °C) for 3 h or paraformaldehyde vapour (80 °C) for 1 h and embedding in wax (Gu *et al.*, 1981). Fixation in Bouin's fluid overnight, in glutaraldehyde (1%) immersion or perfusion fixation for 2 h, in paraformaldehyde (4%) fixation for 4 h or fixation with Carnoy's solution for 4 h retained the antigenicity of various polypeptide hormones, exocrine pancreatic enzymes and cytosolic vitamin D-dependent calcium binding protein (Roth, 1982b; unpublished observations) in sections from paraffin embedded tissues. After fixation with aldehydes, reactive aldehyde groups were blocked by treatment with one of the solutions as described in Section IV.A.1.

Contrary to these results, the choice of the fixative for localization of lectin-binding sites with gold-labelled reagents was of critical importance. A distinct and reproducible staining pattern could be observed only in sections of tissues fixed with either glutaraldehyde (1%, 2 h) or paraformaldehyde (4%, 4 h). The intensity of staining was greatly reduced in sections from Bouin-fixed tissues and a diffuse overall staining together with a strong staining of the nuclei appeared regardless of the lectin used. Fixation with Carnoy's fluid was even worse. An intense diffuse cytoplasmic and nuclear staining appeared in different tissues and cell types with all lectins tested so far. Such a diffuse staining pattern was not observed with Bouin's or Carnoy's solution when lectin-peroxidase conjugates were applied (Stoward *et al.*, 1980).

Semi-thin sections (0·5 μm) from glutaraldehyde or formaldehyde-fixed specimens were prepared after embedding in Epon 812 as conventionally performed for electron microscopy (Roth *et al.*, 1983b). The fixation step with osmium tetroxide has to be omitted. Semithin sections were placed on glass slides and treated with a solution consisting of 2 g KOH, 5 ml of propylene oxide and 10 ml of methanol for 2–5 min at room temperature (Maxwell, 1978). Afterwards, the sections were rinsed in water methanol solution (1:1) and twice in water and PBS and stained by the protein A-gold technique (Roth *et al.*, 1978; Roth, 1982b) or with lectin-gold complexes (Roth *et al.*, 1983b).

3. Protocols for Single and Double Staining

The staining procedure, either performed as a direct (one step) or as an indirect (two step) technique, follows essentially the protocol described for cell surface labelling (Section IV.A.1.). For localization of antigenic sites with the protein A-gold technique (Roth, 1982c), deparaffinized and rehydrated sections or Epon semi-thin sections after removal of the resin were exposed to a solution of 0·5% ovalbumin in PBS for 5 min at room temperature before the first incubation step. Such a treatment could not be performed in labelling with lectins because of the carbohydrate nature of ovalbumin. The staining with protein A-gold complex or lectin-gold complexes which developed gradually as a red colour was monitored under a light microscope and stopped by several rinses of the sections with PBS and distilled water. Sections were then dehydrated through graded alcohols and xylene and mounted in appropriate media (Canada balsam, Eukitt, etc.).

Double staining of tissue antigens can be achieved by the sequential use of the peroxidase anti-peroxidase method and the immunoglobulin-gold staining method (Gu *et al.*, 1981). The PAP technique was carried out as described by Sternberger (1974). Afterwards, the antibody complex from the first staining was removed by treatment of the sections with glycine-HCl solution (pH 2·2) for 2 h. The blue reaction product for peroxidase activity revealed by 4-chloro-1-naphthol was retained by this procedure. The second staining sequence with antibody, followed by immunoglobulin-gold complexes, was then performed and gave a red colouration. Sections could not be dehydrated because of the solubility of the 4-chloro-1-naphthol reaction product in alcohol and were mounted after washing in glycerol jelly.

Roth (1982c) has developed a new type of double labelling technique by using two differently coloured colloids (Plate 8; see Plate section between pp. 148–149). Protein A was bound to colloidal gold to provide a reagent which gave a red colouration. For the first time another novel metal colloid was introduced in cytochemistry, namely colloidal silver which was coated with protein A. The protein A-silver complex resulted in a yellow colouration of positive tissue structures. The double staining protocol consisted of the incubation with the first antibody which was revealed by protein A-gold, followed by the incubation with a second antibody against a further antigen which was visualized with the protein A-silver complex. In this technique no acidic treatment of the sections after the first staining sequence was performed in order to remove the antibody. This was not necessary because of the mode of interaction of protein A predominantly with the Fc-portion of immunoglobulins (Forsgren and Sjöquist, 1966; 1967; Endresen, 1979; Wright *et al.*, 1977). Since both red and yellow are primary colours, an orange colour will develop in cases when the two antigens are present in the same cells. The double stained sections can be dehydrated and mounted. The staining with colloidal silver produces a permanent non-bleaching reaction as is the case with colloidal gold.

4. Cytochemical Controls

In the application of immunoglobulin-gold complexes, protein A-gold or protein A-silver complexes for antigen localization, all types of controls commonly performed in immunohistochemistry have to be done. They include: (a) preabsorption of the specific antibody with its corresponding antigen; (b) replacement of the antibody by buffer solution or non-immune serum; and (c) omission of the antibody step. Details can be found in text books of immunocytochemistry (Sternberger, 1974; Pearse, 1980).

In the direct lectin-gold techniques the following controls must be performed: (a) preincubation of the lectin-gold complex with an inhibitory sugar or glycopeptide; (b) preincubation of the sections with excess amounts of native lectin followed by lectin-gold complex; and (c) treatment of the sections with glycosidases, proteases and other reagents such as periodic acid, etc. For further details the reader is referred to the relevant reviews (Nicolson, 1978; Roth, 1978) and a recent original publication (Roth, 1980).

5. Some Observations (Plate 9; Figs 1, 2)

The techniques for light microscopic demonstration of antigenic sites or glycoconjugates within cells or in the extracellular matrix by the use of the colloidal gold marker are very recent innovations. Nevertheless, the few examples of their application have clearly demonstrated their validity in the localization of single or multiple cellular components. De Mey and coworkers (1981a,b; 1982) succeeded in the visualization of tubulin in interphase and mitotic cells. These investigators claimed that compared with the PAP method, the immunoglobulin-gold complexes provided a clearer picture and allowed them to make new observations. The existence of an elaborate cytoplasmic microtubule complex in interphase endoderm cells which could not be detected by immunofluorescence studies was described. This microtubular network transformed into a spindle-like cage surrounding the nucleus during prophase. Generally, more details could be detected with the use of colloidal gold instead of peroxidase as marker. Roth (1982a; 1983a,b) has now applied a series of lectins with different sugar specificities to various tissues. The resolution obtained was generally superior to that with

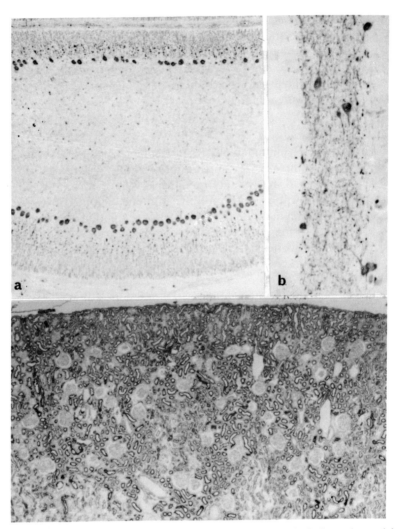

FIG. 1. Chick brain, paraffin sections. Localization of the vitamin D-dependent calcium binding protein in cerebellar Purkinje cells perikarya, dendritic trees and axons (a) and in neurons of the stratum fibrosum superficiale of the tectum opticum (b) with the protein A-gold technique. Same results were obtained in other studies using flourescein or peroxidase-labelled protein A (Roth *et al.* (1981). *Brain Res.* **222**, 452–457). Magnification ×20 (a), ×200 (b).

FIG. 2. (Bottom) Rat kidney, paraffin section. Localization of *Helix pomatia* lectin binding sites. At this low magnification the wide distribution of N-acetyl-D-galactosamine residues in the kidney cortex and adjacent regions of the outer medulla is evident. Magnification ×10.

fluorescein or peroxidase-tagged lectins. For example, in rat kidney (Fig. 2), the *Helix pomatia* lectin-gold complex stained the apical and basolateral plasma membrane of proximal tubular cells whereas in principal cells from distal convoluted tubules the lateral plasma membrane appeared negative. This was later confirmed by electron microscopic investigations (Roth, 1983b).

In summary, there is evidence that the colloidal gold marker system might become a powerful alternative to classical light microscopic markers such as fluorescent dyes and enzymes. The advantages of colloidal gold for light microscopy are obvious. A non-bleaching, permanent staining is obtained. The sections can be dehydrated and mounted in embedding medium. Double staining of antigens with colloidal silver as another contrasting stain can be performed or other cellular constituents can be visualized subsequently by conventional histochemical techniques. No special microscopes are needed. A further important and most interesting aspect is that the same protein-gold complexes can be used also at the electron microscope level for thin section, high voltage, freeze-fracture, shadow-cast replica and scanning electron microscopy. The next section of this chapter deals with these applications.

V. APPLICATIONS IN ELECTRON MICROSCOPY

Owing to the high atomic number of gold, particles of colloidal gold exhibit extremely high density (contrast) when viewed in the transmission electron microscope. Therefore, even particles of about 3 nm and less in diameter can be easily appreciated and clearly differentiated from cellular constituents. Particles of colloidal gold are capable of strong emission of secondary electrons and are, therefore, very useful in scanning electron microscopy, as well. Since gold emits characteristic signals, X-ray microanalysis can be performed on thin sections and quantitative X-ray microanalysis becomes possible with appropriate computer programs.

A. Cell Surface Components, Ligand-induced Redistribution and Endocytosis

1. Incubation Procedures

(a) Labelling of whole plasma membranes and chromosomes mounted on electron microscope grids

The procedure for plasma membranes was first described by Nicolson and coworkers (Nicolson, 1971; Nicolson and Singer, 1971; Nicolson *et al.*, 1971) and involves essentially the preparation of membrane "ghosts" which were mounted on collodion-carbon coated electron microscope grids. Red cell ghosts can easily be prepared by osmotic lysis of unfixed cells which are dropped into a hypotonic buffer or distilled water. The membranes of lysed cells which remained floating at the surface can be picked up by touching them with the carbon side of the grid to which they stick. Membrane ghosts can be prepared from nucleated cells as well. However, the plasma membrane must first be "strengthened" by mild and short fixation with formaldehyde (0·1–0·3% formaldehyde, 2 min) which results in a very limited cross-linking of cytoplasmic structures and does not inhibit lateral movement of membrane components. The fixation is stopped by washing with NH$_4$Cl in isotonic buffer, and finally cells are dropped onto the surface of 0·02 M phosphate buffer. The "cells" which remain at the air-buffer interface are picked up on grids.

Romano *et al.* (1974) applied this procedure to red blood cells which were labelled first with anti-Rh (D) antibodies followed by anti-immunoglobulin-gold complexes and then lysed, or which were lysed after the antibody incubation step, and incubated with the anti-immunoglobulin-gold complex on the grids (Romano *et al.*, 1975). Both procedures gave similar results. With the first protocol, however, the labelling is present at both sides of the membranes since the cells were labelled before lysis, and this superimposition could cause problems of interpretation. To circumvent such problems, "ghosts" from non-labelled cells were used and picked up on grids. The grids were then "conditioned" with a 5% bovine serum albumin solution in buffer in order to reduce or avoid nonspecific adsorption of the markers. Using this method, only the exposed face of the ghosts was labelled. Romano *et al.* (1974; 1975) studied the distribution of A antigenic sites on red blood cells with gold-labelled immunoglobulin.

In general, this method can be used as a simple means to analyze the two-dimensional distribution of cell surface components. The data have to be interpreted with caution since distortions of the membrane can occur and surface components can be released by the hypotonic treatment (Burger, 1968).

Very recently, Hutchinson *et al.* (1982) described the hybridization of DNA or RNA of fixed chromosomes placed on electron microscope grids with biotin-labelled polynucleotide probes (Langer *et al.*, 1981). The biotin-substituted probes were detected via reaction with an antibody against biotin and secondary antibody adsorbed to 20 nm gold particles. The authors mention numerous advantages of this approach over autoradiography such as much higher resolution, the possibility to detect and localize nascent RNA transcripts associated with active transcription units in chromatin spreads, and many others.

(b) Labelling of intact cells for studies on surface topography and endocytosis
It was already mentioned in Section IV.A.1. that labelling can be performed
as a one-step or two-step method with unfixed cells at 4 °C, or with prefixed
cells at room temperature. The same protocols are valid for electron microscopic studies. In order to study ligand-induced redistribution phenomena in
the plane of the plasma membrane and concomitantly appearing endocytosis events, the labelling protocol is performed only with unfixed cells either
as a pulse-chase type experiment or as a continuous exposure experiment.
The latter is important and has to be used when binding of ligands at 4 °C is
hampered due to temperature-induced changes in molecular configuration.
It involves the incubation of cells at 37 °C in isotonic buffered solution
containing BSA and the marker-ligand complexes. Cells are fixed at different time intervals of exposure and processed further as described below.
The pulse-chase type experiments involve the following steps. Incubation of
nonfixed cells with the ligand-marker complexes is performed at 4 °C for
30–60 min. The excess amount of non-bound ligand-marker complexes is
then moved by three rinses with isotonic buffered solution containing BSA
at 4 °C. The cells are finally reincubated in ligand-marker complex-free
medium at 37 °C for different periods of time before fixation with glutaraldehyde.

2. Double-labelling protocols

Simultaneous labelling of two different components on the same cell sample
can be achieved by the use of different markers in combination such as
colloidal gold and peroxidase (Roth and Wagner, 1977a), colloidal gold and
ferritin (Wagner and Wagner, 1977b; Roth and Binder, 1978) and most
efficiently by using gold particles of different sizes (Horisberger *et al.*, 1975;
1978; Horisberger and Von Lanthen, 1978; 1979a; Roth and Binder, 1978).
Such double labelling is not limited to studies of cell surface topography but
also can be used in experiments for redistribution and endocytosis, as first
demonstrated by Roth and Wagner (1977b), and recently applied by Willingham and coworkers (Willingham *et al.*, 1981a,b).

Double labelling can be performed by simultaneous exposure of the cells
to the ligand-marker complexes (Roth and Wagner, 1977a,b; Horisberger *et
al.*, 1978) or by successive incubation steps (Wagner and Wagner, 1977;
Roth and Binder, 1978; Horisberger and Von Lanthen, 1978; 1979a).

Some specific points have to be taken into account in performing double
labelling which are related to the ligands and to the gold particle size. In
experiments with lectin-gold complexes in particular, binding of the lectins
to each other could occur theoretically since most lectins are glycoproteins.
In fact, immobilized Concanavalin A served as an affinity reagent for the

purification of other lectins from soybean and waxbean (Goldstein et al., 1969), or castor bean (Podder et al., 1974). Similarly, the combined use of lectin-gold complexes and immunoglobulin-gold complexes could be problematic. Lectins have been shown to interact with immunoglobulins (Nakamura et al., 1969; Young et al., 1971) and this was used to develop a histochemical affinity technique (Thoss and Roth, 1976).

Among the lectins there are at least three which are not *glyco* proteins, namely Concanavalin A, peanut lectin and wheat-germ lectin and can be combined without problems. In practice, the situation seems to be less troublesome than theoretically expected. No nonspecific colabelling was observed when Concanavalin A, soybean lectin, wheat-germ lectin, *Ricinus communis* lectin I, peanut lectin and *Helix pomatia* lectin were used in various combinations (Roth and Wagner, 1977b; Horisberger et al., 1978; Horisberger and Von Lanthen, 1978; 1979a). Horisberger and Von Lanthen (1978) explained this lack of reactivity between lectin-gold complexes as being due to electrostatic repulsion. It seems that the degree of binding of lectin-gold complexes to the cell surface is also determined by the size of gold particles and steric hindrance occurs above a certain diameter which differs from one lectin to another (Horisberger, 1978; Horisberger et al., 1978).

3. Processing for Thin Section Transmission Electron Microscopy

Postfixation of the samples with buffered osmium tetroxide, alcohol dehydration with or without *en bloc* staining and embedding in a suitable resin are performed according to routine protocols. Thin sections can be counterstained with both uranyl acetate and lead citrate because of the high electron density of the colloidal gold markers.

4. Processing for Surface Replicas

After fixation with osmium tetroxide, samples are dehydrated in a graded series of alcohol, submerged in amylacetate and either air-dried or critical point dried in a critical point drying apparatus. Shadow cast replicas are made by evaporating platinum at 35–45° angle onto the coverslip. The replica is strengthened by further carbon evaporation at a 90° angle. Then, the replicas are cut into small squares using a razor blade or a diamond knife and the coverslip tilted into hydrofluoric acid (4–8%). Floating replica fragments are picked up with platinum wire loops after dilution of the fluoric acid with distilled water and transferred to distilled water and then onto a sodium hypochlorite solution for 1 h. After further rinses with distilled water, the replicas are picked up on grids. The gold particles resist these treatments and remain *in situ* as highly electron dense particles.

5. Processing for Freeze-etch Electron Microscopy

Until now colloidal gold was used only in one freeze-etch study (Wagner *et al.*, 1976) which has proved its applicability for such purposes. Principally, only isolated cells or isolated membranes can be used in order to reveal a gold-labelled probe after freeze-fracturing in the deep-etched cell surface. The labelled and fixed specimens were rinsed in buffer, and in distilled water immediately before rapid freezing in cooled freon. Freeze-fracturing and deep-etching was formed according to established protocols (Bullivant, 1973).

6. Processing for Scanning Electron Microscopy

In their excellent studies Horisberger and his group (Horisberger *et al.*, 1975; for a recent review, see Horisberger, 1981) have shown the extraordinary usefulness of particles of colloidal gold as markers in scanning electron microscopy. This subject is treated in detail in another chapter of this volume by Molday and will not be considered here.

7. Observations (Figs. 3–9)

Lectin-gold complexes, protein A-gold complexes, immunoglobulin-gold complexes and avidin-gold complexes were used in a number of investigations for the detection and localization of surface components on thin sections of material after embedding or on shadow replicas. Most of the investigations with lectins were performed on liver cells or on red blood cells to localize single or multiple lectin binding sites and to investigate their spatial relationship (Horisberger and Rosset, 1976; 1977; Horisberger *et al.*, 1978; Roth and Wagner, 1977a; Roth and Binder, 1978; Wagner and Wagner, 1977). Ackerman and coworkers (Ackerman, 1979; Ackerman and Freeman, 1979; Ackerman *et al.*, 1980a,b) investigated the surface distribution of wheat-germ lectin and Concanavalin A binding sites, of monoganglioside G_{M1}, and of presumptive erythropoetin binding sites on normal bone marrow. Both morphological and quantitative analysis showed that the cell surface labelling was related to cell type, cell lineage and stage of maturation. Similarly, cell type related staining patterns were observed for the monoganglioside G_{M1} on mature human blood cells. Other investigators (Geoghegan *et al.*, 1978; de Mey *et al.*, 1981a,b) localized surface immunoglobulins on B and T lymphocytes. The distribution of epidermal growth factor receptors on ovarian granulosa cells was analysed on surface shadow replicas (Tolson *et al.*, 1981). The same technical approach was applied to reveal virus specific structures on the surface of infected HeLa cell cultures

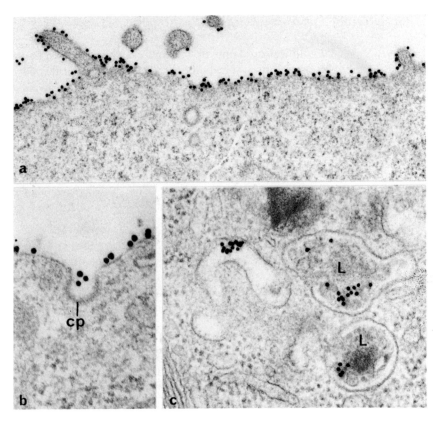

FIG. 3. Demonstration of Concanavalin A binding sites on cultured rat liver cells. Gold particle label is dense and uniform at the cell surface when incubation steps and fixation are performed at 4 °C (a). Internalization via coated pits (CP) occurs when initial cell surface labelling carried out at 4 °C is followed by reincubation of the cells at 37 °C (b). Fusion of endocytotic structures with lysosomes (L) leads to accumulation of gold particles (c). Magnification ×55 000 (a), ×73 000 (b), ×60 000 (c).

(Mannweiler *et al.*, 1982) or fibronectin on the surface of cultured fibroblasts (Fromme *et al.*, 1982). Wagner *et al.* (1976) investigated the number and distribution of A antigenic sites on human red blood cells by freeze-etching and observed no correlation with the number of intramembrane particles.

Beside such static investigations, a number of experiments were aimed to investigate the dynamic behaviour of various cell surface components in relation to membrane mobility. Roth and Wagner (1977b) showed that lectin-gold complexes can be applied to study redistribution and endocytosis phenomena. They observed that redistribution of *Helix pomatia* binding

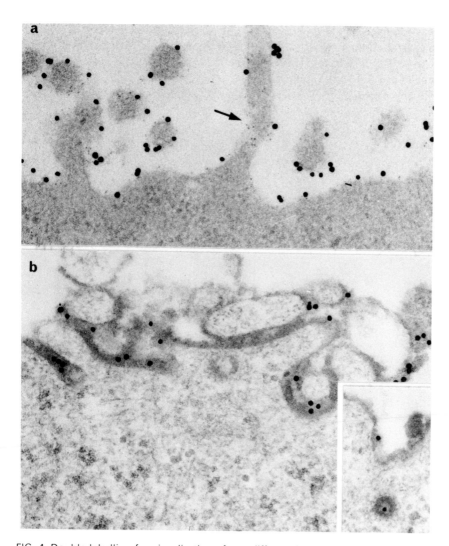

FIG. 4. Double labelling for visualization of two different lectin binding sites on HeLa cells. *Helix pomatia* lectin-gold complex and ferritin conjugated Concanavalin A are applied for labelling of cell surface binding sites at 4 °C (a). Note the difference in electron density of the two markers which is clearly visible in a tangentially cut region of a microvillus structure (arrow). In (b), a double labelling protocol with *Helix pomatia* lectin-gold complex and Concanavalin A-horseradish peroxidase (Bernard and Avrameas (1971) *Exp. Cell Res.* **64**, 232–236) is demonstrated and shows the cointernalization of both lectin binding sites and their presence in the same coated vesicles (inset to b). Magnification ×85 000 (a), ×77 000 (b and inset).

sites also affected rearrangement of Concanavalin A binding sites and this
was followed by co-internalization. More recent investigations using complexes of colloidal gold with insulin (Ackerman and Wolken, 1980; 1981),
low-density lipoprotein (Handley *et al.*, 1981a,b), α_2-macroglobulin (Dickson *et al.*, 1981; Willingham *et al.*, 1981a,b) and bovine serum albumin
(Tartakoff *et al.*, 1981) have shown that the pathway taken by these different

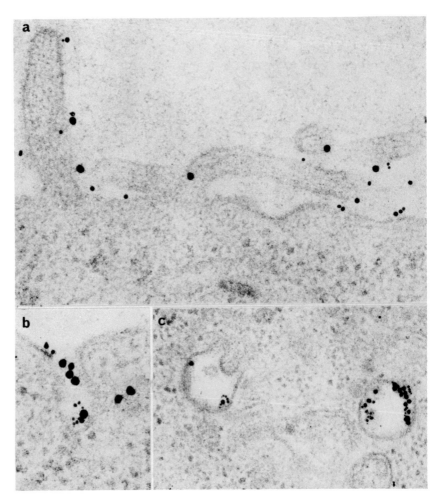

FIG. 5. Double labelling of lectin binding sites with differently sized gold particles. The
bigger gold particles indicate the presence of Concanavalin A binding sites whereas the
smaller ones indicate wheat-germ lectin binding sites (a). Cointernalization of both
lectin binding sites is seen in (b). Finally, both gold particle classes are present in
lysosomal structures (c). Magnification ×84 000 (a), ×98 000 (b), ×54 000 (c).

complexes is similar to that previously described with other markers and involved coated pits and coated vesicles, endosomes and finally lysosomes. The same sequence of endocytotic events was seen with glycoprotein-gold complexes bound to a galactose-specific membrane lectin in Kupffer cells (Kolb *et al.*, 1981; Kolb-Bachofen *et al.*, 1982). Montesano *et al.* (1982) proved the existence of a second distinct pathway for internalization of surface-bound ligands. Tetanus toxin and cholera toxin bound to colloidal gold entered liver cells not through coated pits or coated vesicles but were initially bound and subsequently internalized via non-coated surface micro-invaginations.

B. Localization of Intracellular and Extracellular Components

1. Preembedding Penetration Technique

Until now, this technique was solely applied for tubulin localization in nuclei (de Mey *et al.*, 1981b; 1982; Ochs and Stearns, 1981; Kilmartin *et al.*, 1982). In Section IV.B.1, the procedure of permeabilization of de Mey *et al.*, (1981b) has already been described. Ochs and Stearns (1981) processed cells grown on electron microscope grids for high voltage electron microscopy as follows.

Cells on coverslips were rinsed twice in buffer consisting of 0·1 M PIPES, 1 mM MgCl$_2$, 2 mM EGTA and 4% polyethylene glycol (molecular weight 6000). Detergent treatment with 0·5% Triton X-100 in the same buffer lasted for 1 min. Following extraction and rinses in the buffer, coverslips with the cells were placed in methanol at −20 °C for 5–6 min, rinsed in the above mentioned buffer and finally phosphate buffer.

Incubation with anti-tubulin serum was for 45 min at 37 °C followed by three rinses in PBS and finally protein A-gold complex for 45 min at 37 °C. "Cells" were agitated during the incubations.

Fixation was done with 4% glutaraldehyde (10 min) and 1% osmium tetroxide (3 min).

Dehydration was through graded acetone series followed by critical point drying.

Kilmartin *et al.* (1982) isolated nuclei from yeast and lysed them in 0·1 mM MgCl$_2$. Appropriate fractions obtained after density gradient centrifugation

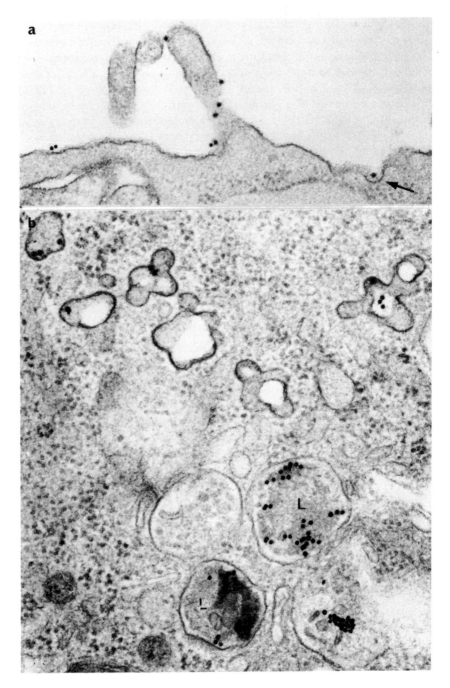

were fixed in glutaraldehyde and reacted with borohydride. Monoclonal antibodies against tubulin were directly bound to colloidal gold and used for labelling.

2. *Postembedding Staining of Thin Sections from Resin-embedded Material*

(a) *Fixation and embedding*

A major problem in postembedding staining procedures is to retain the antigenicity, i.e. the conformation of the cellular material to be studied which is unfortunately altered by all steps needed for tissue processing. The most commonly used fixatives for electron microscopy are glutaraldehyde and formaldehyde and they have proven to be useful for immunocyto-chemical purposes too. However, in most cases, the use of osmium for further fixation of the specimens abolishes the reactivity of the cellular material with antibodies almost completely, with the exception occurring for some polypeptide hormones (Nakane, 1971; Erlandsen *et al.*, 1979).

A recent technical approach to recover antigenicity even after osmium fixation will be reported below. Many investigators have shown that glutar-aldehyde can affect different proteins in their antigenic properties to a varying degree down to complete abolition of antigenicity, (Kyte, 1976; Kraehenbühl *et al.*, 1977). In other words, fixation conditions which are commensurate with adequate stabilization of cellular structures in order to prevent artefactual diffusion, replacement and/or extraction of antigenic material, are generally those which drastically diminish or abolish antigenic properties. A compromise must therefore be reached.

A similar situation exists with respect to dehydration and embedding since organic solvents for water removal and organic substances needed for embedding as well as high temperatures during polymerization all elicit conformational changes of proteins. Our initial investigations on the loca-lization of antigens with the protein A-gold technique (Roth *et al.*, 1978; Roth, 1982b) were performed on thin sections of glutaraldehyde (0·5–4%, 1–2 h fixation time) or formaldehyde (2%, without or with 0·2% glutaral-dehyde, 2–4 h fixation time) fixed tissues which were dehydrated and embedded in Epon 812. Such routine conditions provided, for many anti-gens, a situation in which they could be demonstrated immunocyto-chemically. Other immunocytochemical approaches to localize antigens on thin sections worked similarly well (Garaud *et al.*, 1980; Larsson, 1979).

FIG. 6. Labelling of cultured rat liver cells with tetanus toxin-gold complexes. The inherent distribution of toxin receptors is not random on all surfaces (a). The label is preferentially associated with microvilli and non-coated smooth membrane invagina-tions (arrow). Internalization of complexes occur via non-coated membrane invagina-tions and the label accumulates in lysosomes (L) when cells are reincubated at 37 °C after initial labelling at 4 °C (b). Magnification ×75 000 (a,b).

Recently, Bendayan and Zollinger (1982) reported that they had demonstrated antigens such as exocrine and endocrine pancreatic proteins and polypeptides, a mitochondrial and a peroxisomal enzyme on thin sections or routinely glutaraldehyde *and* osmium tetroxide fixed and Epon-embedded tissues. This was combined with good fine structural preservation. Treatment

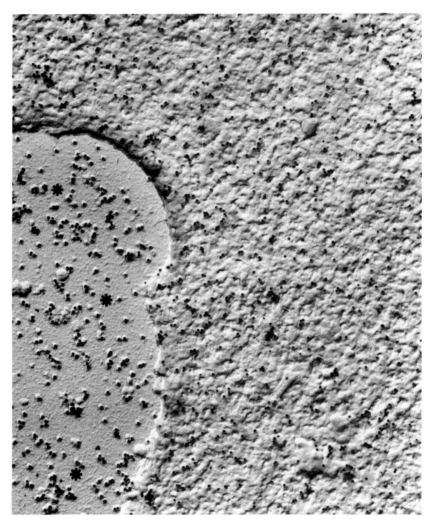

FIG. 7. Shadow cast replica showing a peripheral region of a cultured rat liver cell incubated at 4 °C for localization of *Ricinus communis* lectin I binding sites. The arrangement of the lectin-gold complexes (black particles) at the cell surface appears almost nonclustered and diffuse as it is over the extracellular region (asterisks). Magnification ×33 000.

of the thin sections with a saturated aqueous sodium metaperiodate solution for 30–60 min at room temperature before the immunocytochemical labelling with the protein A-gold technique was the prerequisite to obtain such results. Up to now, no data have been reported on proteins which resisted to glutaraldehyde (and perhaps osmium tetroxide) fixation but not conven-

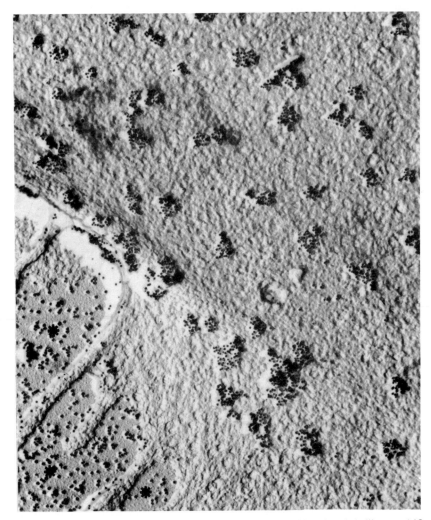

FIG. 8. Same material and labelling as in Fig. 7 but additional to labelling at 4 °C, reincubation at 37 °C for 15 min. The cell surface label (*Ricinus communis* lectin I-gold complexes) is now arranged in clusters whereas the gold particle label over the extracellular region (asterisks) remains diffuse. Magnification ×33 000.

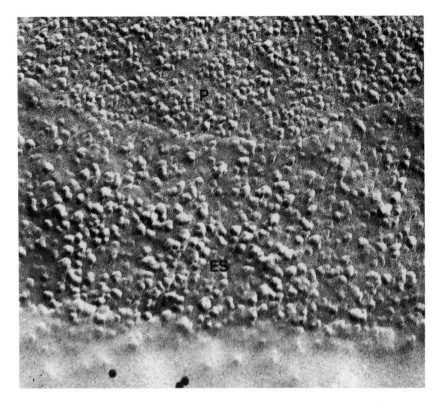

FIG. 9. Freeze-etch replica from a human A red blood cell incubated with *Helix pomatia* lectin-gold complexes. The protoplasmic membrane fracture face (P) exhibits numerous intramembrane particles. The deep etched exoplasmic surface (ES) is separated from the fracture face by a clearly visible step. The distribution of the lectin binding sites on the exoplasmic surface is revealed by the presence of numerous particulate protrusions. In such replica preparations the gold particles do not remain at their initial sites of binding in contrast to shadow cast replicas from whole cells. Magnification ×100 000.

tional Epon embedding. In such cases the recent development of the low temperature embedding procedure using the hydrophilic resin Lowicryl K4M (Carlemalm *et al.*, 1980; 1982; Kellenberger *et al.*, 1980) was of great help. In our first study, we found that the structural preservation of aldehyde-only fixed and low temperature Lowicryl K4M embedded pancreatic tissue was superior to Epon-embedded material (Roth *et al.*, 1981c). In addition, the immunocytochemical staining became more specific due to drastically lowered background staining. Further investigations have shown that these embedding conditions yield more intense specific staining (Bendayan and Shore, 1982). Finally, we succeeded in demonstrating that antigens which were not detectable after Epon embedding became detectable after low temperature Lowicryl K4M embedding (Roth and Berger, 1982; Thorens *et al.*, 1982). All of these data taken together demonstrate that low temperature embedding with Lowicryl K4M allows preservation of fine structural details to a high degree and permits localization of "sensitive" antigens in thin resin sections and this is combined with a high signal-to-noise ratio.

Craig and Goodchild (1982), by the use of a solid radioimmunoassay system, assessed quantitatively the losses in antigenicity of pea seed storage proteins during fixation and processing for embedding. They found that embedding with Lowicryl K4M compared with embedding in Spurr's medium gave a 25% higher labeling with the protein A-gold technique. Therefore, it seems that the theoretical expectations about the protecting effect of low temperature on protein configuration under denaturating environmental conditions (Douzou, 1977; Douzou *et al.*, 1971; Petsko, 1975) are fulfilled by experimental data from immunocytochemical experiments and high resolution investigations on protein structure (Carlemalm and Kellenberger, 1982; Armbruster *et al.*, 1983). A detailed description of how to perform the low temperature embedding with Lowicryl K4M is given by Carlemalm *et al.* (1982). Further practical hints can be found in an Instruction Manual which will be provided, from 1983, with each Lowicryl K4M kit and the "Lowicryl Letters" can be received upon request from Chemische Werke Lowi GmbH, P.O.B., D-8264 Waldkraiburg, FRG.

Whereas numerous investigators could demonstrate antigenic material on thin sections from resin embedded tissues, only a few have succeeded in obtaining positive *and* specific results with labelled lectins. However, drastic treatment of the thin sections was needed, such as partial dissolution of the glycol methacrylate by treatment with alcohol (Gros *et al.*, 1976) or exposure to an alcohol -0.5% KOH solution (Suzuki *et al.*, 1981). In our studies with a battery of lectin-gold complexes, no specific labelling of thin sections was obtained after Epon-embedding regardless of the fixation procedure employed. However, fixation with 1% glutaraldehyde in PBS (1–2 h) or 4% formaldehyde with 0.2% glutaraldehyde in PBS (2–4 h) followed by low temperature embedding with Lowicryl K4M, produced highly satisfactory results. *Without any pretreatment* of the thin sections, highly dense and specific staining was seen with lectins specific for mannose, glucose, fucose, galactose, sialic acid, N-acetyl-D-glucosamine or N-acetyl-D-galactosamine like residues (Roth, 1982a; 1983a,b). Depending on the specificity of the lectins, glycoconjugates could be detected in the rough endoplasmic reticulum. Golgi apparatus, intracellularly stored secretion products, plasma membranes and extracellular connective tissue substances (Roth, 1982a; 1983a,b; Roth *et al.*, 1983b).

(b) Incubation protocols
The staining protocol for the protein A-gold technique has been reported in
detail in Volume 1 of this series (Roth, 1982b). When immunoglobulin-gold
complexes (Garaud *et al.*, 1980; Probert *et al.*, 1981; Schott-Doerr and
Garaud, 1981) or antigen-BSA conjugate-gold complexes (Larsson, 1979)
were used as second-step reagents the method for staining of thin sections
was similar. Briefly, it involves the following steps.

Nickel grids with the attached thin sections were placed on a droplet of 1%
ovalbumin in PBS for 5 min. In the protein A-gold technique no etching
with H_2O_2 is performed. Only when glutaraldehyde-osmium tetroxide
fixed material is used, pretreatment with aqueous saturated sodium
metaperiodate (30–60 min) is performed followed by several rinses with
distilled water. In the two other approaches thin sections were usually
etched with 10% H_2O_2 for 10–15 min.

Grids were then transferred onto drops of the antibody solutions for 1–2 h
at room temperature or 18–48 h at 4 °C and kept in a moist chamber. The
concentration of the antibodies is of critical importance since too high a
concentration results in high background staining. For each antiserum,
the dilution which gives intense specific labelling and low background has
to be determined empirically. Affinity-purified antibodies were used at
20–100 μg ml^{-1} protein concentration in the protein A-gold technique
(Roth and Berger, 1982; Roth *et al.*, 1983a).

The sections were "jet" washed by a mild spray of PBS from a plastic spray
bottle, placed in PBS for 1–2 min and the washing was performed a second
time.

Grids were incubated with one of the above mentioned second-step
reagents for 30–60 min at room temperature.

Grids were washed with PBS as described above and then washed with
distilled water.

Counterstaining of Epon thin sections was done with 2 or 5% aqueous
uranyl acetate (10–20 min) and lead citrate (2–5 min). Thin sections from
Lowicryl K4M embedded specimens were counterstained with 2%
aqueous uranyl acetate (5–7 min) and lead acetate (approximately 1 min).

Staining with lectin-gold complexes involves the following steps.

Nickel grids with the attached Lowicryl K4M thin sections were placed on a droplet of PBS for 5 min at room temperature.

Grids were transferred onto a droplet of lectin-gold complexes for 30 min at room temperature. Depending on the lectin and the tissue or cell type, lectin-gold complexes were used between 3–200 μg ml^{-1} protein concentration.

Grids were "jet" washed by a mild spray of PBS from a plastic spray bottle, placed for 1–2 min in PBS, washed a second time with PBS and finally with distilled water.

Counterstaining with uranyl acetate and lead acetate was performed as described above for Lowicryl K4M sections.

Staining with Concanavalin A and wheat-germ lectin was performed in a two-step technique with horseradish peroxidase-gold and ovomucoid-gold complexes, respectively. Incubation times were 30 min for each step.

Controls for specificity for these techniques have been mentioned already in Section IV.B.4.

In Section V.A.2., double-labelling techniques for demonstration of cell surface components by the use of gold particles of different sizes were used. Colloidal gold particles coated with protein A or antigen-bovine serum albumin conjugates are highly suitable also for localization of different intracellular antigens on the same thin sections. The protein A-gold complexes used for double-labelling studies were from 3 nm and 15 nm gold particles (Roth, 1982d) or from 13 nm and 19 nm gold particles (Bendayan, 1982). This indirect double-labelling protocol with the protein A-gold technique involved four successive incubation steps: first antibody followed by protein A-gold complexes from small gold particles, and then second antibody followed by protein A-gold complexes made with the larger gold particles. Roth (1982d) performed double labelling on thin sections from Lowicryl K4M embedded tissue. An observation of high practical importance was that the protein A-gold complex prepared with 3 nm particles had to be used in the first staining sequence, since otherwise a non-specific co-labelling of the two protein A-gold complexes resulted.

Bendayan (1982) performed double staining on thin sections which were placed on grids without a supporting film so that both faces of the thin sections were exposed and could be labelled. Labelling for the first antigen was done on face "A" of the grids (and thin sections) and the second incubation sequence on face "B" of the grids.

Larsson (1979) used 18 nm gold particles coated with ACTH$_{1-39}$-bovine serum albumin conjugate in combination with 30 nm gold particles stabilized with synthetic human gastrin$_{2-17}$-bovine serum albumin conjugate to demonstrate both antigens in gastric G-cells secretory granules. The staining protocol consisted of four successive incubation steps.

(c) Results (Figs 10–14)

The outstanding advantage of the protein A-gold technique is the replacement of various preparations of anti-species immunoglobulin preparations with a single reagent. It is already well known that protein A in general gives a much lower background (Biberfeld et al., 1975) than anti-species immunoglobulin preparations. Larsson (1979) claimed that his technique detects only specific antibodies and therefore, is superior to the protein A-gold technique with respect to specificity. The use of affinity-purified or monoclonal antibodies in the protein A-gold technique has eliminated such possible sources of nonspecificity. Even though the technique of Larsson (1979) might detect only specifically antigen-directed antibodies, it is still possible to detect specific antibodies nonspecifically bound to the thin sections as with any immunocytochemical approach. Unfortunately, the GLAD technique of Larsson (1979) has found no wide application until now and a real comparison with other techniques has not been performed.

The protein A-gold technique as well as the immunoglobulin-gold staining and the gold labelled antigen technique have allowed the precise localization of various secretory polypeptides in endocrine cells and nerve fibres (Batten and Hopkins, 1979; Doerr-Schott and Garaud, 1981; Garaud et al., 1980; Larsson, 1979; Probert et al., 1981; Ravazzola and Orci, 1980a,b; Ravazzola et al., 1981; Roth et al., 1978; 1980; 1981a; Tanaka et al., 1980; 1981a,b; Warthon et al., 1981; Varndell et al., 1982). The techniques allowed, on the basis of visualized immunoreactive material, precise distinction of cell types with similar secretory granule morphology (Roth et al., 1981a), partly due to the high electron density of the gold particles. The interpretation of results obtained with peroxidase-tagged reagents was difficult due to the inherent density of the secretory granules.

The protein A-gold technique permitted furthermore the detection of various exocrine secretory proteins or storage proteins in plants in all intracellular compartments involved in the biosynthetic pathway (rough endoplasmic reticulum, Golgi apparatus, secretory granules) (Bendayan, 1982; Bendayan and Ørstavik, 1981; Bendayan et al., 1980; Craig and Goodchild, 1982; Roth et al., 1978; 1980; 1981c; Tanaka et al., 1981; Zur Nieden et al., 1981), of enzymes in mitochondria, peroxisomes and granules of eosinophilic granulocytes (Bendayan and Shore, 1981; Reddy et al., 1982; Iozzo et al., 1982), of cytoskeletal elements (Bendayan, 1981b, c; Bendayan et al., 1982), of various collagen types and laminin (Stephens et al., 1982), of

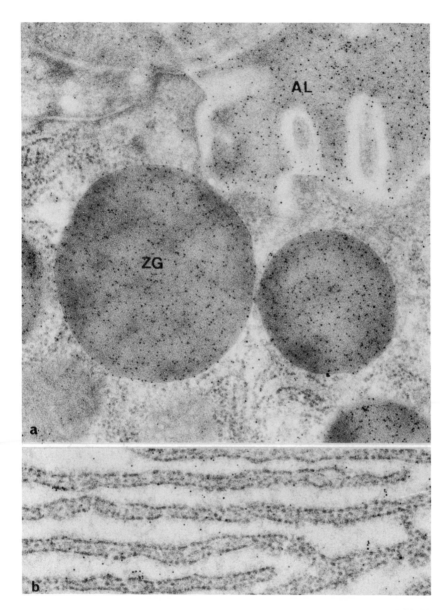

FIG. 10. Localization of amylase by the protein A-gold technique on Lowicryl K4M thin section from rat pancreas. Amylase immunoreactive material is present in the acinar lumen (AL) and zymogen granules (ZG) as indicated by the presence of numerous 3 nm gold particles (a). Amylase can be detected also over the cisternal space of the rough endoplasmic reticulum in basal cell regions (b). Magnification ×43 000 (a), ×53 000 (b).

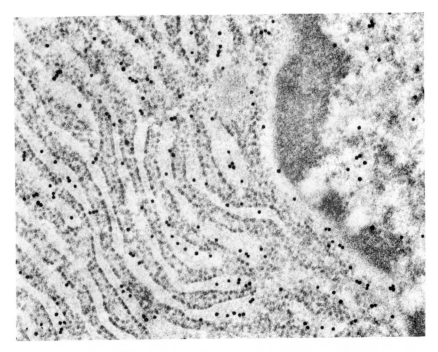

FIG. 11. Thin section from low temperature Lowicryl K4M embedded rat pancreas. Mannose and glucose-containing glycoproteins are revealed with Concanavalin A in the nuclear envelope and rough endoplasmic reticulum. Gold particle label is also present over the nuclear euchromatin. Magnification ×52 000.

albumin in tracer studies (Bendayan, 1980), of soluble cytoplasmic and euchromatic vitamin D-dependent calcium binding protein (Roth *et al.*, 1981b; 1982; Thorens *et al.*, 1982), membrane integral proteins such as galactosyltransferase (Roth and Berger, 1982; Roth *et al.*, 1983a) and other cellular constituents (Nygren *et al.*, 1981).

The immunocytochemical studies on exocrine and endocrine secretory products confirmed the established biochemical data on secretion (Palade, 1975) and also provided further data such as the involvement of the whole Golgi stack in processing of the secretory proteins (Roth *et al.*, 1981c). They also demonstrated directly the presence of various secretory products in the same cellular compartments (Bendayan, 1982; Roth, 1982).

The immunocytochemical localization of the vitamin D-dependent calcium binding protein in its main targets, duodenum and kidney (Roth *et al.*, 1981b; 1982a,b; Thorens *et al.*, 1982) allowed more definite conclusions about its *function*, another advantage of using this methodology.

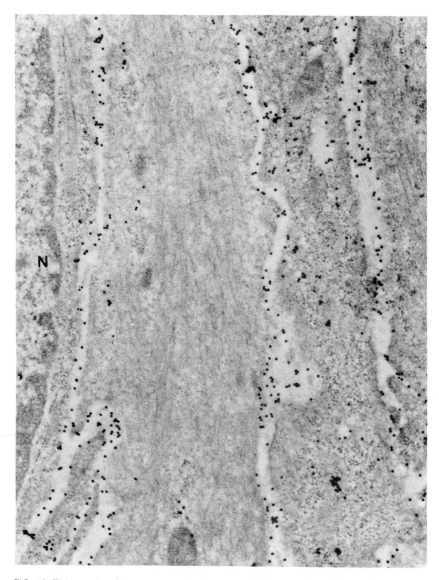

FIG. 12. Thin section from low temperature Lowicryl K4M embedded chick duodenum. The *Ricinus communis* lectin II-gold complexes are preferentially located along the surface of smooth muscle cells in the villus stroma. Intracellular structures such as a part of a nucleus (N), rough endoplasmic reticulum and fibrils are not labelled. Magnification ×27 000.

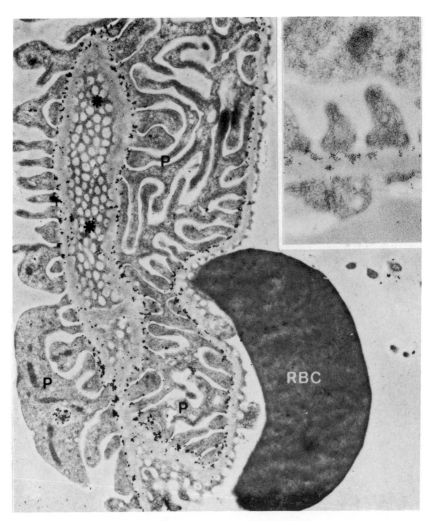

FIG. 13. Thin section (Lowicryl K4M) showing part of a glomerular capillary loop from rat kidney. Distribution of *Helix pomatia* lectin-gold complexes indicates that N-acetyl-D-galactosamine residues are present in the lamina rara externa and lamina densa of the glomerular basement membrane but absent from the lamina rara interna. The inset shows this preferential distribution at a higher magnification with lectin-gold complex prepared from 3 nm gold particles. The gold particle label is absent over any other glomerular structures such as podocytes (P) plasma membrane above the slit diaphragm, red blood cells (the asterisks marks a tangentially cut endothelial cell region). Magnification ×11 000, ×40 000 (inset).

Roth and Berger (1982) and Roth *et al.* (1983a) succeeded for the first time in localizing a glycoslytransferase, the galactosyltransferase. Immunostaining has provided conclusive evidence for the localization of this enzyme in the Golgi apparatus where it was present in a distinct subcompartment which consisted of 2–3 trans Golgi cisternae. The co-distribution of galactosyltransferase with thiamine pyrophosphatase in the same trans Golgi cisternae was demonstrated by a double-staining approach. It

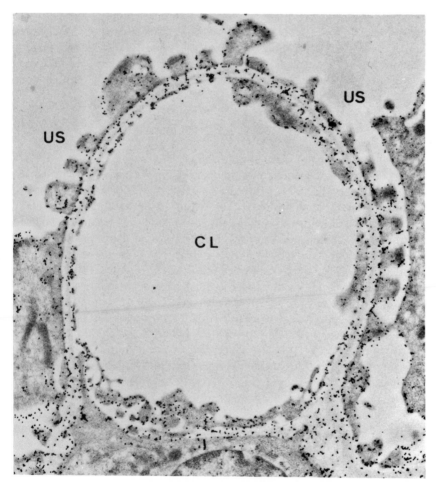

FIG. 14. The distribution of wheat-germ lectin binding sites as indicated by the gold particle label over a cross-sectioned capillary loop is quite different. The label is associated with the plasma membrane of endothelial cells, podocytes and all three layers of the glomerular basement membrane. CL-capillary lumen, US-urinary space. Magnification ×15 000.

involved combination of pre-embedding enzyme cytochemistry with post-embedding immunostaining with the protein A-gold technique. This approach might be very useful in further studies aimed at the elucidation of both enzymatic activities and antigenic composition of cellular organelles.

The development of techniques to localize lectin binding sites on Lowicryl K4M thin sections (Roth, 1982a; 1983a,b) has yielded already highly interesting results. It could be shown (Roth et al., 1983b) that the glycocalyx of renal glomerular podocytes is highly specialized with respect to the presence of terminal, non-reducing N-acetyl-D-galactosamine residues. Such residues as visualized by *Helix pomatia* lectin-gold complexes were seen to be present only at the base of the podocyte foot processes and extending from there in the lamina rara externa and lamina densa of the glomerular basement membrane. The glycocalyx of the podocytes above the slit diaphragm along with other glomerular constituents was not stained.

3. Staining of Ultrathin Frozen Sections

(a) Fixation, sectioning and immunostaining
The problems with respect to retention of antigenicity introduced by fixation by chemical means have been discussed already in Section V.B.2(a) and are the same in cryoultramicrotomy (Tokuyasu, 1980). However, as already mentioned, a wide range of cellular antigens resists such treatment and can be immunocytochemically demonstrated. Despite the use of low concentrations of glutaraldehyde (0·5–1%) in an appropriate buffer or of paraformaldehyde (2%) with varying concentrations of glutaraldehyde (0·1–1%) for 30–60 min, a two-step fixation protocol has been successfully used for the retention of reactivity of "sensitive" antigens. The latter comprises the use of 3% paraformaldehyde with 20 mM ethylacetamide for 2–10 min which is followed by fixation in 3% paraformaldehyde with 0·1% glutaraldehyde for 1 h (Geiger et al., 1981). Problems of distortions of supramolecular structures due to dehydration and embedding in highly polymerized resin are circumvented in the preparation of ultrathin frozen sections. Further improvements in freezing the tissue in adequate solutions (Tokuyasu, 1973) and handling of the thin sections (Tokuyasu, 1978; Tokuyasu and Singer, 1976) have allowed good preservation of cellular fine structural details and have overcome the problems of vulnerability of the frozen thin sections at the time of drying. A full description of the technical steps can be found in the excellent reviews by Tokuyasu (1973, 1980).

The principle of the cryosectioning is as follows.

Small pieces of fixed tissue were immersed in 2·3 M sucrose for 30 min at room temperature. A properly trimmed tissue piece was placed on the specimen holder and was frozen rapidly by plunging in liquid nitrogen. Then it was transferred to the cold chamber of the ultracryotome (Porter Blum, LKB or Reichert).

Sections were cut with a dry glass knife and picked up from the knife by touching them with a small drop of 2·3 M sucrose in a wire-loop. Outside the cryochamber, the sections stretch on the surface of the thawed sucrose solution.

Thin sections on the sucrose were transferred on carbon coated formvar grids and "stored" on drops of PBS or on a layer of 0·3% agarose with 1% gelatine covered with a thin layer of PBS. Blocking of non-specific binding of the immunoreagents was achieved by placing the grids on 2% gelatine in PBS for 10 min. Free aldehyde groups were quenched with glycine (see Section IV.A.).

Grids were placed on drops of antibody solution (75–200 μl^{-1}; Geuze *et al.*, 1981) for 20–30 min at room temperature.

Excess antibody was removed by several rinses with PBS (3–15 min).

Grids were placed on a drop of protein A-gold complexes for 20–30 min at room temperature. Geuze *et al.* (1981b) recommended the inclusion of bovine serum albumin (1%) or IgG-free normal serum to the antibody solution and the protein A-gold complexes to minimize nonspecific interactions.

Sections were thoroughly washed in PBS (4 times 5 min each) and distilled water and positively stained with a solution of 4% uranyl acetate and 0·3 M potassium oxalate (pH 7–8) for 10 min. After rinsing with distilled water, they were stained with 2% aqueous uranyl acetate (5–10 min).

After rinsing with distilled water, grids were placed for a short time on each of three drops of 1·5% methylcellulose and picked up in a wire loop. Excess solution of methylcellulose was removed with filter paper to give a thin and uniform film.

(d) Results (Fig. 15)
Geuze and coworkers (Brands *et al.*, 1980a,b; Geuze *et al.*, 1981a,b) have used the protein A-gold complex (Romano and Romano, 1977; Roth *et al.*, 1978) for staining of antigens on ultrathin frozen sections and also performed double labelling (Geuze *et al.*, 1981b). In the localization of amylase, they

confirmed earlier data on the subcellular distribution of this protein obtained with ferritin-tagged antibodies on ultrathin frozen sections (Geuze *et al.*, 1979), or with the protein A-gold technique on resin-embedded tissue (Bendayan *et al.*, 1980; Roth *et al.*, 1981c). Furthermore, they succeeded in localizing a zymogen granule membrane glycoprotein, named GP-2, which was associated with Golgi membranes and zymogen granule membranes,

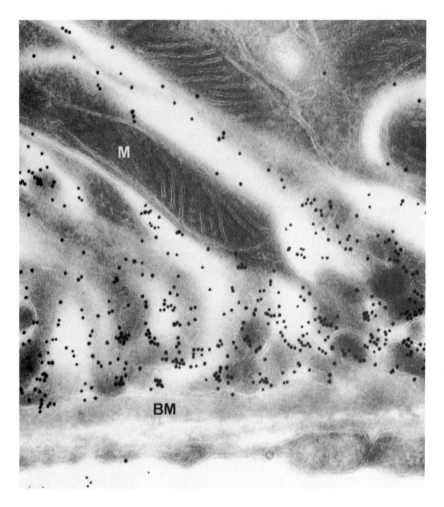

FIG. 15. Ultrathin frozen section from rat kidney incubated with *Helix pomatia* lectin-gold complexes. The gold particle label is associated with the plasma membrane of the basal region of proximal tubular cells. Mitochondria (M) and the basement membrane (BM) are not labelled. From the unpublished work of D. Brown and J. Roth. Magnification×60 000.

but was, at the same time part of the zymogen granule content and released extracellularly by secretion. The same group (Geuze *et al.*, 1982a) also studied the distribution of the asialoglycoprotein receptor in rat liver cells where it was found along the entire hepatocyte plasma membrane. Internalization of the asialoorosomucoid-occupied-receptors occurred rapidly and the dissociation of the ligand-receptor complexes appeared inside vacuoles (Geuze *et al.*, 1982b). Others applied the protein A-gold technique on frozen thin sections to localize clathrin in rat spermatids (Griffiths *et al.*, 1981) or to visualize the passage of Semliki Forest virus protein from the rough endoplasmic reticulum via the Golgi apparatus to the plasma membrane (Green *et al.*, 1981).

4. *Freeze-fracture Cytochemistry*

Freeze-fracture electron microscopy in the classical sense involves the freezing of unfixed or chemically fixed specimens in the hydrated stage, their fracturing under high vacuum in the cold and the production of platinum-carbon replica of the fracture face for subsequent observation (Bullivant, 1973; Bullivant and Ames, 1966; Moor *et al.*, 1961; Sleytr and Robards, 1977). The fracture passes through the cells and seems to split structurally weak regions of the membranes which correspond to their hydrophobic interior (Branton, 1966; Branton and Daemer, 1972; Meyer and Winkelmann, 1966). The result of this process is the appearance of membrane fracture faces which can be investigated in their three-dimensional arrangement. In biological membranes, fracture faces are composed of smooth regions (most probably corresponding to phospholipids) and the so-called intramembrane particles (assumed to be "fractured" integral membrane proteins). This image of the fracture faces is qualitatively similar in all biological membranes. Recently, Pinto da Silva and coworkers (Pinto da Silva *et al.*, 1981a,b) have combined the freeze-fracture technique with cytochemical techniques in order to identify and localize chemical groups and various binding sites on the fracture faces of biological membranes and named this new approach freeze-fracture cytochemistry.

(a) *Processing of cells and tissue for freeze fracturing*
In this technique aldehyde-fixed specimens are processed without dehydration or plastic embedding prior to labelling. Fixation is done with 1% glutaraldehyde at 4 °C for 15–30 min in the case of cells or for 2 h for tissues. Cells are then treated by immersion with 15% or 30% bovine serum albumin which is then solidified by cross-linking with 1% glutaraldehyde for 30 min at room temperature. These gels containing the cells and the fixed tissue pieces are cut into slices of about 1×2×2 mm, impregnated gradually in

30% glycerol, and frozen in freon 22 cooled by liquid nitrogen. The frozen specimens are transferred into a glass container filled with liquid nitrogen and immersed in a slush of liquid nitrogen and solid carbon dioxide. Drops of 30% glycerol and 1% glutaraldehyde in isotonic phosphate buffer (pH 7·4) were frozen in liquid nitrogen and added to the "embedded" cells or tissues in an amount approximately equal to that of the specimens. After all particles sedimented, the material is finally crushed with a glass pestle precooled in liquid nitrogen.

The glass container is then removed from the cooling bath and 2–3 ml of the glycerol-glutaraldehyde buffer (liquid!) are added when the volume of the liquid nitrogen is reduced to about one-tenth. The glass container is immersed briefly in water(30 °C), and, upon thawing of the glycerol, transferred to an ice bucket for 15 min. The fragments of the specimens are then gradually deglycerinated by dropwise addition of 1 mM glycyl-glycine isotonic phosphate buffer (pH 7·4) and washed in isotonic phosphate buffer. Such materials, after being cytochemically labelled, are embedded in Epon 812 for preparation of thin sections. Another possible variation is the preparation of replicas of critical point-dried cells and tissues after fracture label (Pinto da Silva et al., 1981b). For such purposes the frozen specimens are transferred to a Petri dish filled with liquid nitrogen and placed on top of a liquid nitrogen/solid carbon dioxide slush. Fracturing is done with a liquid nitrogen cooled scalpel. Samples are then treated and deglycerinated as described above.

(b) Incubation conditions

Cells or tissues were processed for the localization of Concanavalin A or wheat-germ lectin binding sites with horseradish peroxidase-gold complexes or ovomucoid-gold complexes, respectively (for details, see Sections IV.A.1. and V.A.1.). Antigenic sites were revealed with protein A-gold complexes as described in section V.B.2(b). Incubation with Concanavalin A (1 mg ml^{-1}) and with wheat-germ lectin (0·25 mg ml^{-1}) was for 30 min at 37 °C followed by two rinses with 0·1 M Sorensen phosphate buffer (pH 7·4) containing 4% polyvinylpyrrolidone and incubation with the corresponding glycoprotein-gold complexes for 60 min at room temperature. Other cytochemical procedures using cationized ferritin at pH 7·5 or 4·0 and ferritin conjugated Concanavalin A have been used too.

For the preparation of thin sections, the freeze-fracture labelled cells or tissues were processed as follows. After rinses with Sorensen phosphate buffer containing 4% polyvinylpyrrolidone, the specimens were fixed in 1% osmium tetroxide in veronal acetate buffer (pH 7·6) for 2 h at 4 °C, stained *en bloc* with uranyl acetate (5 mg ml^{-1}), dehydrated in acetone and routinely embedded in Epon 812.

Platinum-carbon replicas of freeze-fracture labelled cells or tissues were prepared in the following way. The specimens were fixed in 1% osmium tetroxide in veronal acetate buffer (pH 7·4) for 30 min, dehydrated in ethanol and critical point dried in ethanol/carbon dioxide. The dried specimens were then placed onto a specimen holder and shadowed with a platinum/carbon electron-gun. The replicas were digested in sodium hypochlorite, rinsed in water and picked up on Formvar coated grids.

(c) Results (Figs 16, 17)

Anionic sites and lectin binding sites were studied on red blood cells, leukocytes, HeLa cells, lymphocytes, liver and spleen by means of cationized ferritin and ferritin conjugated Concanavalin A (Pinto da Silva *et al.*, 1981a,c). Furthermore, gold-labelled probes have been used to study Concanavalin A and wheat-germ lectin binding sites as well as antigenic sites (Pinto da Silva *et al.*, 1981b,d; Pinto da Silva and Torrisi, 1982). So far, these studies have shown the feasibility of the combined use of cytochemical and freeze-fracture techniques to study the topochemistry of plasma membranes, intracellular membranes and the cytoplasm. However, they have also demonstrated that limited reorganization of membrane components occurs during thawing of the fractured probes. Such reorganization most likely involves membrane lipids. Redistribution of membrane integral proteins seems unlikely because of the glutaraldehyde fixation. Perhaps the situation is best characterized by the statement of these authors that

> interpretation . . . appears to involve delicate and subtle problems whose complete solution will ultimately depend on detailed knowledge of the molecular architecture of membranes, of the process of fracture and the nature of reconstitution upon thawing (Pinto da Silva *et al.*, 1981a).

With these precautions in mind novel observations on the distribution of lectin binding sites in fracture faces of membranes from red blood cells and pancreatic cells were made. Wheat-germ lectin binding sites were preferentially labelled in the exoplasmic half of the plasma membrane whereas the protoplasmic face exhibited only a variable and low amount of labelling (Pinto da Silva *et al.*, 1981b; Pinto da Silva and Torrisi, 1982). This partition contrasts with that of Concanavalin A binding sites in red blood cell membrane (Pinto da Silva *et al.*, 1981a,c). The pattern of partition of cell surface binding sites in membrane fracture faces can be best investigated on platinum/carbon replicas of critical point-dried fracture-labelled preparations. Pinto da Silva and Torrisi (1982) point out that partition of Concanavalin A binding sites with the protoplasmic face implies dragging of the entire molecule up to the terminal saccharide across the exoplasmic half of the plasma membrane. However, partition of wheat-germ lectin binding sites with the exoplasmic face does not necessarily imply dragging of some of its

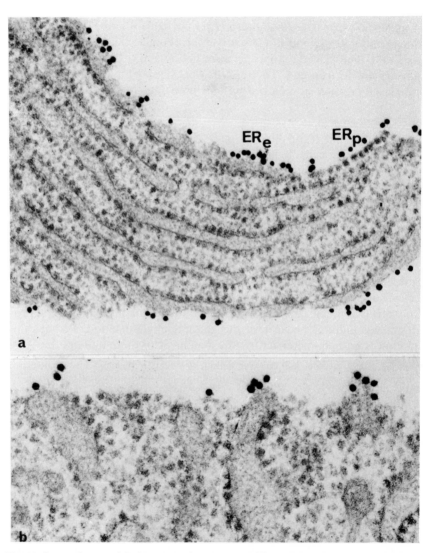

Fig. 16. Freeze-fracture label, rat exocrine pancreas. Mannose and glucose residues are revealed by the labelling with Concanavalin A-horseradish peroxidase-gold complexes. The exoplasmic face of the rough endoplasmic reticulum (ER_e) and the protoplasmic face (ER_p) are labelled (a) as well as material in the lumen of cross-fractured cisternae (b). Magnification ×65 000 (a), ×74 000 (b).

segments through the protoplasmic membrane half since a simple breakage of the amino acid chain could occur and account for such a pattern.

Thin-section and critical-point-drying fracture label was also used to study the distribution and partition of Concanavalin A and wheat-germ lectin binding sites in rat pancreatic tissue. For both lectins, a dense labelling of the exoplasmic halves and a sparse labelling of the protoplasmic face of the plasma membrane was seen. However, wheat-germ lectin resulted in no labelling of rough endoplasmic reticulum and nuclear membranes which

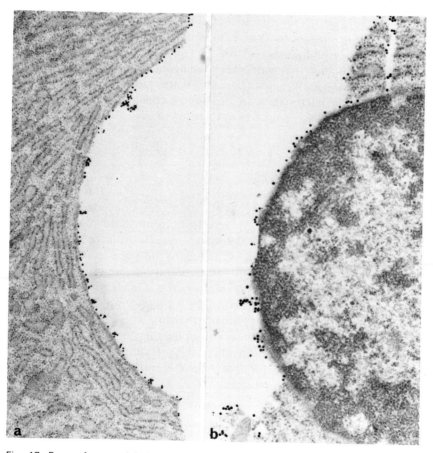

Fig. 17. Freeze-fracture label, rat exocrine pancreas. Labelling of nuclear envelope membranes with Concanavalin A-horseradish peroxidase-gold complexes (a) and (b) represent complementary views and the uneven distribution of the gold particle label in both micrographs can be taken as evidence that most of the label is associated with the exoplasmic halves of the inner and outer nuclear membrane as assumed by Pinto da Silva et al., (1981a). Magnification ×35 000 (a and b).

were strongly positive with Concanavalin A on their exoplasmic halves as expected from biochemical data on glycosylation of proteins.

VI. CONCLUSIONS

The first reported use of colloidal gold as a "staining reagent" comes from the 17th Century. Kunkel manufactured gold ruby glass by adding the purple of Cassius—a colloidal gold—to molten glass. The aim of this chapter was to review the use of colloidal gold as a staining reagent in cytochemistry which started in 1971. Since then colloidal gold has proved to be a versatile and efficient staining reagent for both light and electron microscopy. It can be used as a high resolution marker for the detection of single and multiple antigens or in combination with other cytochemical and immunocytochemical techniques. Beside its application in light microscopy it can be used in all fields of electron microscopy. In this sense, colloidal gold represents a unique, widely applicable marker system for the visualization of cell and tissue constituents.

VII. ACKNOWLEDGEMENTS

I became familiar with colloidal gold by experiments done together with my former colleagues Drs H. W. Meyer (Institute of Pathology, Friedrich-Schiller University Jena) and M. Wagner (Central Institute of Microbiology and Experimental Therapy Jena, Academy of the Sciences of the GDR).

Since 1978 many of the scientific and technical collaborators of the Institute of Histology and Embryology, University of Geneva Medical School, have contributed to different aspects of the work reviewed and I would like to thank all of them. It is a great pleasure to thank Mrs F. Fichard for skilful technical assistance, Mrs M. Müller for typing the various versions of this manuscript and Dr J. Lucocq for reading and correcting the manuscript. The work summarized in this chapter has received continuous support from the Swiss National Science Foundation.

VIII. REFERENCES

Ackerman, G. A. (1979). *Anat. Rec.* **195**, 641–658.
Ackerman, G. A. and Freeman, W. H. (1979) *J. Histochem. Cytochem.* **27**, 1412.
Ackerman, G. A. and Wolken, K. W. (1980). *IRCS Med. Sci.* **8**, 842–843.
Ackerman, G. A. and Wolken, K. W. (1981). *J. Histochem. Cytochem.* **29**, 1137–1149.

Ackerman, G. A., Wolken, K. W. and Gelder, F. B. (1980a). *J. Histochem. Cytochem.* **28**, 1100–1112.
Ackerman, G. A. Wolken, K. W. and Gelder, F. B. (1980b). *J. Histochem. Cytochem* **28**, 1334—1342.
Armbruster, B. L., Garavito, R. M. and Kellenberger, E. (1983). *J. Histochem. Cytochem.* (in press).
Baigent, C. L. and Müller, G. (1980). *Experientia* **36**, 472.
Batten, F. F. C. and Hopkins, C. R. (1979). *Histochemistry* **60**, 317–320.
Bauer, H., Farr, D. R. and Horisberger, M. (1974). *Arch. Mikrobiol.* **97**, 17–26.
Bendayan, M. (1980). *J. Histochem. Cytochem.* **28**, 1251–1254.
Bendayan, M. (1981a). *J. Histochem. Cytochem.* **29**, 531–541.
Bendayan, M. (1981b). *Biol. Cell.* **41**, 157–160.
Bendayan, M. (1981c). *Biol. Cell.* **43**, 153–156.
Bendayan, M. (1981d). *J. Histochem. Cytochem.* **30**, 81–85.
Bendayan, M. and Ørstavik, T. B. (1982a). *J. Histochem. Cytochem.* **30**, 58–66.
Bendayan, M. and Shore, G. C. (1982b). *J. Histochem. Cytochem.* **30**, 139–147.
Bendayan, M., Roth, J., Perrelet, A.and Orci, L. (1980). *J. Histochem. Cytochem.* **28**, 149–160.
Bendayan, M. and Zollinger, M. (1983). *J. Histochem. Cytochem.* **31**, 101–109.
Bendayan, M., Marceau, N., Beaudoin, A. R. and Trifaro, J. M. (1982). *J. Histochem. Cytochem.* **30**, 1075–1078.
Beischer, D. and Krause, F. (1937). *Naturwissenschaften* **25**, 825–829.
Biberfeld, B., Ghetie, V. and Sjöquist, J. (1975). *J. Immunol. Meth.* **6**, 249.
Brands, R., Koninkx-Peeters, R., Slot, J. W. and Geuze, H. J. (1980a). *In* "Proceedings of the 7th European Congress on Electron Microscopy". Vol. 2. pp. 330–331.
Brands, R., Koninkx-Peeters, R., Slot, J. W and Geuze, J. J. (1980b) *Cell Biol. Int. Rep.* **4**, 749.
Branton, D. (1966). *Proc. Natn. Acad. Sci. USA* **55**, 1048–1056.
Branton, D. and Daemer, D. W. (1972). "Membrane Structure". Protoplasmatologia II/E/1. Springer, Wien, New York.
Bullivant, S. (1973). *In* "Advanced Techniques in Biological Electron Microscopy". Vol. 1. pp. 67–112, Springer, Berlin.
Bullivant, S. and Ames, A. (1966). *J. Cell Biol.* **29**, 435.
Burger, M. M. (1968). *Nature* **219**, 499–500.
Carlemalm, E. and Kellenberger, E. (1982). *EMBO J.* **1**, 63–67.
Carlemalm, E., Garavito, M. and Villiger, W. (1980). *In* "Proceedings of the 7th European Congress on Electron Microscopy". Vol. 2. pp. 656–657.
Carlemalm, E., Garavito, R. M. and Villiger, W. (1982). *J. Microscopy* **126**, 123–143.
Cohen, H. J. and Gilbertsen, B. B. (1975). *J. Clin. Invest.* **55**, 84–93.
Craig, S. and Goodchild, D. J. (1982). *Eur. J. Cell Biol.* **28**, 251–256.
De Mey, J., Moeremans, M., De Waele, M., Geuens, G. and De Brabander, M. (1981a). *In* "Protides of the Biological Fluids". Vol. 29. pp. 943–947. Pergamon Press, New York.
De Mey, J., Moeremans, M., Geuens, G., Nuydens, R. and De Brabander, M. (1981b). *Cell Biol. Int. Rep.* **5**, 889–899.
De Mey, J., Lambert, A. M., Bajer, A. S., Moeremans, M. and De Brabander, M. (1982). *Proc. Natn. Acad. Sci USA* **79**, 1898–1902.
De Petris, S. and Raff, M. C. (1972). *Eur. J. Immunol.* **2**, 523–535.

De Waele, M., de Mey, J., Moeremans, M. and van Camp, B. (1982a). *In* "Protides of the Biological Fluids". Vol. 29. pp. 949–953. Pergamon Press, New York.

De Waele, M., de Mey, J., Moeremans, M., Broodtaerts, L., Smet, L. and van Camp, B. (1982b). *J. Clin. Immunol.* (in press).

Dickson, R. B., Willingham, R. C. and Pastan, I. (1981). *J. Cell Biol.* **89**, 29–34.

Doerr-Schott, J. and Garaud, J.-C. (1981). *Cell Tiss. Res.* **216**, 581–589.

Donau (1905). *Monatshefte Chem.* **76**, 525–530.

Dörinkel, F. (1909). *Z. Anorg. Chem.* **63**, 344–348.

Douzou, P. (1977). *Adv. Enzymol.* **45**, 157.

Douzou, P., Sireix, R. and Traves, F. (1971). *Proc. Natn. Acad. Sci. USA* **66**, 787–792.

Endresen, C. (1979) *Acta Path. Microbiol. Scand.* **C87**, 185–187.

Erlandsen, S. L., Parson, J. A. and Rodning, C. B. (1979). *J. Histochem. Cytochem.* **27**, 1286–1289.

Faraday, M. (1857). *Phil. Trans. Royal. Soc. (Lond.)* **147**, 145–181.

Faulk, W. P. and Taylor, G. M. (1971). *Immunochemistry* **8**, 1081–1083.

Faulk, W. P., Vyas, G. N., Phillips, C. A., Fundenberg, H. H. and Chism, K. (1971). *Nature New Biol.* **231**, 101–104.

Feldherr, C. M. and Marshall, J. M. (1962). *J. Cell Biol.* **12**, 640–645.

Forsgren, A. and Sjöquist, J. (1966). *J. Immunol.* **97**, 822-827.

Forsgren, A. and Sjöquist, J. (1967). *J. Immunol.* **99**, 19–24.

Frens, G. (1972). *Kolloid Z. Z. Polymere* **250**, 736–741.

Frens, G. (1973). *Nature Phys. Sci.* **241**, 20–22.

Fromme, H. G., Grote, M., Pfautsch, M., von Figura, K., Voss, B. and Beeck, H. (1982). *Acta Histochem.* **70**, 1–7.

Garaud, J. C., Eloy, R., Moody, A. J., Stock, C. and Grenier, J. F. (1980). *Cell Tiss. Res.* **213**, 121–136.

Geiger, B., Dutton, A. H., Tokuyasu, K. T. and Singer, S. J. (1981). *J. Cell Biol.* **91**, 614–628.

Geoghegan, W. D. and Ackerman, G. A. (1977). *J. Histochem. Cytochem.* **25**, 1187–1200.

Geoghegan, W. D., Scillian, J. J. and Ackerman, G. A. (1978). *Immunol. Commun.* **7**, 1–12.

Geoghegan, W. D., Ambegaonkar, S. and Calvonico, N. J. (1980). *J. Immunol. Meth.* **34**, 11–21.

Geuze, H. J., Slot, J. W. and Tokuyasu, K. T. (1979). *J. Cell Biol.* **82**, 697–707.

Geuze, H. J., Slot, J. W. and Brands, R. (1981a). *Cell Biol. Int. Rep.* **5**, 463.

Geuze, H. J., Slot, J. W., van der Ley, P. A. and Scheefer, R. C. T. (1981b). *J. Cell Biol.* **89**, 653–665.

Geuze, H. J., Slot, J. W., Strous, G. A. M., Lodish, H. F. and Schwartz, A. L. (1982a). *J. Cell Biol.* **92**, 865–870.

Geuze, H. J., Slott, J. W., Strous, G. A. M., Lodish, H. F. and Schwartz, A. L. (1982b). *Biol. Cell* **45**, 191 (Abstr.).

Goldstein, I. J., So, L. L., Yang, Y. and Callies, Q. C. (1969). *J. Immunol.* **103**, 695–698.

Goodman, S. L., Hodges, G. M., Trejdosiewicz, L. K. and Livingston, D. C. (1979). *In* "Scanning Electron Microscopy" (O. Jahari, ed.), pp. 619–628. SEM Inc., O'Hare.

Goodman, S. L., Hodges, G. M. and Livingston, D. C. (1980). *In* "Scanning Electron Microscopy". (O. Jahari, ed.), pp. 133–146. SEM Inc., O'Hare.

Goodman, S. L., Hodges, G. M., Trejdosiewicz, L. K. and Livingston, D. C. (1981). *J. Microscopy* **123**, 201–213.

Green, N. M. (1975). *Adv. Protein Chem.* **29**, 85–133.

Green, J., Griffiths, G., Louvard, D., Quinn, P. and Warren, G. (1981). *J. Mol. Biol.* **152**, 663–698.

Griffiths, G., Warren, G., Stuhlfaut, J. and Jockusch, B. M. (1981). *Eur. J. Cell Biol.* **26**, 52–60.

Gros, D., Obrenovitch, A., Challice, C. E., Monsigny, M. and Schrevel, J. (1977). *J. Histochem. Cytochem.* **25**, 104–114.

Gu, J., de Mey, J., Moeremans, M. and Polak, J. M. (1981). *Regul. Peptides* **1**, 365–374.

Guesdon, J.-L., Ternynck, T. and Avrameas, S. (1979). *J. Histochem. Cytochem.* **27**, 1131–1139.

Gutbier, A. (1902a). *Z. Anorg. Chem.* **31**, 448–450.

Gutbier, A. (1902b). *Z. Anorg. Chem.* **32**, 348–356.

Handley, D. A., Arbeeny, C. M., Witte, L. D. and Chien, S. (1981). *Proc Natn. Acad. Sci. USA* **78**, 368–371.

Handley, D. A., Arbeeny, C. M., Eder, H. A. and Chien, S. (1981b). *J. Cell Biol.* **90**, 778–787.

Havel, R. J., Eder, H. A. and Bragdon, J. H. (1955). *J. Clin. Invest.* **34**, 1345–1353.

Horisberger, M. (1978). *Experientia* **34**, 721–722.

Horisberger, M. (1981). *In* "Scanning Electron Microscopy". (O. Jahari, ed.), Vol. II. pp. 9–31, SEM Inc., O'Hare.

Horisberger, M. and Rosset, J. (1976). *Experientia* **32**, 998–1000.

Horisberger, M. and Rosset, J. (1977). *J. Histochem. Cytochem.* **25**, 295–305.

Horisberger, M. and Von Lanthen, M. (1978). *J. Histochem. Cytochem.* **26**, 960–966.

Horisberger, M. and Von Lanthen, M. (1979a). *J. Microscopy* **115**, 97–102.

Horisberger, M. and Von Lanthen, M. (1979b). *Histochemistry* **64**, 115—118.

Horisberger, M., Rosset, J. and Bauer, H. (1975). *Experientia* **31**, 1147–1148.

Horisberger, M., Roset, J. and Von Lanthen, M. (1978). *Experientia* **34**, 274–276.

Hutchinson, N. J., Langer-Safer, P. R., Ward, D. C. and Hamkalo, B. A. (1982). *J. Cell Biol.* **95**, 609-618.

Iozzo, R. V., MacDonald, G. H. and Wight, T. N. (1982). *J. Histochem. Cytochem.* **30**, 697–701.

Janek, A. (1927). *Kolloid Z.* **41**, 242–243.

Jirgensen, B. and Straumanis, M. E. (1962). "A Short Textbook of Colloid Chemistry", 2nd edn, Pergamon Press, Oxford.

Kausche, G. A. and Ruska, H. (1939). *Kolloid Z.* **89**, 21–26.

Kellenberger, E., Carlemalm, E., Villiger, W., Roth, J. and Garavito, M. (1980). *In* "Low Denaturation Embedding for Electron Microscopy of Thin Sections". pp. 1–59. Chemische Werke Lowi GmbH Waldkraiburg.

Kent, S. P. and Allen, F. B. (1981). *Histochemistry* **72**, 83–90.

Kilmartin, J. V., Wright, B. and Milstein, C. (1982). *J. Cell Biol.* **93**, 576–582.

Kolb, H., Vogt, D. and Kolb-Bachofen, V. (1981). *Biochem. J.* **200**, 445–448.

Kolb-Bachofen, V., Schlepper-Schäfer, J., Vogell, W. and Kolb, H. (1982). *Cell* **29**, 859–866.

Krahenbühl, J. P., Racine, L. and Jamieson, J. D. (1977). *J. Cell Biol.* **72**, 406–423.

Kyte, J. (1976). *J. Cell Biol.* **68**, 304–318.

Lafferty, M. D., Ackerman, G. A., Dunn, C. D. R. and Lange, R. D. (1981). *J. Histochem. Cytochem.* **29**, 49–56.

Langer, P. R., Waldrop, A. and Ward, D. (1981). *Proc. Natn. Acad. Sci. USA* **78**, 6633–6637.

Larsson, L.-J. (1979). *Nature* **282**, 743–746.

Mannweiler, K., Hohenberg, H., Bohn, W. and Rutter, G. (1982). *J. Microscopy* **126**, 145–149.

Maxwell, N. H. (1978). *J. Microscopy* **112**, 253–255.

Meyer, H. W. and Winkelmann, H. (1969). *Protoplasma* **68**, 253–270.

Montesano, R., Roth, J., Robert, A. and Orci, L. (1982). *Nature* **296**, 651–653.

Moor, H., Mühlethaler, K., Walcher, H. and Frey-Wyssling, A. (1961). *J. Biophys. Biochem. Cytol.* **10**, 1–13.

Nakamura, S., Tanaka, K. and Murakawa, S. (1969). *Nature* **188**, 144–145.

Nakane, P. K. (1971). *Acta Endocrinol.* (Suppl. 153), 190–204.

Nicolson, G. L. (1971). *Nature New Biol.* **233**, 244–246

Nicolson, G. L. (1978). *In* "Advanced Techniques in Biological Electron Microscopy". Vol. II. pp. 1–38. Springer Berlin, Heidelberg, New York.

Nicolson, G. L. and Singer, S. J. (1971). *Proc. Natn. Acad. Sci. USA* **68**, 942–945.

Nicolson, G. L., Masouredis, S. P. and Singer, S. J. (1971). *Proc. Natn. Acad. Sci. USA* **68**, 1416–1420.

Nygren, H., Rozell, B., Holmgren, A. and Hansson, H.-A. (1981). *FEBS Lett.* **133**, 145–150.

Ochs, R. L. and Stearns, M. E. (1981). *Biol. Cell* **42**, 19–28.

Palade, G. (1975). *Science* **189**, 347–358.

Pauli, W. (1949). *Helvet. Chim. Acta* **32**, 795–810.

Pearse, A. G. E. (1980). "Histochemistry. Theoretical and Applied". Churchill Livingstone, Edinburgh.

Petsko, G. A. (1975). *J. Mol. Biol.* **96**, 381–392.

Pinto da Silva, P., Parkinson, C. and Dwyer, N. (1981a). *J. Histochem. Cytochem.* **29**, 917–928.

Pinto da Silva, P., Kachar, B., Torrisi, M. R., Brown, C. and Parkinson, C. (1981b). *Science* **213**, 230–233.

Pinto da Silva, P., Parkinson, C. and Dwyer, N. (1981c). *Proc. Natn. Acad. Sci. USA* **78**, 343–347.

Pinto da Silva, P., Torrisi, M. R. and Kachar, B. (1981d). *J. Cell Biol.* **91**, 361–372.

Pinto da Silva, P. and Torrisi, M. R. (1982). *J. Cell Biol.* **93**, 463–469.

Podder, S. K., Surolia, A. and Bachhawat, B. K. (1974). *Eur. J. Biochem.* **44**, 151–160.

Probert, L., De Mey, J. and Polak, J. M. (1981). *Nature* **294**, 470–471.

Ravazzola, M. and Orci, L. (1980a). *Histochemistry* **67**, 221–224.

Ravazzola, M. and Orci, L. (1980b). *Nature* **284**, 66–67.

Ravazzola, M., Perrelet, A., Roth, J. and Orci, L. (1981). *Proc. Natn. Acad. Sci. USA* **78**, 5661–5664.

Reddy, J. K., Bendayan, M. and Reddy, M. K. (1982). *Ann. N.Y. Acad. Sci.* **381**, 495–498.

Romano, E. L., Stolinski, C. and Hughes-Jones, N. C. (1974). *Immunochemistry* **11**, 521–522.

Romano, E. L., Stolinski, C. and Hughes-Jones, N. C. (1975). *Brit. J. Haematol.* **30**, 507–516.

Romano, E. L. and Romano, M. (1977). *Immunochemistry* **14**, 711–715.

Roth, J. (1978). *Exp. Path.* (Suppl.) **3**, 1–187.
Roth, J. (1980). *Acta Histochem.* (Suppl. XXII), 113–121.
Roth, J. (1982a). *In* "Electron Microscopy". Vol. 3. pp. 245–252.
Roth, J. (1982b). *In* "Techniques in Immunochemistry" (G. R. Bullock and P. Petrusz, eds.), Vol. 1. pp. 107–134, Academic Press, London.
Roth, J. (1982c). *J. Histochem. Cytochem.* **30**, 691–696.
Roth, J. (1982d). *Histochem. J.* **14**, 791–801.
Roth, J. (1983a). *J. Histochem. Cytochem.* **31**, 547–552.
Roth, J. (1983b). *J. Histochem. Cytochem.* (In press).
Roth, J. and Wagner, M. (1977a). *J. Histochem. Cytochem.* **25**, 1181–1184.
Roth, J. and Wagner, M. (1977b). *Exp. Path.* **14**, 311–320.
Roth, J. and Binder, M. (1978). *J. Histochem. Cytochem.* **26**, 163–169.
Roth, J. and Berger, E. G. (1982). *J. Cell Biol.* **93**, 223–229.
Roth, J., Bendayan, M. and Orci, L. (1978). *J. Histochem. Cytochem.* **26**, 1074–1081.
Roth, J., Bendayan, M. and Orci, L. (1980). *J. Histochem. Cytochem.* **28**, 55–57.
Roth, J., Ravazzola, M., Bendayan, M. and Orci, L. (1981a). *Endocrinology* **108**, 247–253.
Roth, J., Thorens, B., Hunziker, W., Norman, A. W. and Orci, L. (1981b). *Science* **214**, 197–200.
Roth, J., Bendayan, M., Carlemalm, E., Villiger, W. and Garavito, M. (1981c). *J. Histochem. Cytochem.* **29**, 663–671.
Roth, J., Brown, D., Norman, A. W. and Orci, L. (1982), *Am. J. Physiol.* **243**, F243–F252.
Roth, J., Lentze, M. J. and Berger, E. G. (1983a). *Science* (in press).
Roth, J., Brown, D. and Orci, L. (1983b). *J. Cell Biol.* (in press).
Scherrer, P. (1920). *In* "Kolloidchemie" (R. Zsigmondy, ed.), 3rd ed, p. 387.
Scherrer, P. and Staub, H. (1931). *Z. Physik. Chem.* **A154**, 309–321.
Schott-Doerr, J. and Garaud, J.-C. (1981). *Cell Tiss. Res.* **216**, 581–589.
Schwab, M. E. and Thoenen, H. (1978). *J. Cell Biol.* **77**, 1–13.
Sleytr, W. B. and Robards, A. W. (1977). *J. Microscopy* **111**, 77–100.
Slot, J. W. and Geuze, H. J. (1981). *J. Cell Biol.* **90**, 533.
Stathis, F. C. and Fabrikanos, A. (1958). *Chem. Ind. (London)* **27**, 860–861.
Stephens, H., Bendayan, M. and Silver, M. (1982). *Biol. Cell* **44**, 81–84.
Sternberger, L.A. (1980). *In* "Immunocytochemistry", Prentice Hall Inc., New Jersey.
Stoward, P. J., Spicer, S. S. and Miller, R. (1980). *J. Histochem. Cytochem.* **28**, 979.
Suzuki, S., Tsuyama, S., Suganuma, T., Yamamoto, N. and Murata, F. (1981). *J. Histochem. Cytochem.* **29**, 946.
Tanaka, T., Gresik, E. W., Michelakis, A. M. and Barka, T. (1980). *J. Histochem. Cytochem.* **28**, 1113–1118.
Tanaka, T., Gresik, E. W. and Barka, T. (1981a). *J. Histochem. Cytochem.* **29**, 1189–1195.
Tanaka, T., Gresik, E. W. and Barka, T. (1981b). *J. Histochem. Cytochem.* **29**, 1229–1231.
Tartakoff, A., Vassalli, P. and Montesano, R. (1981). *Eur. J. Cell Biol.* **26**, 188–197.
Taylor, H. S. (1926). *J. Phys. Chem.* **30**, 145.
Taylor, R. B., Duffus, W. P. H., Raff, M. C. and de Petris, S. (1971). *Nature New Biol.* **233**, 225–229.
Thiessen, P. A. (1924). *Z. Anorg. Chem.* **133**, 393–408.

Thiessen, P. A. (1942). *Kolloid Z.* **101**, 242–248.
Thorens, B., Roth, J., Norman, A. W., Perrelet, A. and Orci, L. (1982). *J. Cell Biol.* **94**, 115–122.
Thoss, K. and Roth, J. (1976). *Histochemistry* **49**, 67–72.
Tokuyasu, K. T. (1973). *J. Cell Biol.* **57**, 551–565.
Tokuyasu, K. T. (1978). *J. Ultrastruct. Res.* **63**, 287–307.
Tokuyasu, K. T. (1980). *Histochem. J.* **12**, 381–403.
Tokuyasu, K. T. and Singer, S. J. (1976). *J. Cell Biol.* **71**, 894–906.
Tolson, N. D., Boothroyd, B. and Hopkins, C. R. (1981). *J. Microscopy* **123**, 215–226.
Vanino, L. (1905). *Ber. Dt. Chem. Ges.* **38**, 463–466.
Varndell, I. M., Tapia, F. J., de May, J., Rush, R. A., Bloom, S. R. and Polak, J. M. (1982). *J. Histochem. Cytochem.* **30**, 682–690.
Wagner, M. and Wagner, B. (1976). *Z. Immun. Forsch.* **151**, 117–125.
Wagner, M. and Wagner, B. (1977). *Z. Immun. Forsch.* **153**, 450–456.
Wagner, M., Roth, J. and Wagner, B. (1976). *Exp. Path.* **12**, 277–281.
Weisser, H. B. (1933). "Inorganic Colloid Chemistry", Vol. I. John Wiley, New York.
Wharton, J., Polak, J. M., Probert, L., de Mey, J., McGregor, G. P., Bryant, M. G. and Bloom, S. R. (1981). *Neuroscience* **6**, 969–982.
Willingham, M. C., Pastan, I. H., Sahagian, G. G., Jourdian, G. W. and Neufeld, E. F. (1981a). *Proc. Natn. Acad. Sci. USA* **78**, 6967–6971.
Willingham, M. C., Rutherford, A. V., Gallo, M. G., Wehland, J., Dickson, R. B., Schlegel, R. and Pastan, I. H. (1981b). *J. Histochem. Cytochem.* **29**, 1003–1013.
Wright, C., Willan, K. J., Sjödahl, J., Burton, D. R. and Drock, R. A. (1977). *Biochem. J.* **167**, 611–668.
Young, N. M., Leon, M. A. and Takahashi, T. (1971). *J. Biol. Chem.* **246**, 1596–1601.
Zsigmondy, R. (1898). *Liebigs Ann.* **301**, 29–54.
Zsigmondy, R. (1901). *Z. Analyt. Chem.* **40**, 697–719.
Zsigmondy, R. (1905). "Zur Erkenntnisse, der Kolloide". G. Fischer, Jena.
Zsigmondy, R. (1924). *Mikrochemie* **2**, 50.
Zsigmondy, R. and Thiessen, P. A. (1925). "Dass Kolloidale Gold". Akadem. Verlagsgesellschaft, Leipzig.
Zur Nieden, U., Neumann, D., Mantenffel, R. and Weber, E. (1981). *Eur. J. Cell Biol.* **26**, 228–233.

Subject Index